Recent Advances in Atmospheric-Pressure Plasma Technology

Recent Advances in Atmospheric-Pressure Plasma Technology

Editor

Bogdan-George Rusu

MDPI • Basel • Beijing • Wuhan • Barcelona • Belgrade • Manchester • Tokyo • Cluj • Tianjin

Editor
Bogdan-George Rusu
"Petru Poni" Institute of
Macromolecular Chemistry
Romania

Editorial Office
MDPI
St. Alban-Anlage 66
4052 Basel, Switzerland

This is a reprint of articles from the Special Issue published online in the open access journal *Applied Sciences* (ISSN 2076-3417) (available at: https://www.mdpi.com/journal/applsci/special_issues/atmospheric_pressure_plasma).

For citation purposes, cite each article independently as indicated on the article page online and as indicated below:

LastName, A.A.; LastName, B.B.; LastName, C.C. Article Title. *Journal Name* **Year**, *Volume Number*, Page Range.

ISBN 978-3-0365-6880-5 (Hbk)
ISBN 978-3-0365-6881-2 (PDF)

Contents

About the Editor vii

Bogdan-George Rusu
Recent Advances in Atmospheric-Pressure Plasma Technology
Reprinted from: *Appl. Sci.* **2022**, *12*, 10847, doi:10.3390/app122110847 1

Vanesa Rueda, Rafael Diez, Nicolas Bente and Hubert Piquet
Combined Image Processing and Equivalent Circuit Approach for the Diagnostic of Atmospheric Pressure DBD
Reprinted from: *Appl. Sci.* **2022**, *12*, 8009, doi:10.3390/app12168009 5

Muhammad Jehanzaib Khan, Vojislav Jovicic, Ana Zbogar-Rasic and Antonio Delgado
Enhancement of Wheat Flour and Dough Properties by Non-Thermal Plasma Treatment of Wheat Flour
Reprinted from: *Appl. Sci.* **2022**, *12*, 7997, doi:10.3390/app12167997 21

Viktoras Papadimas, Christos Doudesis, Panagiotis Svarnas, Polycarpos K. Papadopoulos, George P. Vafakos and Panayiotis Vafeas
SDBD Flexible Plasma Actuator with Ag-Ink Electrodes: Experimental Assessment
Reprinted from: *Appl. Sci.* **2021**, *11*, 11930, doi:10.3390/app112411930 41

Yuma Suenaga, Toshihiro Takamatsu, Toshiki Aizawa, Shohei Moriya, Yuriko Matsumura, Atsuo Iwasawa and Akitoshi Okino
Plasma Gas Temperature Control Performance of Metal 3D-Printed Multi-Gas Temperature-Controllable Plasma Jet
Reprinted from: *Appl. Sci.* **2021**, *11*, 11686, doi:10.3390/app112411686 55

Yuma Suenaga, Toshihiro Takamatsu, Toshiki Aizawa, Shohei Moriya, Yuriko Matsumura, Atsuo Iwasawa and Akitoshi Okino
Influence of Controlling Plasma Gas Species and Temperature on Reactive Species and Bactericidal Effect of the Plasma
Reprinted from: *Appl. Sci.* **2021**, *11*, 11674, doi:10.3390/app112411674 65

Ibrahim A. AlShunaifi, Samira Elaissi, Imed Ghiloufi, Seham S. Alterary and Ahmed A. Alharbi
Modelling of a Non-Transferred Plasma Torch Used for Nano-Silica Powders Production
Reprinted from: *Appl. Sci.* **2021**, *11*, 9842, doi:10.3390/app11219842 75

Michał Chodkowski, Iryna Ya. Sulym, Konrad Terpiłowski and Dariusz Sternik
Surface Properties of Silica–MWCNTs/PDMS Composite Coatings Deposited on Plasma Activated Glass Supports
Reprinted from: *Appl. Sci.* **2021**, *11*, 9256, doi:10.3390/app11199256 93

Atif H. Asghar and Ahmed Rida Galaly
The Effect of Oxygen Admixture with Argon Discharges on the Impact Parameters of Atmospheric Pressure Plasma Jet Characteristics
Reprinted from: *Appl. Sci.* **2021**, *11*, 6870, doi:10.3390/app11156870 111

Mária Domonkos, Petra Tichá, Jan Trejbal and Pavel Demo
Applications of Cold Atmospheric Pressure Plasma Technology in Medicine, Agriculture and Food Industry
Reprinted from: *Appl. Sci.* **2021**, *11*, 4809, doi:10.3390/app11114809 133

About the Editor

Bogdan-George Rusu

Bogdan-George Rusu, PhD. Phys., is researcher at the "Petru Poni" Institute of Macromolecular Chemistry, Iasi, Romania. He graduated from the Faculty of Physics, University "Al. I. Cuza", Iași, Medical Physics section. He also has an M.Sc. degree in Plasma Physics, Spectroscopy and Polymer Physics and a PhD in Physics at the University Al. I. Cuza, Faculty of Physics, Iași and at the Institut Européen des Membranes, Université de Montpellier II, Montpellier, France.

Plasma technology diagnosis, plasma treatment, and plasma polymerizations have been the focus of Rusu Bogdan-George's research for more than 15 years. As his main scientific interest, he mentions: the processing of materials with plasma (dielectric barrier discharge DBD at atmospheric pressure plasma treatment, plasma polymerization, and physical and photochemical changes induced by the UV–polymer laser interaction); the deposition of thin layers (using various techniques such as magnetron discharge sputtering, hollow cathode deposition, and pulsed laser deposition); and the preparation of nanoparticle suspension solutions (C, Si, and ZnO) using laser ablation in different liquids and testing them in biomedical applications.

The scientific results in these fields were realized through 33 scientific articles, of which 24 were published in specialized journals rated by ISI; and 47 communications at national/international conferences, including 10 oral presentations.

applied sciences

MDPI

Editorial

Recent Advances in Atmospheric-Pressure Plasma Technology

Bogdan-George Rusu

"Petru Poni" Institute of Macromolecular Chemistry, 41 A Gr. Ghica Voda Alley, 700487 Iasi, Romania; rusu.george@icmpp.ro

1. Introduction

In recent years, plasma technology has presented an alternative in the processing and development of new materials. Of the plasma processing methods developed thus far, atmospheric pressure plasma is the most economically accessible, due to the low costs of this technology. Among the first applications of plasmas in atmospheric pressure was the treatment of various polymeric materials. Plasma treatment efficiently improves the surface wettability and adhesion properties of different types of materials. This is possible because plasma parameters such as particle density, collision frequency, mean kinetic energy of the particles, and the presence of chemical active species will cause a large variety of elementary processes both within the plasma volume and on the plasma–material interface. Consequently, the quality and magnitude of the polymer surface treatment, including etching, functionalization, and crosslinking, might also be controlled [1]. Generally, the plasma used in material processing can be generated in different gases, pressure ranges, or discharge geometries.

Another technique developed later was that of a plasma polymerization technique. Plasma polymerization is a versatile method for the deposition of films with functional properties, which are suitable for a range of applications. These plasma polymers have different properties than those fabricated via conventional polymerization: the plasma-polymerized films are usually branched, highly cross-linked, insoluble, and adhere well to most substrates [2].

In the last decade, new applications of plasmas at atmospheric pressure have been developed, such as: plasma medicine, plasma agriculture, plasma used in food industry, in 3D printing technology, textile industry, and so on. This Special Issue attempts cover all these applications, publishing both target applications of the atmospheric pressure plasma and also the fundamental aspects that appear in the case of these types of discharge.

Citation: Rusu, B.-G. Recent Advances in Atmospheric-Pressure Plasma Technology. *Appl. Sci.* **2022**, *12*, 10847. https://doi.org/10.3390/app122110847

Received: 18 October 2022
Accepted: 24 October 2022
Published: 26 October 2022

2. Review of Special Issue Contents

Contributions to this Special Issue focus on different aspects of Atmospheric-Pressure Plasma Technology, giving valuable examples of applied research in the field. This Special Issue of *Applied Sciences*, "Recent Advances in Atmospheric-Pressure Plasma Technology", includes one review [3] and eight original papers [4–11], providing new insights into the application of atmospheric pressure plasma technology.

Domonkos et al [3] discussed the application of cold atmospheric pressure plasma (CAPP) technology in different configurations. Their manuscript outlines the application of CAPP in medicine for the inactivation of various pathogens (e.g., bacteria, fungi, viruses, sterilization of medical equipment, and implants) in the food industry (e.g., food and packing material decontamination), agriculture (e.g., disinfection of seeds, fertilizer, water, soil). In medicine, plasma also holds great promise with regard to direct therapeutic treatments in dentistry (tooth bleaching), dermatology (atopic eczema, wound healing), and oncology (melanoma, glioblastoma).

Asghar et al. [4] discussed the changes induced in the atmospheric pressure plasma jets (APPJs) characteristics of the gas mixture; more precisely, argon/oxygen (Ar/O_2) mixture.

The voltage–current waveform signals of APPJ discharge, gas flow rate, photo-imaging of the plasma jet length and width, discharge plasma power, axial temperature distribution, optical emission spectra, and irradiance were investigated.

Chodkowski et al. [5] focused on fabrication and physicochemical properties investigations of silica-multiwalled carbon nanotubes/poly(dimethylsiloxane) composite coatings deposited on the glass supports activated by cold plasma in air or argon. They found that the type of plasma influences the surface properties of the deposited coating.

AlShunaifi et al. [6] realized a two-dimensional numerical model to simulate operation conditions in the non-transferred plasma torch, used to synthesis nanosilica powder. The numerical results showed good correlation and good trends with the experimental measurement. This study allowed us to obtain more efficient control of the process conditions and better optimization of this process in terms of the production rate and primary particle size.

Suenaga et al. [7] realized an evaluation of the effect of plasma gas species and temperature concerning the reactive species produced and the bactericidal effect of plasma. Nitrogen, carbon dioxide, oxygen, and argon were used as the gas species, and the gas temperature of each plasma varied from 30 to 90 oC. The results demonstrate that the plasma gas type and temperature have a significant influence on the reactive species produced, and the bactericidal effect of plasma and the disinfection process could be improved by properly selecting the plasma gas species and temperature.

Suenaga et al. [8] design and build a multi-gas temperature-controllable plasma jet that can adjust the gas temperature of plasmas with various gas species and evaluated its temperature control performance. By varying the plasma jet body temperature from −30 °C to 90 °C, the gas temperature was successfully controlled linearly in the range of 29–85 °C for all plasma gas species.

Papadimas et al. [9] realized a single dielectric barrier discharge (SDBD)-based actuator. The consumed electric power was measured, and the optical emission spectrum was recorded in the ultraviolet–near infrared (UV–NIR) range. The average temperature of the neutral species over the actuator was found to be around 410 K at the maximum power level.

Khan et al. [10] reported a dielectric barrier discharge (DBD) plasma rotational reactor for the direct treatment of wheat flour. The primary research goal was to determine the effects of short-period cold plasma treatment of DBD type on flour and dough properties. The obtained results showed a 6–7% increase in flour hydration due to cold plasma treatment, which also contributes to hydrogen bonding due to changes in the bonded and free water phase.

Rueda et al. [11] report a study which is focused on gas treatments (NOx abatement) by dielectric barrier discharge (DBD) at atmospheric pressure. Two diagnostic methods are considered to evaluate the discharging ratio on the reactor surface: an image processing method and a DBD equivalent circuit analysis, both presented in this paper. The experimental results show good agreement between the two methods. These two strategies work very well and provide remarkably coherent results under different intensity conditions.

This Special Issue has attracted 38 citations and received more than 8700 views, demonstrating the growing interest in this topic.

The Editor would like to express his appreciation to the contributors for their dedication and excitement during the process of compiling their individual essays for this Special Issue. The Multidisciplinary Digital Publishing Institute (MDPI) editorial team members also deserve praise for their professionalism and commitment to publishing this Special Issue. We hope that the readers will enjoy this collection of papers and will be motivated to envision fresh concepts for future developments in plasma research technology.

Funding: This research received no external funding.

Conflicts of Interest: The author declares no conflict of interest.

References

1. Keidar, M.; Weltmann, K.D.; Macheret, S. Fundamentals and Applications of Atmospheric Pressure Plasmas. *J. Appl. Phys.* **2021**, *130*, 080401. [CrossRef]
2. Jang, H.J.; Jung, E.Y.; Parsons, T.; Tae, H.-S.; Park, C.-S. A Review of Plasma Synthesis Methods for Polymer Films and Nanoparticles under Atmospheric Pressure Conditions. *Polymers* **2021**, *13*, 2267. [CrossRef] [PubMed]
3. Domonkos, M.; Tichá, P.; Trejbal, J.; Demo, P. Applications of Cold Atmospheric Pressure Plasma Technology in Medicine, Agriculture and Food Industry. *Appl. Sci.* **2021**, *11*, 4809. [CrossRef]
4. Asghar, A.; Galaly, A. The Effect of Oxygen Admixture with Argon Discharges on the Impact Parameters of Atmospheric Pressure Plasma Jet Characteristics. *Appl. Sci.* **2021**, *11*, 6870. [CrossRef]
5. Chodkowski, M.; Sulym, I.; Terpiłowski, K.; Sternik, D. Surface Properties of Silica–MWCNTs/PDMS Composite Coatings Deposited on Plasma Activated Glass Supports. *Appl. Sci.* **2021**, *11*, 9256. [CrossRef]
6. AlShunaifi, I.; Elaissi, S.; Ghiloufi, I.; Alterary, S.; Alharbi, A. Modelling of a Non-Transferred Plasma Torch Used for Nano-Silica Powders Production. *Appl. Sci.* **2021**, *11*, 9842. [CrossRef]
7. Suenaga, Y.; Takamatsu, T.; Aizawa, T.; Moriya, S.; Matsumura, Y.; Iwasawa, A.; Okino, A. Influence of Controlling Plasma Gas Species and Temperature on Reactive Species and Bactericidal Effect of the Plasma. *Appl. Sci.* **2021**, *11*, 11674. [CrossRef]
8. Suenaga, Y.; Takamatsu, T.; Aizawa, T.; Moriya, S.; Matsumura, Y.; Iwasawa, A.; Okino, A. Plasma Gas Temperature Control Performance of Metal 3D-Printed Multi-Gas Temperature-Controllable Plasma Jet. *Appl. Sci.* **2021**, *11*, 11686. [CrossRef]
9. Papadimas, V.; Doudesis, C.; Svarnas, P.; Papadopoulos, P.; Vafakos, G.; Vafeas, P. SDBD Flexible Plasma Actuator with Ag-Ink Electrodes: Experimental Assessment. *Appl. Sci.* **2021**, *11*, 11930. [CrossRef]
10. Khan, M.; Jovicic, V.; Zbogar-Rasic, A.; Delgado, A. Enhancement of Wheat Flour and Dough Properties by Non-Thermal Plasma Treatment of Wheat Flour. *Appl. Sci.* **2022**, *12*, 7997. [CrossRef]
11. Rueda, V.; Diez, R.; Bente, N.; Piquet, H. Combined Image Processing and Equivalent Circuit Approach for the Diagnostic of Atmospheric Pressure DBD. *Appl. Sci.* **2022**, *12*, 8009. [CrossRef]

applied sciences

Article

Combined Image Processing and Equivalent Circuit Approach for the Diagnostic of Atmospheric Pressure DBD

Vanesa Rueda [1,2], Rafael Diez [2,*], Nicolas Bente [1] and Hubert Piquet [1,*]

[1] LAPLACE Laboratory, Université de Toulouse, CNRS, INPT, UPS, 2 rue Charles Camichel, BP 7122, CEDEX 7, 31071 Toulouse, France
[2] Department of Electronics Engineering, Pontificia Universidad Javeriana, Bogota 110231, Colombia
* Correspondence: rdiez@javeriana.edu.co (R.D.); hubert.piquet@laplace.univ-tlse.fr (H.P.)

Abstract: The framework of this paper is the study of gas treatments (NOx abatement) by dielectric barrier discharge (DBD) at atmospheric pressure. To investigate the impact of various solutions for electrical energy injection on the treatment process, two diagnostic methods are considered to evaluate the discharging ratio on the reactor surface: an image processing method and a DBD equivalent circuit analysis, both presented in this paper. For the image analysis, the discharge area is first translated into gray levels, then segmented using the Otsu's method in order to perform the discharging ratio diagnostic. The equivalent circuit approach, derived from the classical Manley's diagram analysis, includes the behavior of the part of the reactor in which no discharge is happening. The identification of its parameters is used to estimate the discharging ratio, which evaluates the percentage of the reactor surface covered by the discharge. Experimental results with specifically developed power supplies are presented: they show a good agreement between the two methods. To allow a quantitative comparison of the discharge uniformity according to the operating conditions, the statistical analysis of gray level distribution is performed: non-uniform discharges with intense energy channels are shown to be clearly distinguished from more diffuse ones.

Keywords: dielectric barrier discharge; partial surface discharging; discharging ratio; image processing; equivalent circuit; Manley diagram; NOx abatement; DBD diagnostic; atmospheric pressure; discharge uniformity

Citation: Rueda, V.; Diez, R.; Bente, N.; Piquet, H. Combined Image Processing and Equivalent Circuit Approach for the Diagnostic of Atmospheric Pressure DBD. *Appl. Sci.* **2022**, *12*, 8009. https://doi.org/10.3390/app12168009

Academic Editor: Bogdan-George Rusu

Received: 8 July 2022
Accepted: 8 August 2022
Published: 10 August 2022

1. Introduction

Non-Thermal Plasma (NTP) are broadly used for applications such as ozone generation, treatment of surfaces, medical treatments, disinfection, and UV production [1–6]. In recent years, NTP has also become a rising technology for environmental protection. Many studies have reported effective removal of pollutants such as nitrogen oxides (NOx), sulfur dioxide (SO_2), carbon dioxide (CO_2), particulate matter, and volatile organic compounds (VOC) [1,7], with treatments usually processed at atmospheric pressure.

Dielectric Barrier Discharges (DBDs) are NTP produced in reactors, including at least one insulating layer between two metallic electrodes. In comparison with other NTP reactors, such as corona discharges and electron beams, DBDs are characterized by the absence of sparks, thanks to the dielectric barriers which limit the local current rise and by the possibility of obtaining uniform discharges, where the NTP covers the entire surface of the reactors, guaranteeing a quality treatment.

DBDs operate in filamentary or homogeneous mode [8,9]. In the homogeneous mode, the plasma is uniform and diffuse [1,8] and it presents a glowing aspect. For some applications, it has been proven to improve the process: for instance, thin films deposit requires homogeneous discharges in order to obtain a uniform treatment and prevent local damage on the treated surface [2]. The filamentary mode is characterized by streamers, intense energy channels distributed over the electrodes surface, randomly, or sometimes following geometrical patterns [10]. Ozone generation, UV emission for instance, benefits from this mode. At atmospheric pressure, DBD generally operates in filamentary mode, and offer capabilities to initiate very valuable chemical transformations. According to their highly desirable characteristics, DBDs and packed-bed DBDs are widely used for pollutant removal applications. This is the case for the prospective application of our studies (NOx abatement) [7].

Experimental conditions such as the reactor geometry, materials, gas mixture, pressure, and electrical supply waveforms not only influence the discharge mode, but also the characteristics of the power injection into the plasma and the full or partial coverage of the reactor's surface by the NTP. Obtaining operating conditions where the surface of the reactor is fully covered by the plasma is indeed highly desirable for gas treatments: it means that each volume of the gas injected into the reactor will receive the effect of NTP treatment, contrary to the situation where only part of the reactor's surface is covered by the NTP, and thus part of the flowing gas may not receive the expected treatment. Such opposite situations are shown in Figure 1 (side view of a cylindrical reactor, detailed in Section 2, showing the streamers distribution seen through the transparent walls made with quartz).

Figure 1. Typical discharge appearance with partial discharging and different β percentages (white frame showing the limits of the reactor).

The partial discharging is quantified by the β (no units) percentage, which takes the 1 value when the surface is fully covered and 0 value when the discharge is OFF [8,11,12]. Among the diagnostic criteria used for the diagnostic of NTP delivered by DBD, this β discharging ratio is very important to improve the understanding of the efficiency of the gas treatments (NOx abatement in our case).

Different diagnostic methods of the discharge mode, based on its appearance, have been proposed. Ref. [9] introduced a simple method that detects the homogeneous glow discharge using the Manley figure and the voltage and current waveforms. This method is based on a definition of the homogeneous APGD (Atmospheric Pressure Glow Discharge), where only one current pulse per voltage half-cycle is generated. Other diagnostic methods include Intensified Charge-Coupled Device (ICCD), high-speed imaging, optical emission spectrum, numerical simulations, and image processing [13].

Given that the image processing method is effective, simple, and does not require expensive equipment, it is a good solution to analyze the discharges under different experimental conditions. However, if the aim is to detect the conventional glow discharge (APGD), it can only be used with short exposure time (~10 ns, which requires an expensive camera). When higher exposure times are used, the filaments cannot be always distinguished. Nevertheless, the image processing can be still used to analyze the uniformity of the discharge: in this paper an image processing algorithm is set up to study the uniformity of the discharges rather than the discharge mode (homogeneous or filamentary). This analysis of the discharge uniformity is based on the image gray level histogram [13] and produces, as a result, an estimation of the β partial discharging ratio. Additional statistical analysis of the images also allows a quantified comparison of the uniformity of the discharges.

Other diagnostics of DBD systems can be also achieved on the basis of measured electrical waveforms. Using these measurements, it is possible to identify the parameters of the well-known Manley diagram [14] and its associated DBD's equivalent circuit [15].

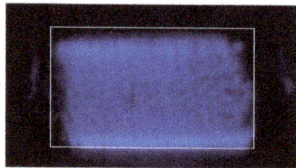

Originally based on the assumption that the discharge is uniform (with parameters of the equivalent circuit corresponding to a full use of the surface of the electrodes, i.e., $\beta = 1$), this approach can be simply extended [8,16] to consider partial discharging situation.

In order to implement complementary approaches for diagnostic of the discharges obtained in a DBD reactor for NOx abatement studies, the two aforementioned approaches (image processing and equivalent circuit) are considered in this paper. The article is organized as follows: Section 2 presents first the reactor, the power supply and the experimental test-bench, for which measurements are used in this paper. Then, the image processing algorithm for diagnostic with estimation of the β percentage of the surface covered by the discharge is detailed. Finally, the equivalent circuit, considering partial discharging phenomenon and the identification of its parameters (chiefly the β ratio) using the electrical measured waveforms, is presented.

In Section 3, the application of the two methods at different operating conditions obtained with the test-bench is proposed and the correspondence between the obtained β percentage values is discussed.

2. Materials and Methods

2.1. Experimental Setup

The schematic diagram of the experimental setup is presented in Figure 2. The system consists of a DBD reactor, a gas blending system, a power supply, measurement instruments, and the control interface:

- The reactor has a coaxial cylindrical geometry made up of quartz. The inner electrode is a stainless-steel foil, and the outer electrode is a metallic mesh (knitted thin wires made of tinned copper steel, usually used for EMI/RFI shielding of cables [17]) wrapped around the quartz tube. The diameter of the outer dielectric is 28 mm, and the diameter of the inner dielectric is 22 mm. The length of the mesh is 60 mm. Detailed dimensions are given in Figure 2.
- The feed-gas stream is composed of NO and N_2 and flows through the DBD reactor. The gas composition and total flow rate are adjustable. Two mass flow controllers (Bronkhorst EL-FLOW Prestige) are used to measure and regulate them. Presented results are for 3 lpm flow, with a NO concentration of 800 ppm.
- The DBD voltage is measured with a 200 MHz digital oscilloscope (LeCroy HDO4024) connected through a 1000:1 voltage probe (Testec TT-SI 9010), and the current is measured using a current probe (LeCroy AP015). The NO and NO_2 concentrations are obtained by the gas analyzer (Testo 350).

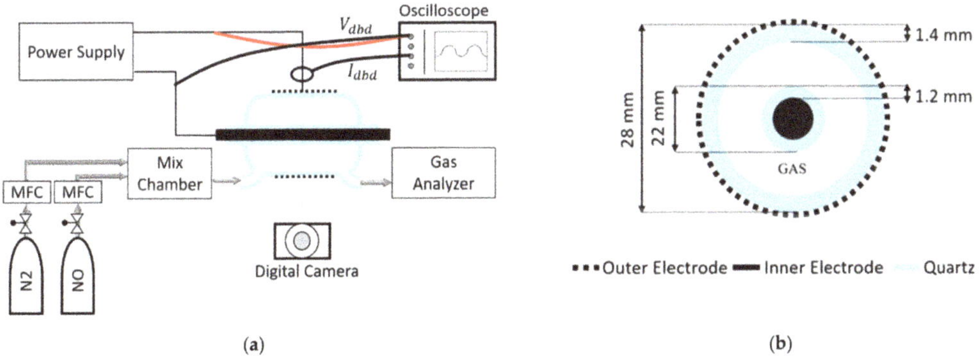

Figure 2. Experimental setup (**a**) and reactor dimensions (**b**).

Two different electrical supplies are used for the experimentations: a sinusoidal voltage source and a square current source. The sinusoidal voltage waveforms (Figure 3b) are generated by a function generator connected to an audio amplifier. Since the output voltage of the amplifier is too low to ignite a discharge, the amplifier output is connected to a high-voltage transformer. Frequency and peak voltage are the degrees of freedom made available by this supply: a maximum frequency of 20 kHz and a maximum voltage of 12 kV can be generated.

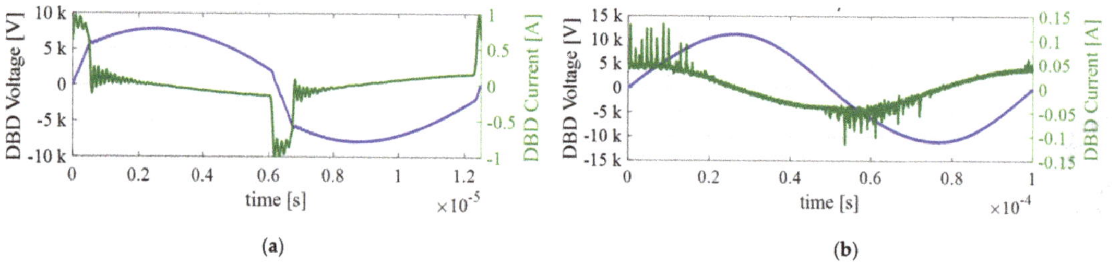

Figure 3. Typical electrical waveforms (v_{DBD}, blue and i_{DBD}, green): (**a**) Square Current Source: here, fsw = 80 kHz, J = 1 A, d = 10%. (**b**) Sinusoidal Voltage Source: here, v_{DBD_peak} = 11.2 kV, f = 10 kHz.

A specific power supply has been also developed to create the plasma and to control the energy injected into the NTP. This one delivers square current waveforms (Figure 3a), which is generated by the power converter presented in [18,19]. This converter consists of a DC current source connected in cascade with a full-bridge current inverter and a step-up transformer. The converter delivers current pulses, whose shape is controlled by three degrees of freedom: frequency fsw, current amplitude J, and pulses duration Δtp. ($\Delta tp = d/(fsw^*2)$, d being the duty cycle, in the range 5–95%). The maximum output current J is 1.2 A, and the maximum voltage is 11 kV. The frequency fsw can be varied from 80 kHz to 200 kHz. In order to control the rise of the reactor temperature, this supply is operated in "Burst mode" [1]: pulses trains are separated by power injection pauses; the durations of both bursts and pauses are fully controlled.

Side view images of the discharge are acquired by a digital camera (Logitech C920), with an interval of 20 s and an exposure time of 1/128 s. This camera is installed 40 cm from the axis of reactor and provides images such as the ones displayed in Figure 1. The area of interest is 28 mm high (outer diameter of the reactor) and 60 mm long (length of the metallic mesh). The camera acquires images with 2304 × 1536 pixels; once cropped for the area of interest, these values reduce to 437 × 248 (the difference in proportions results from a very slight misalignment of the camera with respect to the reactor axis). Despite such a device having an exposure time much longer than the lifetime of the streamers, as will be shown below, very interesting information concerning the distribution of the plasma can be drawn from the analysis of these images.

2.2. *Image Processing Algorithm*

The aim of the image processing is to calculate the β discharging ratio, which defines the surface covered by the plasma. The algorithm is achieved in two main steps:

- a geometrical transformation, which achieves a cylindrical projection.
- a segmentation process, used to calculate the surface of the area covered by the discharge.

The initial image captured by the camera (Figure 4) first receives basic manipulations, which makes the file lighter and speeds up further treatments.

First of all, the image is cropped (Figure 5a), so as to keep only the reactor (useful region) with the same dimensions as its side view: L width and 2.R height. Then, in order to reduce the size of the file containing the picture and speed up its manipulation, the true-color RGB image is converted into a grayscale image. Each element of the resulting matrix contains only the gray level, ranging from 0 to 255, calculated as a weighted sum of the corresponding red, green and blue pixels. The gray level (GL) is calculated with the Python coded function (1), which implements recommendation Rec.709 [20]; these weights are considered to better represent human perception of red, green, and blue than equal weights.

$$GL = 0.2125 \times R + 0.7154 \times G + 0.0721 \times B \quad (1)$$

The obtained image is presented on Figure 5b; in all the pictures presented in this paper, for better readability, the grayscale images are shown with a color scale from violet (background), the lowest intensity, to yellow, the highest.

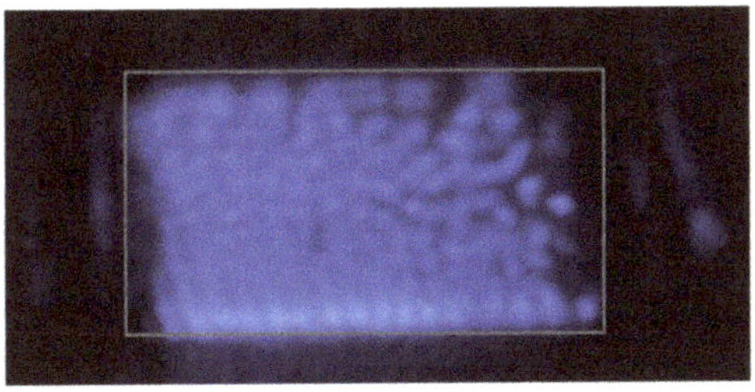

Figure 4. Initial image, acquired by the camera.

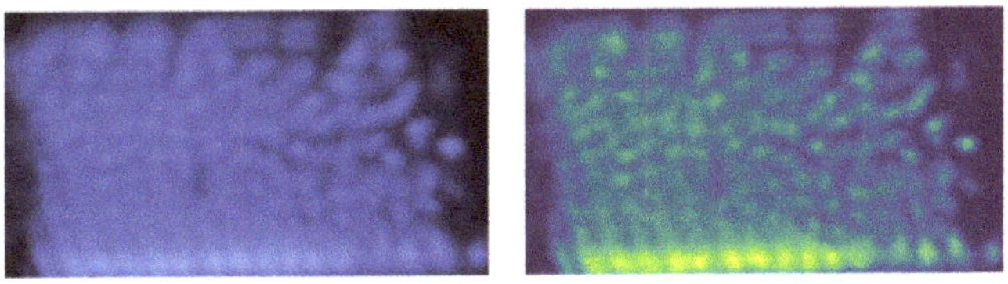

(**a**) (**b**)

Figure 5. Initial cropped image (**a**), and grayscale transformed (**b**).

2.2.1. Geometrical Transformation

The geometrical transformation is introduced in order to compensate the deformation of the discharge representation, which is caused by the cylindrical shape of the reactor, captured on the flat sensor of the camera. For that purpose, the Abel transformation [21–23] initially considered has been finally withdrawn, because the plasma distribution around the gas gap does not present the cylindrical invariance which is mandatory. A new method for calculation is proposed below.

On the taken image, the reactor cylindrical shape is flattened by the camera, as shown on Figure 6. The reactor has length L and is placed along the Z axis; the camera's optical axis is on the X axis. The plane (X, Y) is an orthogonal cross-section of the reactor (Figure 6b). The points $m(y_p)$ cover the external surface of the reactor, at outer radius r, for θ ranging from −90° to 90°. The point M(y), with y ranging from −R to +R, is the orthogonal projection, captured by the camera, of the points $m(y_p)$. Only the outer electrode is shown. Several geometrical assumptions are made:

(a) The streamer distribution is symmetrical to the plane X = 0 (the hidden face of the reactor is assumed to present the same aspect as the captured one). Therefore, only the front face is analyzed.
(b) The camera plane (Y, Z) is far enough from the reactor that the light rays reach it in parallel. This ensures that the points M(y) and $m(y_p)$ are aligned parallel to the optical axis of the camera (X axis). Therefore, the height of the image captured by the camera (Figure 6c) is equal to 2.R.
(c) Only the external surface of the reactor is considered—no depth of the plasma volume is considered (it means that possible streamers are seen as spots on the outer surface).

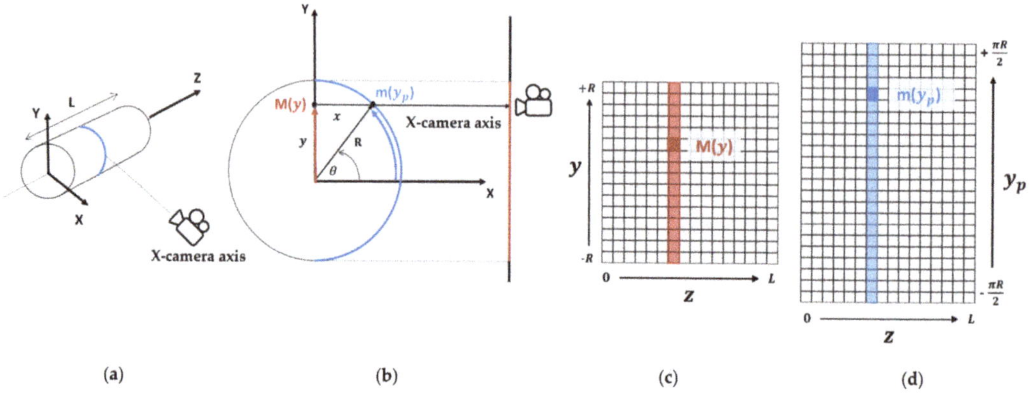

Figure 6. Principle of the geometrical transformation (projection): (**a**) 3D view of the reactor and the camera. (**b**) Orthogonal cross-section of the reactor. (**c**) Acquired picture. (**d**) Transformed picture.

Starting from the captured image, the goal of the geometrical transformation is to build the projected output image (Figure 6d): it is the rollout of the DBD reactor external surface. The height ratio between the captured image (Figure 6c) and the projected one (Figure 6d) is therefore equal to $\pi/2$. The width is the same for both images and equal to the length L of the reactor.

In order to build Figure 6d, each M(y) point of the acquired image is used to define the $m(y_p)$ point at vertical position y_p; if a streamer appears on the original picture as a spot with $\Delta z \Delta y$ size, on the transformed image it is spanned into $\Delta z \Delta y_p$ with:

$$y_p = R \times \theta = R \times \sin^{-1}\left(\frac{y}{R}\right) \quad (2)$$

$$\Delta y_p = \frac{\Delta y \times R}{\sqrt{R^2 - y^2}} = \frac{\Delta y}{\cos(\theta)} \quad (3)$$

Equation (2) is obtained by a basic trigonometric manipulation: the length y_p, which is also a circle segment, is equal to the radius R multiplied by the θ angle. The ratio $\Delta y_p / \Delta y$ from Equation (3) is a first-order approximation obtained with first y-derivative of Equation (2). Using these equations, the image is projected to cylindrical coordinates and rolled out. This process is repeated along the Z axis in all planes (X, Y) of the reactor to obtain the full picture. Figure 7b shows the obtained image in cylindrical coordinates.

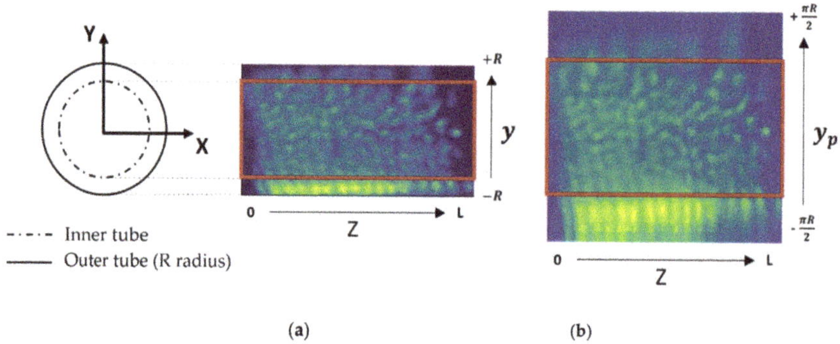

Figure 7. Projected unrolled image of the outer surface of the reactor: (**a**) Acquired grayscale image—Cylindrical coordinates output image (**b**). Red rectangle highlights the inner tube of the reactor.

2.2.2. Image Segmentation

Step 1—area of interest: as can be seen in the unrolled picture Figure 7b, the lower and upper parts of the discharge look brighter than the central part of it. The coaxial geometry of the reactor and the transparent quartz walls cause this effect. In the central part of the discharge, the inner electrode creates a solid background for the pictures, whereas in the upper and lower parts, the gas gap between the two electrodes and quartz barriers produces an optical effect that intensifies the discharge. To avoid biased results due to this optical effect and according to the assumption (c) that the plasma volume has no depth, the image is cropped again, erasing the parts which do not present a solid background. They correspond to the gas gap and only the central part of the picture, which has the height of the diameter of the inner tube (red frame figure below), is kept (Figure 8b)—one should notice that this figure is different from the original one, Figure 7a.

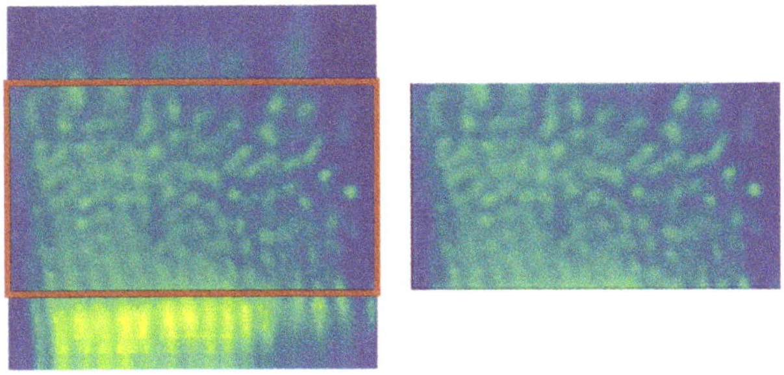

(**a**) (**b**)

Figure 8. Cylindrical coordinates output image (**a**), and its cropped central region with solid background (**b**).

Step 2—image segmentation: the discharge area is segmented using a thresholding technique, as shown in Figure 9. It means that a gray-level value called "threshold value" is used as the delimiter between the background and the discharge area. All pixels with values less than the threshold value are considered as background, and pixels with values greater than the threshold are considered as the discharge area. In order to find the threshold value, Otsu's method is used [24]: this method chooses a threshold value that minimizes the variance of the thresholded background and discharge pixels. The ability of this method to segment the image even with low intensity discharges (operating points at low power) of uniform appearance is remarkable (as will be shown in Section 3).

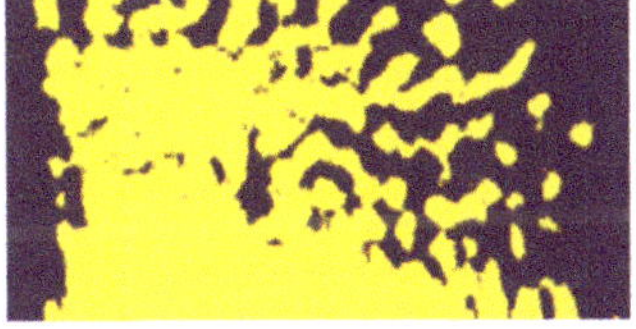

Figure 9. Segmented Discharge area (violet is background, yellow is discharge area).

Step 3—image analysis: the calculation of the β percentage is achieved with the ratio between the number of pixels of the discharge, obtained with the segmentation, and the total number of pixels. Other statistical results quantifying the discharge's uniformity are also presented in Section 3.3.

2.3. Partial Surface Discharging Analysis via the Electric Model

The DBD is commonly modelled in the literature by the electric circuit shown in Figure 10. C_d represents the capacitive behavior of the dielectric barrier(s), in this case the series equivalent capacitance of the two quartz cylinders. The gas is modeled as a dielectric (C_g) as long as it is not conductive ($|v_{gas}| < Vth$, thus $i_{gas} = 0$), and after breakdown it is represented with a constant voltage ($v_{gas} = \pm Vth$), the sign of which depends on the direction of the gas current [15,18,19].

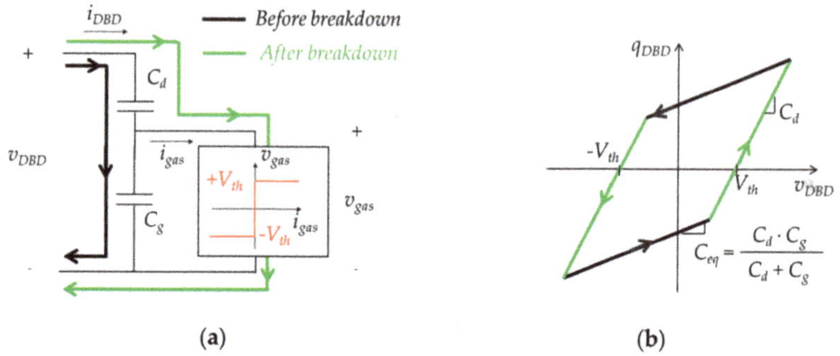

Figure 10. Simplified electric circuit model of the DBD, with current paths in ON–green and OFF–black plasma states (**a**) and its Manley's diagram (**b**).

The parameters of this model (C_d, C_g and Vth) are found with experimental waveforms for voltage and current on the DBD, then tracing the electrical charge vs. voltage diagram (known as Manley's diagram) as shown in Figure 10.

The slopes of the parallelogram are used to define the dielectric and series equivalent capacitances (respectively, C_d for the ON state and C_{eq} for the OFF state—C_{eq} being the value of the series connection of C_d and C_g). From the latter, the gas capacitance (C_g) is calculated. The zero-cross with the voltage axis determines the threshold voltage (Vth). The area enclosed by the parallelogram is equal to the energy injected during one period to the DBD, so it can be used to determine the average power.

It is well known that Vth, C_g, and C_d are physical parameters determined by the gas composition, pressure, dielectric material, and geometry; these three values define the behavior of the equivalent circuit, which remains predictive as long as the surface covered by the plasma on the electrodes, remains stable. Indeed, variations in the identified parameters as a function of the electric conditions given by the power supply are common, even if the reactor geometry does not change [11,12]. As shown in Figure 11, this can be observed in the case of the DBD reactor used in this work: here, the electrical energy injected into the plasma, controlled by the power supply, is changed. Accordingly, the discharge covers the whole surface of the reactor ((a), $\beta = 1$) or only part of it ((b), $\beta < 1$). Note that, concerning the identified parameters of the equivalent circuit (Figure 10), C_{eq} is similar for both cases, however, identified C_d and Vth change significantly: being physical parameters of the reactor, such changes are not acceptable.

As observed in the pictures beside the Manley's diagrams, this phenomenon in the model identification takes place when the discharge occurs in a partial area of the available electrode surface (Figure 11b). Depending on the operating conditions of the power supply, the discharge area extends until it fully covers the electrodes, and the values measured using Manley's diagram coincide with the theoretical ones. In that scenario, the classic DBD electric model, shown in Figure 10, completely represents the load. Nonetheless, for the partial surface discharging case, a modified model is proposed in the literature [8,11,25]. In consequence, a different equivalent electric model has to be used, where C_d, and C_g are both split into the non-discharging and discharging area (α and β percentages respectively, which fulfil: $\alpha + \beta = 1$), as displayed in Figure 12.

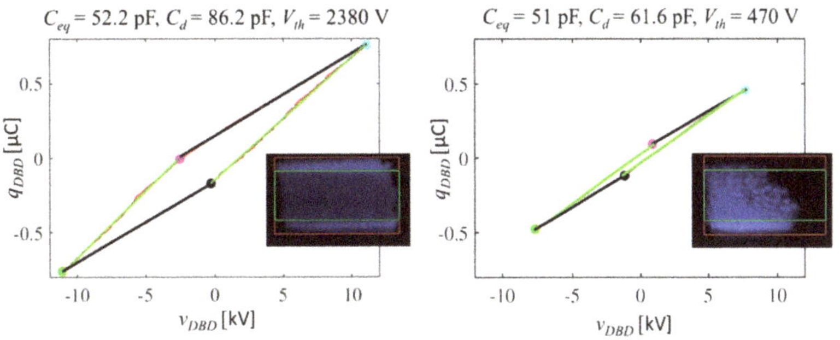

(a) (b)

Figure 11. Change of the DBD identified model parameters (C_{eq}, C_d and Vth) for the same reactor, with different supply conditions, leading to different discharging ratio: β = 1 (**a**) and β < 1 (**b**).

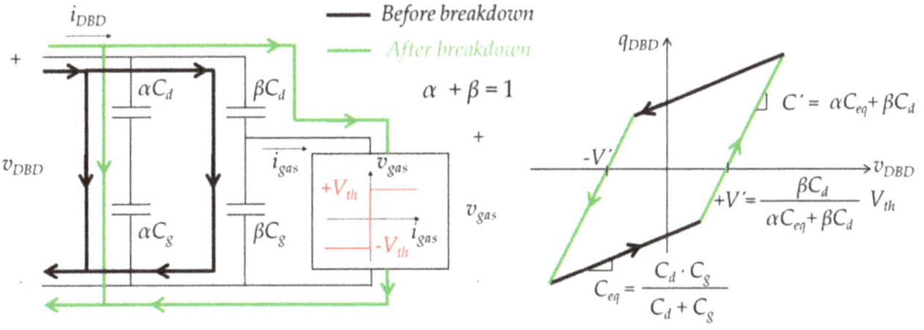

(a) (b)

Figure 12. DBD electrical model for partial discharging area (**a**), proposed in [11], along with its modified Manley's diagram (**b**).

In this case, the α and β parameters are calculated having previously identified C_d, C_{eq}, C_g, and Vth, using the Manley's diagram for a discharge covering all the surface. For the partial discharging area condition, C_{eq} does not change, as the series capacitor of the two equivalent circuits is the same when there is no discharge (Figures 10 and 12): this is proven experimentally in the example of Figure 11, with an error below 2.4% between the two measurements.

The percentage of the discharge area (β) can be found with the slope when the discharge has been established (C'), as follows:

$$\beta = \frac{C' - C_{eq}}{C_d - C_{eq}} \tag{4}$$

The breakdown voltage, Vth, can be verified according to Equation (5), using the charge variation in the OFF state, $\Delta Qdbd_{OFF}$ (black segments on Figure 12)

$$V\text{th} = \frac{\Delta Qdbd_{OFF}}{2 \times C_g}, \text{OFF state} \tag{5}$$

3. Results

The application of the two diagnostic methods for β discharging ratio, described in the previous section, is now presented and discussed.

3.1. *Agreement of the Circuit Analysis Method and Image Processing for β Ratio Diagnostic*

Two operating points obtained at 5 kHz with the sine voltage generator, corresponding to two different power levels (10 W and 25 W), are selected. Figure 13 presents the obtained results in each column (top-down): the electrical waveforms (voltage—blue, and current—green), the Manley diagram build with these data, the acquired reactor's pictures, the segmented and cropped (area of interest) grayscale image together with the β discharging ratio obtained from the equivalent circuit approach and with the image processing. The last data is associated with the margin error (the difference between the maximum and minimum values) estimated through repeated calculations using three different images acquired in steady state conditions (see below) during three different experiments.

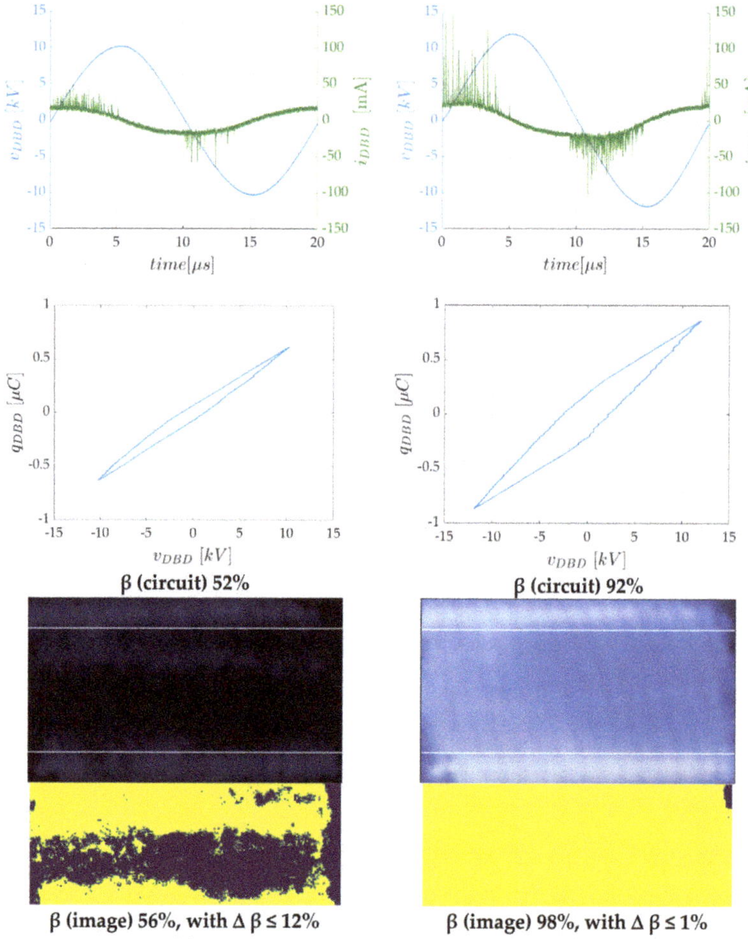

(a) (b)

Figure 13. Application of both diagnostic methods: (**a**) low power level (10 W). (**b**) high power (25 W). Measures are acquired in steady state.

It should be mentioned that the coverage of the discharge area varies from the time the system is started, with a typical transient shown in Figure 14. Here, the record starts when the power supply is turned ON, with a gas flow already stabilized (see Figure 2). For the presented operating conditions (f = 10 kHz, P = 30 W), one can observe during the transient the rise of the discharging surface (and accordingly the β ratio), which definitively stabilizes only after approximatively 120 s. For steady-state process analyses, data should only be acquired after this system time constant.

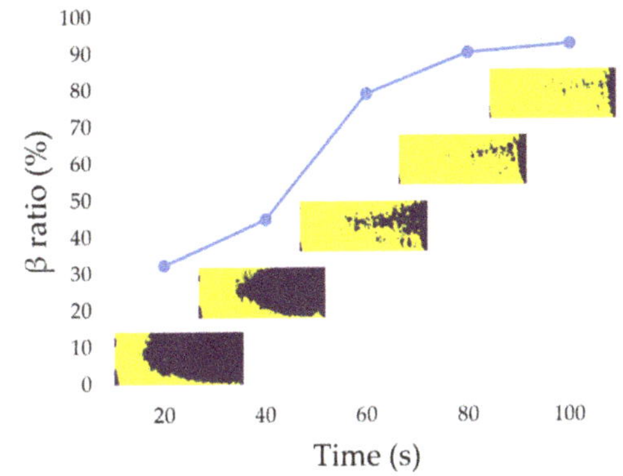

Figure 14. Partial discharging ratio β variation during the startup transient.

The two methods described in the previous section are now applied on a set of measures acquired with operating points covering a large domain (sine voltage power supply). This diversity of considered conditions is aimed at comparing the results of the two methods, whose results are presented on Figure 15: for each operating condition, three measurements are acquired in steady state during different experiments. The displayed value is the average of these three results, and the error bar indicates the maximum and minimum values. One can notice the very good agreement with a difference which remains generally below 10%. In most cases, the β discharging ratio obtained with the electrical circuit approach remains in the error range of the image processing method. The latter is obtained, using several images repeatedly acquired for each operating point; this systematic uncertainty remains below 12%.

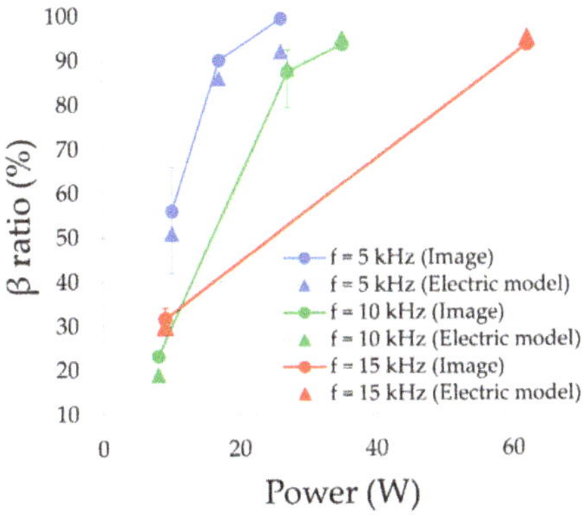

Figure 15. Partial discharging ratio β obtained with image processing and equivalent circuit analyzes. Results are grouped by values of supply frequency; adjustments of injected power are achieved with the peak value of imposed v_{DBD} voltage. Displayed values are obtained in steady state.

3.2. Application to Rectangular Current Power Supply Operated in Burst Mode

As shown in Figure 16, results obtained with the rectangular current power supply are difficult to analyze through the equivalent circuit approach: indeed, each burst of current pulses injected into the DBD creates an electrical transient (see voltage and current waveforms on Figure 16a), which has no time to vanish before the end of the burst. As a result, the Q-V Manley diagram exhibits a poorly trapezoidal shape, as can be appreciated in Figure 16b: this makes it very difficult to select the slopes to be used for the calculation of the circuit's parameters.

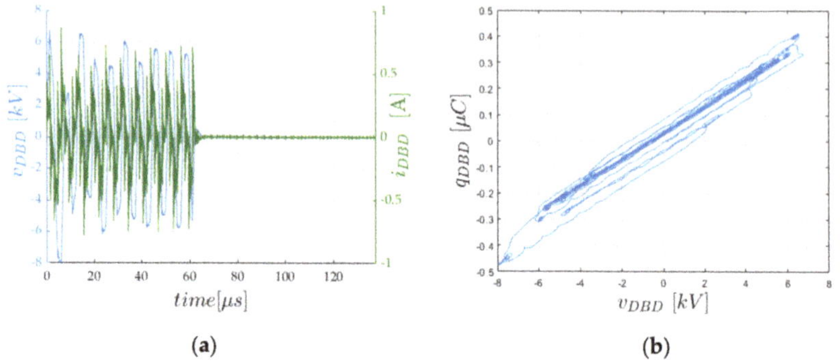

Figure 16. Rectangular current supplied system: electrical measurements of a whole burst (**a**), with DBD voltage (blue) and current (green), and associated Q-V Manley diagram (**b**).

Taking advantage of the very good convergence of both methods for β ratio diagnostic highlighted on Figure 15, it is proposed to admit:

- the parameter set (C_d, C_g, Vth), acquired thanks to previously achieved experiment, where the discharge fully covers the surface of the reactor (β = 100%), sketched by the equivalent circuit of Figure 10;
- the β ratio obtained by the image processing.

Using Equations (4) and (5), which translate the behavior of the equivalent circuit of Figure 12, it becomes possible to build and to draw the parallelepipedal figure, which should be considered.

Note that the image acquisition shows an averaged behavior of the system. As for the β value provided by the analysis of this image, therefore, this approach provides an equivalent average behavior over the burst. The image processing of the acquired picture shown in Figure 17a gives: β = 56%. Together with already known circuit parameters (C_d = 90 pF, C_g = 135 pF, Vth = 2585 V, independent from operating conditions), Figure 17b shows the Manley figure (red).

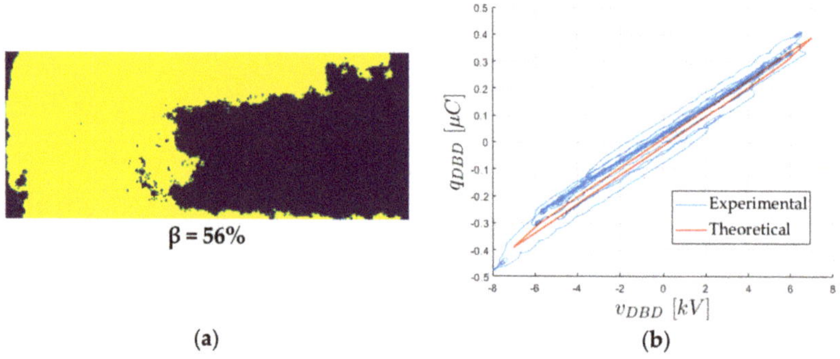

Figure 17. Rectangular current supplied system: processed image corresponding to Figure 16 (**a**), giving a value: β = 56% experimental Manley diagram (**b**), blue and the theoretical one (red), obtained with the known parameter set for the equivalent circuit: C_d = 90 pF, C_g = 135 pF, Vth = 2585 V.

3.3. Effect of the Supply Waveform on the Discharge Uniformity: Additional Diagnostic Provided by the Image Processing

In addition to the segmentation process, other statistical diagnostics of the images can provide very useful information about the discharge. We now consider the operating conditions obtained with the electrical waveforms shown in Figure 3, with two different generators; the waveforms are completely different but, in fact, they have the same power level (approx. 40 W).

The appearance of the discharges [26] shown in Figure 18 are very different: the discharge obtained with the sinusoidal voltage source (column (b)) appears much more diffuse than the one pumped with the rectangular current source (column (a)): in the original picture (column (a)), the spots which can be related to the streamers are clearly visible.

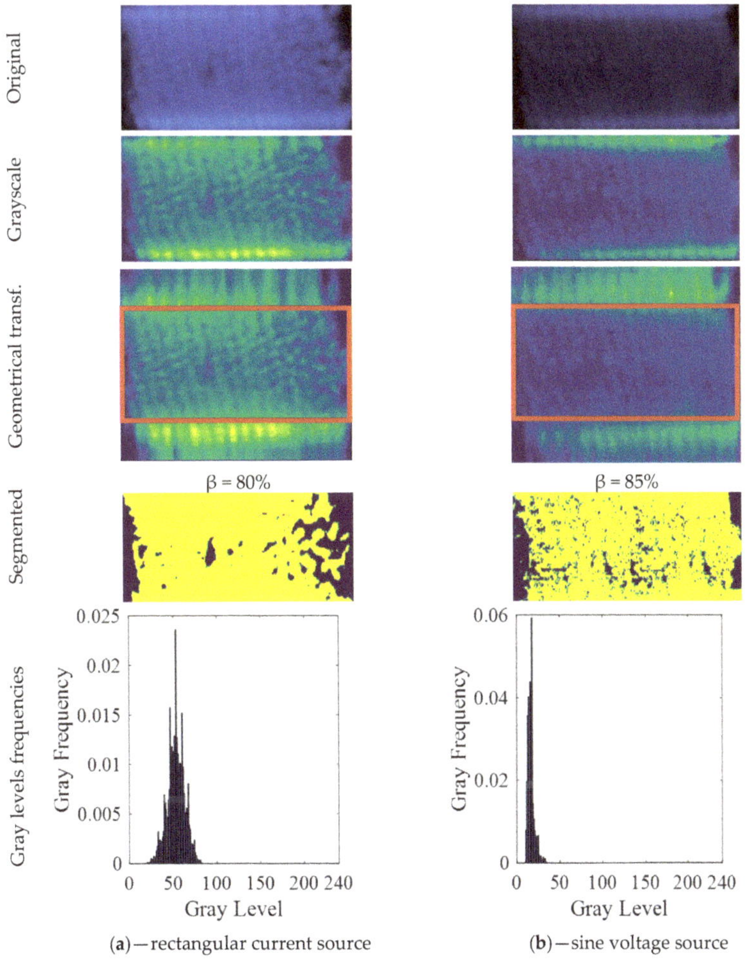

Figure 18. Image diagnostic of operating conditions obtained with square current source (column (**a**)) and sine voltage power supply (column (**b**))—electrical waveforms presented in Figure 3—from top to bottom: original image, grayscale, result of geometrical transformation, segmented image (central area), gray levels frequency.

The gray-levels histograms of the last row in Figure 18 present the result of a statistical analysis, which presents good matching with the discharge appearance and offers a quantification solution to translate the visual effect into a number. This analysis was proposed by [13] and is achieved as previously on the only central part of the image (red frame); it is carried out after the translation of the image into gray levels and its geometrical transformation (before the segmentation): the horizontal axis of the histogram presents the gray level (from 0 to 255), and the vertical axis presents the frequency of pixels for each level. Based on the histogram results, statistical measures as the mean gray level and the standard deviation are used to characterize the discharge. Below, the parameters of this analysis are commented:

- Mean Gray Level (μgray): It is the mean of the gray-level value (in the central discharge area). This indicates the mean brightness of the discharge. In order to be able to compare the discharges obtained under different operating conditions, care must be taken to deactivate all automatic settings of the camera.
- Gray Level Intensity: It is the sum of the gray-level values of the pixels in the area of interest.
- Discharge Intensity/mm^2: It is the Gray Level Intensity divided by the area covered by the discharge.
- Standard Deviation (SD): the SD measures the dispersion of the data from its mean value, and it is a crucial parameter to determine the discharge uniformity quantitatively [27]. In an ideal uniform discharge, all the reactor pixels should have the same gray-level value; thus, the SD is zero in this case. The SD value will rise if the gray level takes increasingly different values on the surface. In general, the lower the standard deviation, the data points tend to be closer to their mean, meaning a more uniform discharge. The value of SD is calculated considering each pixel of the image, as defined in [27].

Table 1 presents the resulting parameters of the image processing for both cases shown in Figure 18.

Table 1. Grayscale images statistical properties (electrical waveforms presented on Figure 3 and images in Figure 18).

Pict.	β [%]	Discharge Area [mm^2]	Mean Gray Level—μgray	Gray Level Intensity	Gray Level Intensity/mm^2	Standard Deviation—SD
Rectangular current—column (a)	80	1659	52.73	1,787,099	1077	10.12
Sinusoidal voltage—column (b)	85	1762	15.83	576,172	327	3.88

As can be seen, the SD of the case obtained with the rectangular current source is significantly higher than cases with the sine voltage. Despite the fact that cases worked with similar electrical power, the intensity of the first case is higher than for the second. Accordingly, the discharges obtained by the sinusoidal voltage source are more uniform, diffuse, and weak than the discharges obtained by the square current source. This observation has been verified with a set of different operating points in a wide range of the β parameter.

The Manley figures of both supply conditions showed that DBD works in a filamentary mode, even if diffuse and uniform discharges appeared with the sinusoidal voltage source.

One can notice that the image (a) is much more luminous than the (b) one—this is confirmed by the difference of the values of the Gray level Intensity/mm^2. Nevertheless, the Otsu's algorithm has been clearly able to differentiate the background and the area covered by the discharge. In this way, the discharge segmentation process is validated under different image conditions.

4. Conclusions

Two methods to evaluate the β discharging ratio of a dielectric barrier discharge are proposed in this paper. The equivalent circuit-based method uses recorded waveforms of voltage and current of the DBD reactor to build the Manley's diagram and to identify the equivalent circuit parameters and the β ratio. The image processing method uses pictures of the discharge captured through the transparent walls of the reactor. A two-step algorithm is presented and validated. First, a geometrical transformation compensates the distortion due to the shape of the reactor. Second, the segmentation of the images based on the Otsu's method is used to identify the discharge area and then to analyze it, based on the gray-level histograms.

These two methods were proved to work very well and to provide remarkably coherent results, under different intensity conditions of the discharge, when pumped with different electrical waveforms obtained with two very different power supplies. Additionally, a comparison between the discharges produced by a square current source and a sinusoidal voltage source with similar power levels has shown that more uniform discharges are obtained with the sinusoidal voltage source, and more intense discharges are obtained with the square current source. These observations have been correlated with statistical properties of the gray level acquired images, which provide a quantified appreciation of the discharge uniformity, very useful for achieving the comparison of the performances.

Author Contributions: Conceptualization, R.D. and H.P.; Investigation, V.R., R.D., N.B. and H.P.; Software, V.R. and N.B.; Supervision, R.D. and H.P.; Validation, V.R.; Visualization, V.R. and N.B.; Writing—original draft, V.R., R.D. and H.P.; Writing—review & editing, R.D., N.B. and H.P. All authors have read and agreed to the published version of the manuscript.

Funding: This research received no external funding.

Data Availability Statement: Not applicable.

Acknowledgments: The authors thank the French-Colombian cooperation program ECOS Nord—Colciencias-ICETEX, as well as Javeriana University project 10035.

Conflicts of Interest: The authors declare no conflict of interest.

References

1. Kogelschatz, U. Dielectric-barrier discharges: Their History, Discharge Physics, and Industrial Applications. *Plasma Chem. Plasma Process.* **2003**, *23*, 1–46. [CrossRef]
2. Massines, F.; Sarra-Bournet, C.; Fanelli, F.; Naudé, N.; Gherardi, N. Atmospheric Pressure Low Temperature Direct Plasma Technology: Status and Challenges for Thin Film Deposition. *Plasma Process. Polym.* **2012**, *9*, 1041–1073. [CrossRef]
3. Fridman, G.; Friedman, G.; Gutsol, A.; Shekhter, A.B.; Vasilets, V.N.; Fridman, A. Applied Plasma Medicine. *Plasma Process. Polym.* **2008**, *5*, 503–533. [CrossRef]
4. Ivankov, A.; Capela, T.; Rueda, V.; Bru, E.; Piquet, H.; Schitz, D.; Florez, D.; Diez, R. Experimental Study of a Nonthermal DBD-Driven Plasma Jet System Using Different Supply Methods. *Plasma* **2022**, *5*, 75–97. [CrossRef]
5. Wiesner, A.; Diez, R.; Florez, D.; Piquet, H. System for experimental investigation of DBD excilamps in view of control and optimization of UV emission. *Math. Comput. Simul.* **2019**, *165*, 92–106. [CrossRef]
6. Lomaev, M.I.; Sosnin, E.A.; Tarasenko, V.F.; Shits, D.V.; Skakun, V.S.; Erofeev, M.V.; Lisenko, A.A. Capacitive and barrier discharge excilamps and their applications (Review). *Instrum. Exp. Tech.* **2006**, *49*, 595–616. [CrossRef]
7. Talebizadeh, P.; Babaie, M.; Brown, R.; Rahimzadeh, H.; Ristovski, Z.; Arai, M. The role of non-thermal plasma technique in NOx treatment: A review. *Renew. Sustain. Energy Rev.* **2014**, *40*, 886–901. [CrossRef]
8. Fang, Z.; Qiu, Y.; Zhang, C.; Kuffel, E. Factors influencing the existence of the homogeneous dielectric barrier discharge in air at atmospheric pressure. *J. Phys. D Appl. Phys.* **2007**, *40*, 1401–1407. [CrossRef]
9. Okazaki, S.; Kogoma, M.;Ueharaÿ, M.; Kimura, Y. Appearance of stable glow discharge in air, argon, oxygen and nitrogen at atmospheric pressure using a 50 Hz source. *J. Phys. D Appl. Phys.* **1993**, *26*, 889–892. [CrossRef]
10. Belinger, A.; Naudé, N.; Ghérardi, N. Transition from diffuse to self-organized discharge in a high frequency dielectric barrier discharge. *Eur. Phys. J. Appl. Phys.* **2017**, *79*, 10802. [CrossRef]
11. Peeters, F.J.J.; van de Sanden, M.C.M. The influence of partial surface discharging on the electrical characterization of DBDs. *Plasma Sources Sci. Technol.* **2014**, *24*, 015016. [CrossRef]
12. Peeters, F.; Butterworth, T. Electrical Diagnostics of Dielectric Barrier Discharges. In *Atmospheric Pressure Plasma-from Diagnostics to Applications*; IntechOpen: London, UK, 2018. [CrossRef]

13. Wu, Y.; Ye, Q.; Li, X.; Tan, D. Classification of dielectric barrier discharges using digital image processing technology. *IEEE Trans. Plasma Sci.* **2012**, *40*, 1371–1379. [CrossRef]
14. Manley, T.C. The Electric Characteristics of the Ozonator Discharge. *Trans. Electrochem. Soc.* **1943**, *84*, 83–96. [CrossRef]
15. Pipa, A.; Brandenburg, R. The Equivalent Circuit Approach for the Electrical Diagnostics of Dielectric Barrier Discharges: The Classical Theory and Recent Developments. *Atoms* **2019**, *7*, 14. [CrossRef]
16. Kriegseis, J.; Moller, B.; Grundman, S.; Tropea, C. Capacitance and power consumption quantification of dielectric barrier discharge (DBD) plasma actuators. *J. Electrost.* **2011**, *69*, 302–312. [CrossRef]
17. Dubois, J. EMI/RFI Shielding Products & Smart Electronics Systems. Available online: https://www.jacquesdubois.com/ (accessed on 1 August 2022).
18. Rueda, V.; Wiesner, A.; Diez, R.; Piquet, H. Power Estimation of a Current Supplied DBD Considering the Transformer Parasitic Elements. *IEEE Trans. Ind. Appl.* **2019**, *55*, 6567–6575. [CrossRef]
19. Florez, D.; Schitz, D.; Piquet, H.; Diez, R. Efficiency of an Exciplex DBD Lamp Excited Under Different Methods. *IEEE Trans. Plasma Sci.* **2018**, *46*, 140–147. [CrossRef]
20. The International Telecommunication Union. *Basic Parameter Values for the HDTV Standard for the Studio and for International Programme Exchange*; ITU-R Recommendation BT.709, [formerly CCIR Rec. 709]; The International Telecommunication Union: Geneva, Switzerland, 1990.
21. van der Schans, M. Characterization of a Dielectric Barrier Discharge with a Square Mesh Electrode. Master's Thesis, Eindhoven University of Technology, Department of Applied Physics, Eindhoven, The Netherlands, 2014. Available online: https://pure.tue.nl/ws/portalfiles/portal/46997630/784532-1.pdf (accessed on 1 August 2022).
22. Keefer, D.R.; Smith, L.M.; Sudharsanan, S.I. Abel inversion using transform techniques. In Proceedings of the International Congress on Applications of Lasers & Electro-Optics, Arlington, VA, USA, 10–13 November 1986; pp. 50–58. [CrossRef]
23. Dribinski, V.; Ossadtchi, A.; Mandelshtam, V.A.; Reisler, H. Reconstruction of Abel-transformable images: The Gaussian basis-set expansion Abel transform method. *Rev. Sci. Instrum.* **2002**, *73*, 2634–2642. [CrossRef]
24. Otsu, N. A Threshold Selection Method from Gray-Level Histograms. *IEEE Trans. Syst. Man. Cybern.* **1979**, *9*, 62–66. [CrossRef]
25. Zhang, Q.; Zhao, H.; Lin, H.; Wu, J. A Novel Electrical Model of Dielectric Barrier Discharge for Quasi-Homogeneous Mode and Filamentary Mode. In Proceedings of the 21st International Conference on Electrical Machines and Systems (ICEMS), Jeju, Korea, 7–10 October 2018; pp. 865–870. [CrossRef]
26. Radu, I.; Bartnikas, R.; Wertheimer, M.R. Frequency and Voltage Dependence of Glow and Pseudoglow Discharges in Helium Under Atmospheric Pressure. *IEEE Trans. Plasma Sci.* **2003**, *31*, 1363–1378. [CrossRef]
27. Ye, Q.; Yun, D.; Yang, F.; Tan, D. Application of the gray-level standard deviation in the analysis of the uniformity of DBD caused by the rotary electrode. *IEEE Trans. Plasma Sci.* **2013**, *41*, 540–544. [CrossRef]

applied sciences

MDPI

Article

Enhancement of Wheat Flour and Dough Properties by Non-Thermal Plasma Treatment of Wheat Flour

Muhammad Jehanzaib Khan [1,*], Vojislav Jovicic [1,*], Ana Zbogar-Rasic [1] and Antonio Delgado [1,2]

[1] Institute of Fluid Mechanics (LSTM), Friedrich-Alexander-University Erlangen-Nuremberg (FAU), 91054 Erlangen, Germany
[2] German Engineering Research and Development Center LSTME Busan, Busan 46742, Korea
* Correspondence: muhammad.j.khan@fau.de (M.J.K.); vojislav.jovicic@fau.de (V.J.)

Abstract: Demand to improve food quality attributes without the use of chemicals has risen exponentially in the past few years. Non-thermal plasma (NTP) (also called 'cold plasma') is becoming increasingly popular for this purpose due to its unique low-temperature and non-chemical nature. In the present research, the concept of in situ dielectric barrier discharge (DBD) plasma treatment inside a rotational reactor for the direct treatment of wheat flour was experimentally analyzed. The primary research goal was to determine the effects of short-period NTP treatment of DBD type on flour and dough properties. For this purpose, the influence of different operating parameters was tested, i.e., treatment time, the amount of flour placed in the reactor and the environmental (air) temperature. Changes in the structural attributes of the most commonly used flours (type 550 and 1050) and their respective doughs were studied using a set of analytical techniques. Rheological analysis demonstrated the ability of NTP to significantly intensify the visco-elastic properties of dough produced from wheat flour type 550 that was treated for less than 180 s. This indicated that plasma treatment enhanced intermolecular disulphide bonds in gluten proteins, which resulted in stronger protein–starch network formations. However, longer treatment times did not result in a significant increase in the visco-elastic properties of wheat dough. The obtained results showed a 6–7% increase in flour hydration due to NTP treatment, which also makes a contribution to hydrogen bonding due to changes in the bonded and free water phase. Experimental findings further confirmed the dependence of NTP treatment efficiency on environmental air temperature.

Keywords: wheat flour; dough; rheology; non-thermal plasma; dielectric barrier discharge; wheat functionality; hydration properties; microstructure

Citation: Khan, M.J.; Jovicic, V.; Zbogar-Rasic, A.; Delgado, A. Enhancement of Wheat Flour and Dough Properties by Non-Thermal Plasma Treatment of Wheat Flour. *Appl. Sci.* **2022**, *12*, 7997. https://doi.org/10.3390/app12167997

Academic Editor: Bogdan-George Rusu

Received: 28 June 2022
Accepted: 8 August 2022
Published: 10 August 2022

1. Introduction

Cereals and grains are abundantly used worldwide, constituting a major part of human food consumption. Cereals and their products are energy sources for humans and animals, and contain carbohydrates, proteins, fiber and vitamins (such as E and B), along with magnesium and zinc [1–3]. Grains are consumed either whole or in powder form, which forms exist in different granulations and have different chemical compositions [4]. Generally, a grain consists of three parts: (1) bran, i.e., the outer layer, mostly rich with dietary fiber; (2) germ, i.e., the inner layer, consisting of lipids and proteins; and (3) endosperm, i.e., the bulk of a kernel, full of starch, proteins and minerals [5]. A powder form, i.e., flour, is a blend of these parts in different proportions, leading to different flour classifications.

Plant-based foods are often subjected to thermal or chemical processing prior to consumption [6]. However, nowadays, the customer requirement to preserve nutrient ratios by reducing the treatment temperatures for preserving food quality and reducing the use of chemical treatment agents have urged food engineers to search for other, suitable, non-chemical food processing methods. Modern consumers demand rich organoleptic, additive-free food, environmentally friendly processing, freshness and high sensory and nutritional attributes [7,8]. On the other hand, insufficient processing of food products can lead to the proliferation of bacterial, parasitic and pathogenic infections in humans [9]. Food-borne illnesses have significantly increased in recent years due to consumption of food that has been inadequately processed and therefore correct storage is additionally important to prevent mould formation, pest infestation and grain germination [6]. Microorganisms and pathogens occur in grains stored in humid environments, in which bran absorbs a significant amount of water, thus lowering the concentration of gluten and starch in the kernel and ultimately affecting end product quality [5,10].

Conventional thermal processing measures for food, for boosting shelf life, hygiene and structural properties, can be very detrimental to food nutrient ratios and sensory and organoleptic qualities [11]. Currently employed sterilization and processing techniques, such as chemical preservation [12,13], addition of bio-preservatives [14], mild heat treatments [15], microwave processing [16], ultrasound processing [17], reduction of water activity [18], high hydrostatic pressure technology [19,20] and vacuum and hurdle techniques [21], provide limited benefits in comparison with their adverse alterations of food properties, such as shape, color, taste, smell, structure, nutrient degradation, formation of toxic byproducts, etc. [9,22].

Wheat is one of the most important and the world's leading staple crop, which is full of nutrients [3]. The main factors affecting the quality of wheat-based products are gluten proteins, which are responsible for the visco-elastic properties of end products [23]. Their properties affect the rheological behavior and the gas-holding capability of a dough, as well as the texture and final volume of baked products. Wheat kernels are composed of 70–75% starch, 10–14% proteins, with the remainder constituted by minerals [24]. Wheat proteins are divided into two groups, i.e., non-gluten and gluten proteins. Gluten proteins comprise around 80–85% of the total protein contents of wheat flour and are further divided into gliadins and glutenins. Gliadins are monomeric proteins, which are mainly responsible for viscous and extensibility behavior during dough network formation. Glutenins are polymeric or aggregative proteins which influence the elastic and cohesiveness properties of dough networks.

The number and distribution of sulphur–sulphur (S-S) bonds, which are formed due to the presence of cysteine residues in gliadins and glutenins, significantly influence dough properties. However, S-S bonds are formed differently in two protein types: in gliadins, they lead to the formation of intramolecular S-S bonds, while in glutenins intermolecular S-S bonds are formed [25]. The S-S bonds for dough network formation start to activate during the kneading process, as soon as the wheat flour is hydrated due to the addition of water. During the network formation, these S-S bonds are in the form of fibrils. Macrofibrils of protein aggregates are formed by the formation of intermolecular S-S bonds. These fibrils then transform to a continuous film, which finally forms a homogeneous and fine gluten matrix [26,27]. On the other hand, several low-molecular weight thiols, containing a free SH group, are present in wheat flour, and have strong dough-weakening effects. The tripeptide glutathione (GSH) has the biggest impact; it is present in reduced (GSH) and oxidized, glutathione disulfide (GSSG) forms. A free SH group reacts with glutenin and forms glutathionylated protein (PSSG), which negatively affects the formation of intermolecular S-S bonds.

Wheat flour is normally processed not only to improve hygiene, shelf life and texture-related properties, but also to minimize the negative effects of GSH and GSSH [28]. A common industrial practice is to use chemical additives, e.g., ascorbic acid (i.e., vitamin C) as a reducing agent, which is extensively used to improve wheat flour textural properties (e.g., elastic and viscous properties). Its oxidized form dehydroascorbic acid (DHA) is responsible for the removal of free SH groups in flour, hence preventing the glutathione to create PSSG. The reaction mechanism is shown in Equations (1) and (2). Ascorbic acid easily converts to DHA in the presence of an enzyme and is limited by the availability of atmospheric oxygen during kneading. DHA reacts with GSH to form ascorbic acid and

GSSG, thus limiting the formation of PSSG. As a result, the number of S-S intermolecular bonds increases.

$$\text{Ascorbic acid} + 0.5\ O_2 \rightleftharpoons \text{Dehydroascorbic Acid} + H_2O \quad (1)$$

$$\text{Dehydroascorbic Acid} + \text{GSH} \rightleftharpoons \text{Ascorbic acid} + \text{GSSG} \quad (2)$$

Although many other chemicals (KIO_3, $KbrO_3$, chlorine, etc.) and oxidizing bacteria have been used to modify wheat flour functionality, the food industry is moving towards restricting the use of chemicals, and therefore the need for non-chemical treatment methods increases. Ozone is an example of an oxidizing agent, acceptable for use in the food industry [29]. Mei et al. [30] and Desouky et al. [31] investigated the effects of ozone on both wheat flour and grain functionality and suggested it as a good alternative to chemicals for improving wheat flour characteristics. The key features that are responsible for the superiority of ozone over commonly used chemicals are its high oxidation potential and the fact that no residues are left after the treatment [32].

Non-thermal plasma (NTP) has emerged as a new and effective method in food processing that retains food quality better than conventional methods [33]. Corona discharge (CD) and dielectric barrier discharge (DBD) are two forms of atmospheric non-thermal plasmas that can produce abundant amounts of ozone together with some other active species [34]. In contrast to ozone generators, DBD and CD can produce ozone in situ and create a ground for a direct reaction between reactive oxygen species and wheat proteins. Plasma is a an overall neutral gas, mainly composed of positively and negatively charged particles, neutrons, ions and particles that are heavy and with high energies [35]. Plasma is the fourth state of matter and is abundantly present in the universe. It was first discovered in the 18th century by William Crookes and named by Irving Langmuir and Levy Tonks in 1929 [36]. Based on electron temperature and thermodynamic equilibrium, plasma can be classified as high-temperature (thermal) or low-temperature (non-thermal) plasma [37]. Ionization degree may vary from partial ionization, in the case of NTP, to full ionization, in the case of thermal plasma [38].

Thermal plasmas with high electron densities ($>10^{22}\ m^{-3}$) and temperatures (4000 to 20,000 K) can be produced by electric discharge to reach high current flow through a fully ionized gas [39]. Electron temperature in NTP is much higher compared to the temperature of the bulk gas molecules, leading to a much lower temperature of the overall plasma, in the range of 30–50 °C [7]. NTP is thus quite suitable for the treatment of living cells, tissues and heat-sensitive materials [38].

Numerous researchers ([4,34,40–45] have studied the interaction of DBD plasma with wheat flour and have found that ozone and active species ($H^\bullet$, $O^\bullet$, $OH^\bullet$, $HO_2^\bullet$) generated during gas ionization can promote structural changes in starch and protein macromolecules (e.g., promoting cross-linking, depolymerization between molecules and the formation of new functional groups) similar to the changes induced by the use of chemicals. Mishra et al. [46] studied the influence of NTP treatment on wheat flour structural properties and determined an increase in the elastic and viscous modulus of the prepared dough. Modifications to biological characteristics and surface properties were confirmed by Bahrami et al. [34]. They reported no change in the total aerobic bacterial count and non-starch lipids. No visible change in the total protein amount was reported; however, there was a trend towards higher-molecular weight fractions, which resulted in thicker dough.

NTP, which is produced in a gas phase, is rich in high-energy species and the contact between the surfaces of flour particles and plasma species is crucial for its structural changes. The reactor design for flour treatment with NTP is of vital importance, as it influences the uniform exposure to plasma species and thus allows for optimal effects of plasma treatment in terms of flour functionality [47].

This study introduces a novel concept of a cylindrical, rotational reactor for wheat flour treatment with in situ produced NTP. Ease of scaling up was considered as a key factor during the development of the concept. The research focus was on defining the optimal operating conditions (e.g., the minimal treatment time) to reach the maximum dough strength, as well as understanding the influence of reactor capacity and the influence of environmental air temperature change (often variable from day to day) on the efficiency of the NTP treatment process.

2. Materials and Methods

Germany's wheat flour type 550 (equivalent to all-purpose flour) and type 1050 (equivalent to high-gluten flour) were used in this study to investigate the effects of non-thermal plasma. The main difference between the two flour types lies in their protein contents. Flour analysis demonstrates protein contents of 11.10 g and 12.68 g per 100 g of flour in the types 550 and 1050, respectively. A change in the hydration properties and the microstructure of wheat flour was determined before and after the NTP treatment. The effects of NTP treatment in terms of change in dough strength were analyzed in detail by means of rheological analysis.

2.1. Experimental Setup

The experimental setup for a batch treatment of flour samples using NTP, as shown in Figure 1, consists of three parts: (1) a plasma generator (HVG 80-3000, company Diener, Germany) [48]; (2) a cylindrical, rotational reactor, for the treatment of flour samples with DBD plasma; and (3) a control and data acquisition system (DAQ) system.

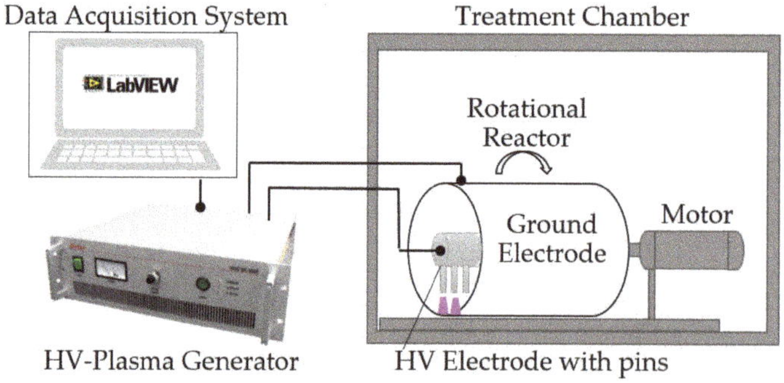

Figure 1. Experimental setup for Non-thermal plasma (NTP) treatment of wheat flour.

DBD plasma type was produced under atmospheric conditions using a high-voltage plasma generator (power: 120 W, frequency: 80 kHz, voltage: 7 kV). Air was used as plasma gas. The reactor has a capacity between 50 and 500 g of flour. It is designed as a rotational cylindrical vessel, made of stainless steel, and contains two concentric electrodes (Figure 2): (1) an outer (ground) electrode, which is in the form of a hollow, rotating cylinder (D = 150 mm, L = 300 mm, wall thickness = 2 mm) made of stainless steel and mounted axially on a rotating shaft. A dielectric barrier (thickness = 2 mm), made of Plexiglas (Polymethyl-methacrylate, PMMA), was attached to the inner side of the outer electrode. To ensure a uniform mixing during the NTP treatment, baffles (made of plastic, height = 30 mm and thickness = 3 mm) were placed on the inner wall of the outer cylinder. The outer electrode is connected to a motor, in order to provide its rotation; and (2) an inner (high-voltage) electrode (D = 50 mm, made of stainless steel), which is stationary and is positioned coaxially to the outer electrode. In order to reduce the electric power needed to induce DBD, a row of thin pins (made of aluminum, height = 43 mm and thickness = 5 mm) are attached to the high-voltage electrode, with a discharge gap of 2 mm between the pin tips and the dielectric layer (Figure 2). The reactor is closed with a cap from one side, and the other side is left open to the atmosphere.

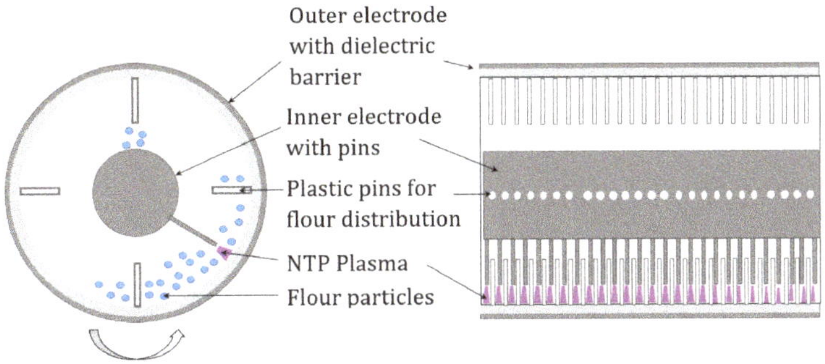

Figure 2. Test reactor for dielectric barrier discharge (DBD) plasma flour interaction.

At the beginning of each experiment, flour is added to the reactor and partially fills the annular gap between the electrodes. During the treatment, the reactor rotates at a constant speed of 10 RPM. Although the reactor is open to the environment, a low rotational speed was selected to avoid the formation of flour clouds that might lead to an explosive atmosphere. Since plasma-generated reactive species, including ozone, have very short half-lives, the described configuration enables a direct contact between these species and the target flour. After the treatment, flour samples were analyzed using a set of analytical techniques which will be described further in the text.

2.2. Dough Preparation

Doughs were prepared from untreated and treated flour samples in order to identify and compare the changes induced by the plasma treatment.

A standard approach to keep flour stable at room temperature for the purpose of packing and storing is to keep its moisture content at 14%. This standard moisture content may vary when flour is exposed to air, depending on its humidity. A compensation for this change in moisture content was used to modify the basic recipe. The correct amounts of flour and water for dough sample preparation were determined according to Equations (3) and (4), respectively.

$$\text{Flour mass (corrected)} = (100 - 14) \times M/(100 - x) \tag{3}$$

$$\text{Water mass (corrected)} = (\text{WAM} \times M) + (M - \text{corrected flour mass}) \tag{4}$$

where M (g) is the initial amount of flour (250 g), x (%) is the amount of moisture in flour (for this flour batch, determined to be 13.4%) and WAM (%) is the water-absorption capacity, for the default moisture content of 14%. Flour, water (25 °C) and salt (1 g) were mixed in a dough preparation machine (MUM48A1, Bosch). After 10 min of kneading, the dough was stored in a plastic bag to avoid drying and left to rest for 30 min at 25 °C. Afterwards, rheological analysis was performed to determine the dough's visco-elastic properties.

2.3. Analysis of Flour and Dough

2.3.1. Flour Hydration Properties

Water plays an important role in wheat dough strength due to the ability of protein matrixes to absorb and retain bound, capillary and physically entrapped water against gravity [49]. At lower hydration levels, water bonds flour proteins and starch granules via hydrogen bonds. Free water phase starts to appear at higher hydration levels (water fraction from 0.23 to 0.35), where chemical reactions (i.e., development of gluten matrix) occur during the dough development process [50]. Hence, small changes in both bonded and free water levels result in considerable variation in dough visco-elastic properties.

For this reason, the water-holding capacity (WHC) and the water-binding capacity (WBC) of untreated (control) and treated flour samples were measured and compared. The

WHC is the amount of water retained by flour particles without any stress conditions. For this purpose, 1 ± 0.05 g wheat flour was mixed with 10 mL of deionized water and left for 24 h. Afterwards, the supernatant was filtered and the wet wheat flour sample was weighed again. The WBC is the amount of water retained by flour after centrifugation. The samples were prepared according to the WHC procedure, and after 24 h centrifuged at 2000 revolutions for 10 min. Both WHC and WBC were measured according to the procedure described by Chaple et al. [41].

2.3.2. Dough Rheology

Rheological testing is a method commonly employed in the analysis of food-related substances; it is used to study the deformation and flow behavior (i.e., visco-elastic behavior) of test samples. Frequency and amplitude sweeps are two common practices used to study visco-elastic behavior. The former shows the influence of angular frequency on visco-elastic properties, while keeping the deformation amplitude constant. It is usually used to study frequency and time-dependent behavior within a non-destructive deformation range of materials. The latter demonstrates the influence of stress amplitude (at a constant frequency) on dough rheological properties.

The current investigation is based on an amplitude sweep study, by means of which G' (storage modulus), G'' (loss modulus), the linear visco-elastic region (LVE) and the yield and flow point can be determined. A rheometer (UDS-200, Anton Paar, Germany) [51] was used for the rheological study. A dough sample (10 g) was placed between the probe (MP31) and the bottom plate of the rheometer. Sandpaper (No. 60) was used on the probe and on the bottom plate, to avoid wall slip during the analysis. The frequency was set to 0.5 Hz and the amplitude gamma was set from 0.001 to 200% log to observe the visco-elastic region. The total number of measurement points was 40 and the time interval between each point was 20 s. Storage and loss moduli were plotted as functions of deformation on a log–log graph to study dough behavior.

2.3.3. Scanning Electron Microscopy (SEM)

Scanning electron microscopy (SEM) is a technique that allows analysis of the microstructures of wheat dough samples. The development of a wheat dough microstructure is a complex process which depends on time, the addition of water and the input of mixing energy. The microstructure and the rheological properties of a dough are connected to the properties of the individual flour components, their behavior after the addition of water, the free water phase and the mobility of water [52].

The microstructural changes in the wheat flours and the respective doughs were followed by SEM (Auriga, Carl-Zeiss, Jena, Germany). The analysis was performed with an accelerating voltage of 1 kV and a working distance of 5 mm. Prior to SEM analysis, both flour and dough samples were placed in an oven at 30 °C for 24 h and then cooled in a desiccator in order to remove moisture from the samples without destroying their structures.

2.4. Experimental Procedure

In the scope of this research, the influence of process parameters, i.e., treatment time, treated flour amount and air temperature, on changes in wheat flour and dough was determined and quantified. In the first set of experiments, the influence of treatment time (1, 3 and 5 min) on dough functional properties was determined. For this purpose, wheat flour samples with a mass of 50 g were treated by NTP. In the second set of experiments, the effect of the treatment reactor design (i.e., reactor volume vs. mass of the treated flour) on dough strength was investigated. The reactor was filled with flour (50, 150, 250, 350 and 450 g) and treated for 3 min. The third set of experiments included the effects of NTP, produced at different air temperatures (10, 20, 30 and 40 °C), on dough strength (flour amount: 50 g, treatment time: 3 min).

3. Results and Discussion

3.1. Effects of Non-Thermal Plasma Treatment Time on Wheat Flour and Dough Properties

3.1.1. Hydration Properties of Flour

The variation in the moisture content of wheat flour samples with treatment time (1, 3 and 5 min) is shown in Figure 3. It was determined five times per sample, based on which the standard deviation was calculated. The obtained results showed a general trend towards a decrease in moisture content with respect to treatment duration. A low moisture content (i.e., 12–15%) keeps the flour stable at room temperature. A decrease in the moisture content of wheat flour is also connected to change in physically "bounded" water amount and has a decisive influence on rheological, physical and chemical properties. There are certain indications in the literature that a lowering of moisture content results in mechanical rigidity and the complex viscosity of a dough [53,54], which characteristics are directly related to the stronger visco-elastic properties of wheat dough.

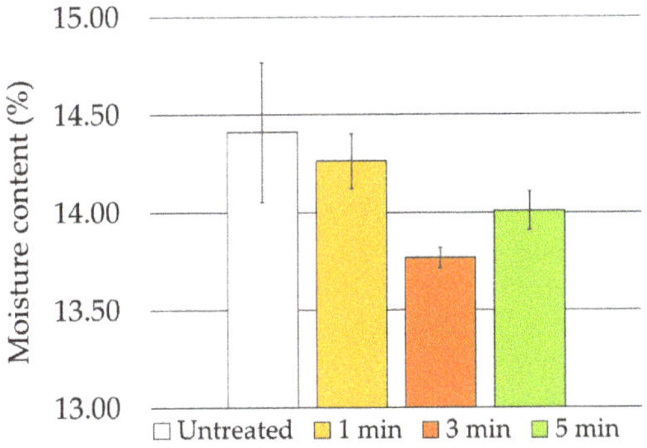

Figure 3. Change in the moisture content of wheat flour (type 550) as a function of NTP treatment time.

The dependence of the WHC on treatment time (1, 3 and 5 min), as shown in Figure 4a, was determined five times per sample, based on which the standard deviation was calculated. The WHC of the untreated sample was 168% ± 5% water retained per one gram of flour, which increased slowly with treatment time to reach its maximal value of 173% ± 4%, corresponding to 3 min of plasma treatment time. This corresponds to the finding shown in Figure 3, i.e., that as the moisture content decreases with treatment time, the water-holding ability of the flour increases. Still, no firm conclusion could be drawn at this point, as the standard deviation of this measurement was high compared to the observed change in WHC values.

The WBC dependence on treatment time, shown in Figure 4b, was also determined using five measurements per sample. The WBC level for untreated flour was measured to be 73% ± 3%. The maximum increase, just under 80% ± 1%, was observed for the NTP treatment of 3 min. Longer treatment resulted in decrease in WBC. Higher hydration values (WHC, WBC) were observed in the case of the untreated type 1050 flour (92% ± 1%) due to its higher protein content. However, no significant differences in the tendencies relating to hydration properties between the flour types 550 and 1050 were observed; thus, these were not separately presented.

Both the WHC and WBC of the tested wheat samples (types 550 and 1050) increased with plasma treatment time. The treatment time of three minutes resulted in a maximum enhancement (7% ± 3%) of the WBC of type 550 flour. It is postulated that this increase in WHC can be due to the hydrolytic depolymerisation of starch [41]. In addition, the surface modifications (increase in surface energy due to the addition or exchange of functional groups [55,56]) of flour particles due to the plasma treatment could be another important factor that influences the hydration properties of flour. It has also been reported in the literature that plasma treatment results in a decrease in water contact angle, leading to higher water permeability, which results in an increased affinity of flour particles towards water [57].

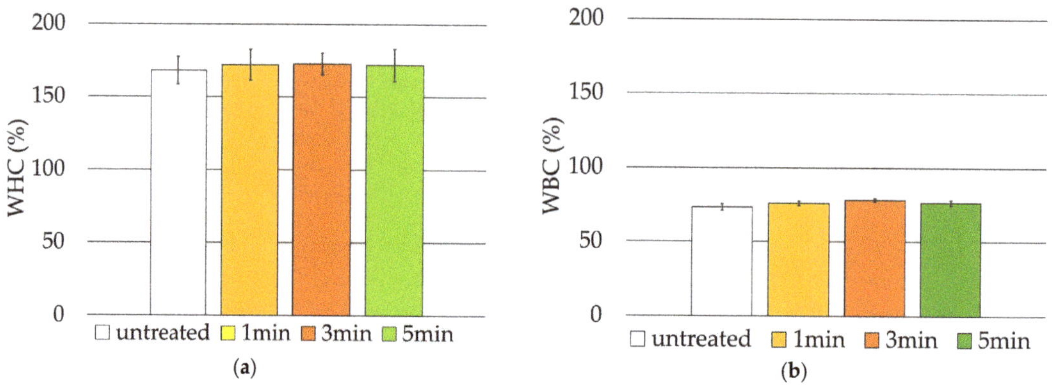

Figure 4. Change in the water-holding (**a**) and water-binding (**b**) capacity of wheat flour (type 550) as a function of NTP treatment time.

3.1.2. Visco-Elastic Properties of Dough

Changes in the functional properties of doughs produced with untreated and treated wheat flour were tested as a function of flour treatment duration. These properties were determined by rheological measurements, where the dependence of the storage and loss moduli (G' and G'') of doughs were plotted against the induced deformation. The modulus G' represents the elastic properties and the modulus G'' represents the viscous properties of a wheat dough. These two parameters, together with their combination, contribute to the functional properties of wheat dough, defining it as a visco-elastic material.

The change in the G' and G'' values of doughs made from the two flour types (550 and 1050) as a function of deformation and treatment time on a logarithmic scale are presented in Figure 5a,b.

A rheological behavior diagram for wheat dough has three parts: (1) a linear visco-elastic region, where the elastic properties prevail. This lies between zero deformation and the deformation at which the yield point (i.e., the end of the elastic behavior and the start of plastic behavior) has been reached. This is the point at which the strain corresponds to a ~5% drop in the storage modulus [58]; (2) a plastic region, where the increasing deformation starts to permanently destroy the dough (or protein–starch) structure and cannot be regained. This is the region between the yield point and the flow point (i.e., the threshold of shear stress, above which solid material will start to flow); and (3) the region above the flow point, where a solid behaves as a liquid, since the deformation potential is so huge that all the forces responsible for holding the material structure are overruled.

Figure 5a,b shows that G' is higher than G'', as is characteristic of visco-elastic materials. The experimental results demonstrate that the changes caused by the NTP treatment of flour, reflected by increases in the G' and G'' values of the formed dough, initially increased as the treatment time was prolonged. This increase reached its maximum value for the treatment time of 3 min for both flour types, after which the values of G' and G'' sank.

Figure 5a and Table 1 demonstrate that the NTP treatment showed its maximum potential for the type 550 flour, with a two-fold increase in the visco-elastic properties (G' = 85–130% and G'' = 76–111%) for the treatment duration of 3 min. This finding corresponds to the maximum change in hydration properties of flour with the three minutes treatment, as shown in Figure 4. On the other hand, the moduli of the untreated high-protein flour (type 1050) were already significantly higher compared to those of the flour type 550, i.e., 200–400% for G' and 200–330% for G''. Thus, the corresponding maximum changes in G′ and G″ in the plasma-treated samples of type 1050 were low to mild (G′ = 0–28% and G″ = 0–16%) (Figure 5b and Table 1). This finding also confirms the limited enhancement of the hydration properties of the type 1050 flour.

(a)

(b)

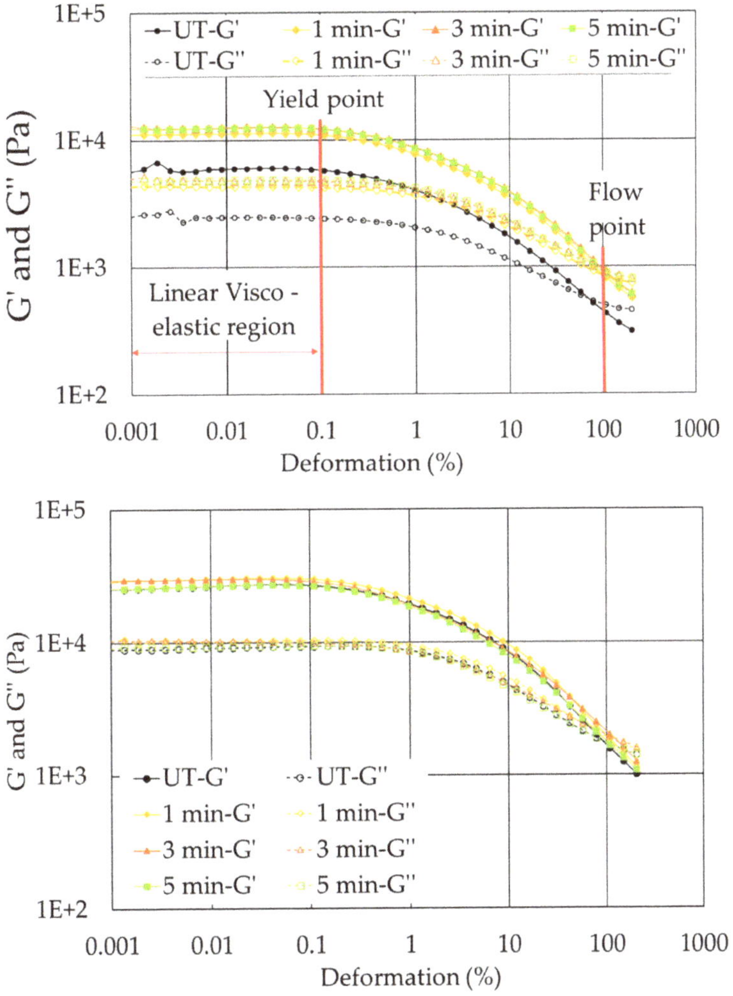

Figure 5. Change in the storage (G′) and loss (G″) moduli of wheat dough as a function of NTP treatment time: (**a**) for the flour type 550; (**b**) for the flour type 1050.

Table 1. Increase in G′ and G″ for the doughs produced with NTP-treated flour samples (presented as minimum-to-maximum increase) in comparison to doughs produced with untreated flour samples) as a function of treatment time.

Increase (%)	1 min		3 min		5 min	
Flour Type	G′ (%)	G″ (%)	G′ (%)	G″ (%)	G′ (%)	G″ (%)
550	67–105	57–88	85–130	76–111	81–123	72–110
1050	10–17	8–19	0–28	0–16	0–8	0–5

Analysis of variance (ANOVA) [59] was used in order to determine significant statistical differences between the samples. The obtained results for the type 550 flour ($p < 0.05$) (provided in the Supplementary Materials S1) confirmed the existence of significant statistical differences between untreated and treated samples, i.e., the effect of non-thermal plasma treatment on flour properties was statistically significant. However, in the case of type 1050, the obtained p-value was larger than 0.05. This implies that the effect of NTP treatment on type 1050 flour was not statistically significant, i.e., the influence of treatment cannot be established.

A general trend towards an increase in the yield points of the doughs produced with plasma-treated flour samples can be noticed, representing an increase in the linear visco-elastic (LVE) region. Increased elastic properties further indicate an increase in dough strength. The results presented in Figure 5a demonstrate that the flow point value increased by 51% and the yield point value by 75% when the flour type 550 was treated for 3 min in comparison to the untreated (control) sample. Chittrakorn et al. [60] explained an increase in dough strength in terms of an increase in the number of disulphide bonds within the protein matrix in the dough, i.e., the higher the number of disulphide bonds, the higher the storage and loss moduli. The properties of the dough made from flour type 1050 (Figure 5b) showed similar qualitative behaviors under the same plasma conditions; however, the quantitative change was much lower than for that made with type 550 flour.

Some other authors ([53,61,62]) have suggested that change in visco-elastic behavior could be connected to the hydration properties of wheat flour. The changes in moisture content, WHC and WBC, as shown in Figures 3 and 4, reflect the change in bonded and free water content levels, which directly affect gluten–starch and starch–starch bonding through hydrogen bonds. These bindings, enhanced by the plasma treatment, started to dominate the dough characteristics, making the treated samples stronger than the control samples.

Based on the presented results, it can be concluded that a plasma treatment time of 5 min will result in decreased structural strength of wheat dough, which could be connected to the weakening of disulphide bonds in the protein matrix and to the decrease in the WHC and WBC of wheat flour. Further, it can be concluded that NTP-induced intensification of visco-elastic properties is inversely proportional to the amount of protein present in the flour, i.e., with a higher protein content, the change in the visco-elastic properties of dough due to NTP is lower.

3.1.3. Wheat Dough Microstructure

Bechtel et al. [63] studied dough development with light and transmission electron microscopy and revealed that starch granules in dough are usually bigger particles, having an average size of 10–20 μm, while the protein components are in the form of sheets and fibrils which surround the starch particles. The gluten (protein) network structure is affected by gluten quantity, quality and the number of intermolecular disulphide bonds. Similar SEM analyses of starch and protein structures can be found in the literature [52,63,64].

The SEM images of doughs with untreated and treated (1, 3 and 5 min treatment time) flours (type 550) are shown in Figure 6. As claimed above, proteins create a smooth structure that surrounds the round starch particles. Further, two classes of starch granules can be noticed which differ with respect to their average diameters. It has been reported that type A starch granules (with a flattened shape and about 25 microns in diameter) contribute to malting yield, while type B granules (spherical in shape and about 6 microns in diameter) are responsible for water absorption due to their large surface-to-volume ratios [65].

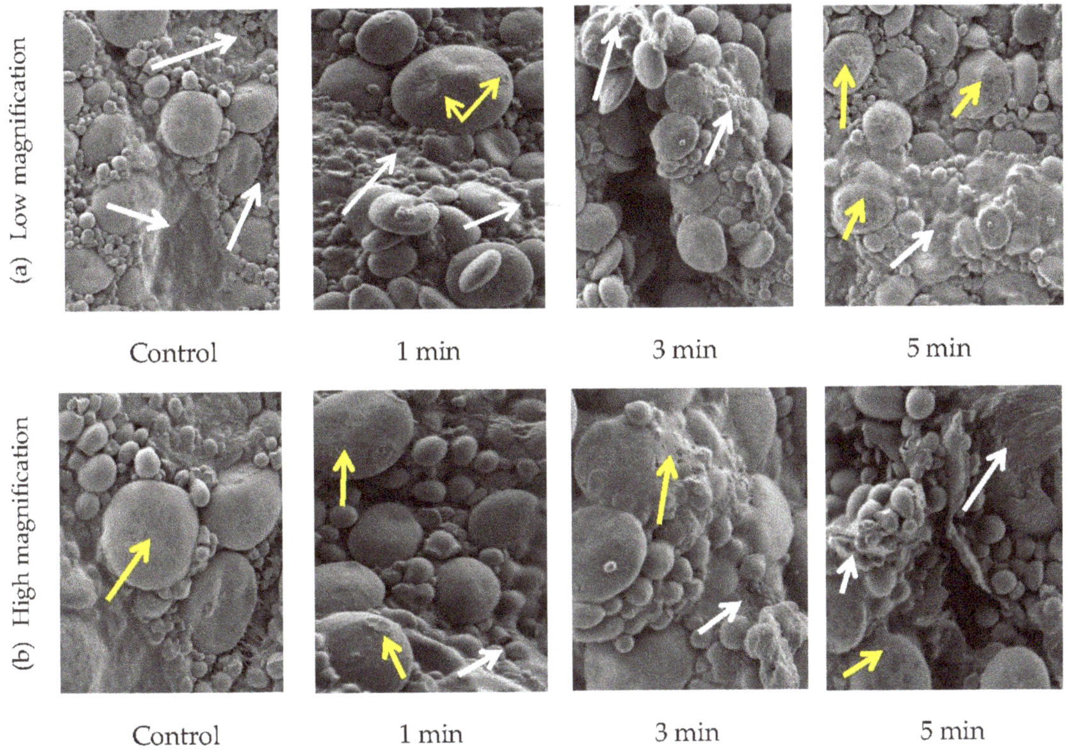

Figure 6. SEM Images of the wheat dough samples prepared with untreated and plasma-treated (1 min, 3 min, 5 min) flour under (**a**) low and (**b**) high magnifications (corresponding to 1000× and 2000× magnifications in the current SEM set-up). White arrows—gluten network; yellow arrows—changes to starch particles.

In the case of the control sample (Figure 6a), the gluten matrix was non-homogeneous, i.e., it was a discontinuous network in which large and small fragments of gluten could be observed (indicated by arrows). Starch granules are covered with thin gluten layers. However, the starch granules were not fully embedded in the protein matrix, which corresponds to the findings of Bajic et al. [66,67]. In comparison to that prepared with untreated flour, the SEM images of the dough prepared with plasma-treated flour (Figure 6a,b) showed a well-developed gluten matrix network in which starch particles were uniformly embedded, i.e., a well-developed gluten matrix could be observed. This resulted in a stronger dough, consistent with the rheological analysis presented in Figure 5.

The SEM images for increased treatment times showed only minor differences in the developed gluten network characteristics. However, when the treatment time was equal to 5 min, damage to starch granules was observed (Figure 6a,b), which led to the weakening of gluten networks. This negatively affects the storage and loss moduli of wheat dough [68,69], as confirmed by the results presented in Figure 5.

Comparison of the results presented in Figures 5 and 6 indicated an optimal plasma treatment time of 3 min to enhance dough rheological properties. If this time is exceeded, negative effects might occur as a result of the NTP treatment, leading to the weakening of dough networks.

SEM images for type 1050 samples are visually similar with respect to gluten and protein particles. However, no significant differences between the developed gluten networks of the NTP-treated samples were observed.

3.2. Effects of Non-Thermal Plasma-Treatment Reactor Filling on Wheat Flour and Dough Properties

As a next step, the role of flour mass in the plasma reactor on changes in flour properties was investigated. The reactor was filled with different amounts (50, 150, 250, 350 and 450 g) of wheat flour (type 550 and 1050), which are equivalent to 2, 6, 10, 13 and 17% occupancy of the reactor volume (flour density ρ = 593 kg/m^3 [70]).

3.2.1. Hydration Properties of Flour

Similar to the findings for moisture content, presented in Figure 3, the moisture content also remained close to 14% with varying flour masses and therefore the results are not discussed further here.

Figure 7a,b shows the dependence of WHC and WBC on wheat flour mass (type 550). Even though a stronger effect of NTP in a less full reactor would be expected, a general trend of increase in WHC and WBC values with increase in flour mass was observed. The WHC and WBC values generally increased for dough prepared with treated flour, with the maximal increase for the flour mass of 150 g, i.e., 6% filling of the reactor volume.

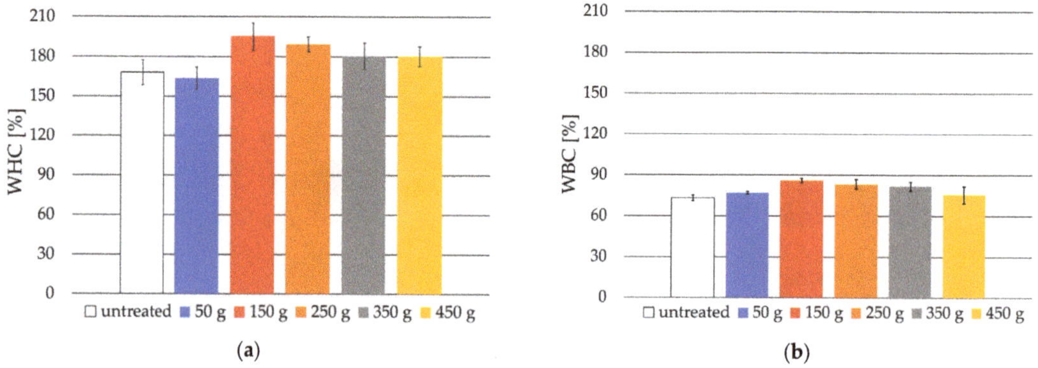

Figure 7. Effects of reactor filling on the WHC (**a**) and WBC (**b**) values of untreated and NTP-treated flour (type 550; treatment time: 3 min).

The above observation could be attributed to the fact that, during the flour treatment, a proportion of the flour particles stick to the reactor wall and to the HV pins. According to Chaple et al. [41], sample surface area exposed to plasma treatment is an important factor that influences the hydration properties of flours. At a lower flour mass (50 g, equivalent to 2% of reactor volume), a bigger share of the treated flour mass is immobilized and thus the treatment is not uniform. At a moderate mass (150–350 g, i.e., 6–13% of reactor volume), a smaller proportion of flour particles are 'glued' to the reactor surfaces and thus a more intensive mixing takes place, contributing to more effective contact between the plasma species and the flour particles. At higher mass (450 g, i.e., 17% of reactor volume), the contact between the flour mass and the plasma species decreases, hence contributing to a decrease in hydration properties. In the case of type 1050, the change in hydration properties lay within the standard deviation range, hence no conclusion could be drawn and the results are not shown here.

3.2.2. Visco-Elastic Properties of Dough

Equivalent to the analysis shown in Figure 5 and Table 1, Figure 8 and Table 2 describe the influence of flour mass (i.e., reactor filling) on wheat dough visco-elastic properties. Independent of the treated flour quantity, the results demonstrate an increase in visco-elastic properties of doughs made with treated flour samples in comparison to doughs prepared with untreated wheat flour.

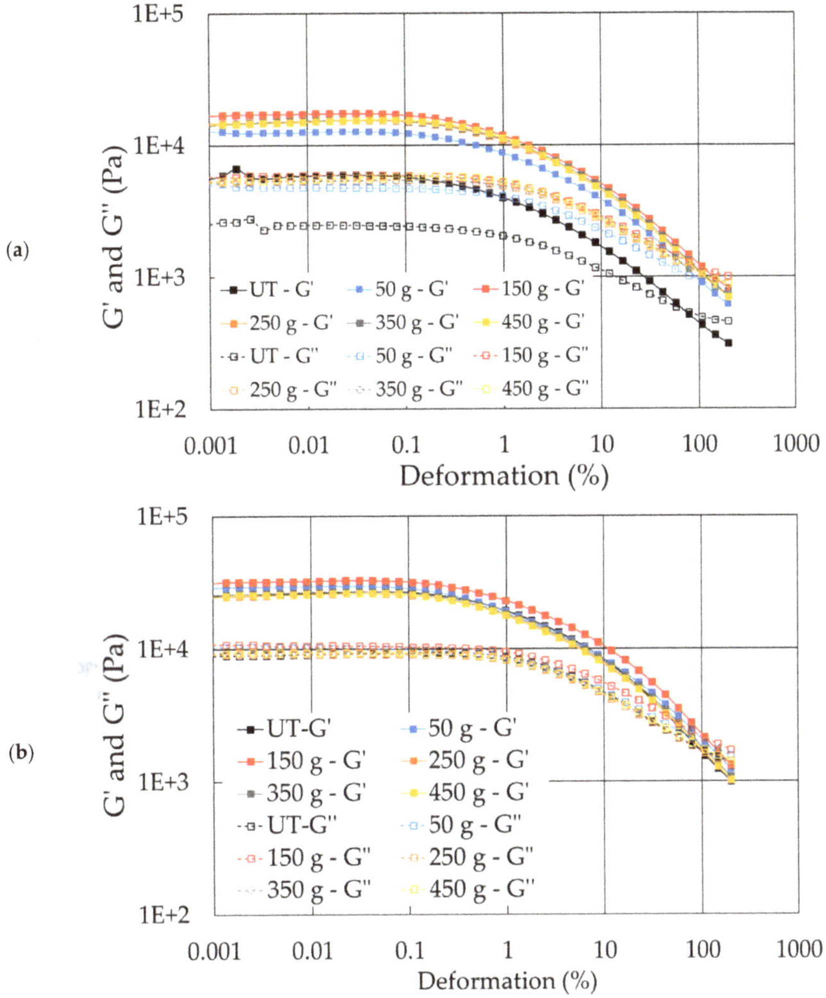

Figure 8. Change in the storage (G′) and loss (G″) moduli of wheat dough as a function of NTP treatment at different reactor fillings (50, 150, 250, 350 and 450g, at 10 RPM): (**a**) type 550; (**b**) type 1050.

Table 2. Increase in the G′ and G″ values of the doughs produced with plasma-treated flour samples (presented as minimum-to-maximum increase in comparison to doughs produced with untreated flour samples) as a function of reactor filling (i.e., flour mass).

Increase (%)	50 g		150 g		250 g		350 g		450 g	
Flour Type	G′ (%)	G″ (%)	G′ (%)	G″ (%)	G′ (%)	G″ (%)	G′ (%)	G″ (%)	G′ (%)	G″ (%)
550	85–130	76–111	155–203	114–158	119–172	94–141	119–184	91–150	115–183	93–159
1050	0–28	0–17	19–40	8–29	0–5	0–4	0–10	0–6	0–4	0–6

The experimental results demonstrate that when a too small (50 g) or a too large (450 g) amount of flour is placed inside the treatment reactor, the rheological properties of the formed dough are only mildly increased. G′ and G″ reach their maximum values with a flour mass of 150 g and then slowly decline again. Such a limitation is not observed in the case of rheological property enhancement using chemicals, such as Vitamin C or ascrobic acid, L-Cysteine and Azodicarbonamide (ADA) [71–73]. A few milligrams of such chemicals (e.g., 10–20 mg of ADA) per kilogram of wheat flour is enough to improve wheat flour properties [74]. Similar to the findings in Figure 5, the results shown in Figure 8 also confirm the previous findings about the limited influence of NTP treatment on the properties of dough made with flour type 1050. This can be connected to the changes in WHC and WBC values shown in Figure 7. It has also been reported that chemical improvers, e.g., vitamin C, also generally improve the visco-elasticity of low-gluten flour as compared with high-gluten flour [75]. Statistical analysis again confirmed p-values less than 0.05 in the case of type 550 and greater than 0.05 in the case of type 1050.

The presented results demonstrate the significance of flour particle–plasma species contact, which depends on the percentage of the reactor volume that is filled with flour. This factor can significantly limit the effect of NTP on flour functional properties. In order to achieve better effects of NTP treatment, the threshold for the reactor volume in this set-up is in a range of 6–13%.

3.3. Effects of Environmental Temperature during NTP Treatment on Dough Properties

Further, the effect of environmental air temperature on the NTP treatment of flour was investigated. A lower voltage demand for plasma formation and an earlier air breakdown due to increased air temperature was reported in the literature [76–78].

A flour sample (type 550, mass 50 g) was treated in the rotational reactor. The air temperature in the plasma reactor chamber was increased using an air heater in 10 °C steps from 10 °C to 40 °C while keeping the relative humidity at 50% ± 10%. The experimental results, shown in Figure 9, demonstrate the dependence of the visco-elastic properties of wheat dough produced at various air temperatures on the non-thermal plasma treatment. Statistical analysis (ANOVA) confirmed the existence of significant statistical differences between the untreated and treated samples, with p-values obtained less than 0.05. Independent of air temperature, the results demonstrated an increase in the visco-elastic properties of the dough produced with NTP-treated flour.

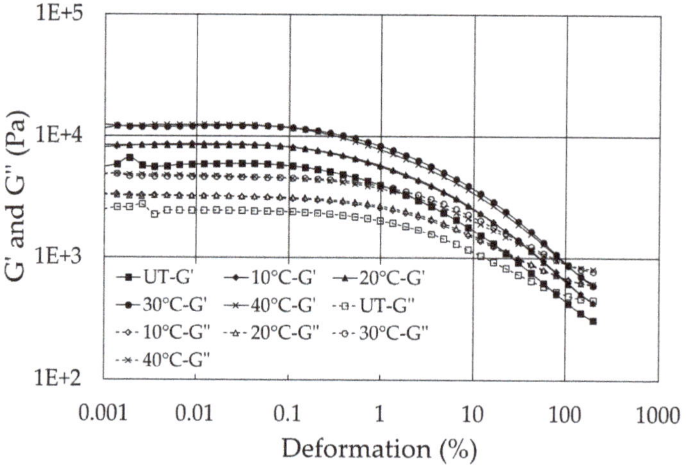

Figure 9. Change in the storage (G′) and loss (G″) moduli of wheat dough as a function of environmental (air) temperature.

The results presented in Table 3 demonstrate the change (in percentage) in visco-elastic properties (G′ and G″) of wheat doughs produced with plasma-treated flour samples at air temperatures between 10 °C and 40 °C in comparison to the control sample. When

NTP was generated at an air temperature up to 20 °C, the visco-elastic properties of dough increased maximally between 25 and 53%. When the air temperature increased to 30 °C, the change in visco-elastic properties almost doubled. A further increase in air temperature (i.e., 40 °C) did not further affect the values of visco-elastic properties significantly.

Table 3. Increase in G′ and G″ values for the doughs produced with plasma-treated flour samples (presented as minimum-to-maximum increase in comparison to doughs produced with untreated flour samples) as a function of environmental temperature.

Increase (%)	G′	G″
@ 10 °C vs. UT	25–53%	20–44%
@ 20 °C vs. UT	26–51%	17–43%
@ 30 °C vs. UT	80–121%	71–105%
@ 40 °C vs. UT	81–120%	75–110%

The breakdown voltage demand is strongly influenced by the gas temperature, as it is inversely proportional to the temperature of the gas, as shown in Equation (5) [78]:

$$U = (T_r/T_g) \times U_o \quad (5)$$

where U (V) and U_o (V) are the breakdown voltage at the desired gas temperature and gas breakdown voltage at room temperature, respectively; T_r is the ambient room temperature (300 K); and T_g is the gas temperature.

If the temperature of the gas is increased, the breakdown voltage demand decreases and vice versa. It has been reported that air warmed to a certain temperature impairs its insulating power and makes it dielectrically weak, resulting in the formation of the arc at longer distances [79]. This means that if the discharge gap and supply voltage is constant (as is the case here; i.e., if a 2 mm discharge gap and a constant maximum voltage of 7 kV is supplied to the system), then at lower temperatures (in this case, an air temperature of 10 °C) the gas is partially ionized, leading to the production of a limited number of active species. This limit is overruled by the increase in the gas temperature (in this case, 30 °C), as at that constant voltage and discharge gap, the gas is more easily ionized (decrease in air dielectric strength) due to higher temperatures. Further increase in temperature leads to a decrease in breakdown voltage demand; however, the number of active species stays constant, as the gas is already fully ionized at lower temperatures. This was the reason why a strong increase in visco-elastic properties in wheat flour was noticed as the air temperature was increased from 10 °C to 30 °C. However, no further increase in visco-elastic properties was detected when the air temperature was increased to 40 °C.

4. Conclusions

The key findings of the presented research are:

- Due to the non-thermal nature of the generated plasma, the moisture content of treated wheat flour (type 550 and 1050) does not change significantly and stays close to 14%.
- Three minutes was identified as an optimal NTP treatment time for all test cases, with which the changes in visco-elastic properties reached their maximum values.
- Increase in the hydration properties (WHC and WBC) of wheat flour with an increase in NTP treatment time was determined. A maximum increase in WBC value of approximately 6% was observed for the NTP treatment time of 3 min. Longer treatment times resulted in decreases in WBC values.
- Rheological analysis demonstrated the effectiveness of NTP in enhancing the visco-elastic properties of wheat dough. In the case of doughs formed using NTP-treated flour type 550, the visco-elastic properties, i.e., the storage (*G*′) and loss (*G*″) moduli, increased, on average, by more than 100%. A maximum increase of 130% was detected for the dough made with flour treated with NTP for three minutes.

- For doughs produced with flour type 550 treated by NTP for three minutes, the yield and the flow point increased by 75 and 51%, respectively.
- Based on the rheological measurements, NTP treatment was found to be effective in enhancing the visco-elastic properties G′ and G″ of the flour type 550 samples (the G′ and G″ values more than doubled), while for the type 1050 samples its influence was less noticeable.
- The amount of treated flour, i.e., the extent of reactor volume filling, was identified as an important factor that significantly influences the effects of the NTP treatment of flour. Based on the hydration and rheological properties of the obtained doughs, it was concluded that for the presented reactor the optimal fill is in the range of 6 to 13% of the reactor volume.
- A wheat flour mass of 150 g (equivalent to 6% of the reactor volume) was identified as an optimal mass for the present geometry for which the maximum enhancement in rheological properties (type 550: G′ ≥150%, G″ ≥200%; type 1050: G′ = 40% and G″ = 30%) was observed.
- Environmental (air) temperature has a significant effect on the visco-elastic properties of doughs produced with NTP-treated flour, indicating the importance of air temperature on plasma formation. The biggest difference (>100%) was noticed when the air temperature changed from 20 °C to 30 °C. Further increase did not contribute significantly to dough rheological properties.
- Analysis of variance (ANOVA) was performed in order to detect statistical differences among the samples due to NTP treatment. In the case of type 550 flour, the *p*-value was less than 0.05, confirming the existence of significant statistical difference and thus an influence of the non-thermal plasma treatment on flour properties. On the other hand, in the case of flour type 1050, the *p*-value was greater than 0.05, leading to the conclusion that no significant statistical difference existed between the untreated and treated samples.

NTP treatment has the potential to replace the use of chemicals in order to enhance the functional properties of wheat dough. However, as an outlook of this work, it is vital to investigate the effects of NTP on flour and dough structural network attributes, e.g., proteins, starch, microorganisms, color, etc., before further implementation of the treatment. Future scaling, involving such considerations as the processing efficiency, cost and control of the NTP process, could also be challenging. In the next phase of this research, the aim is to further study the effects of NTP on wheat network structural attributes in more detail.

Supplementary Materials: The following supporting information can be downloaded at: https://www.mdpi.com/article/10.3390/app12167997/s1, manuscript-supplementary.

Author Contributions: Conceptualization, M.J.K., A.Z.-R. and V.J.; methodology, M.J.K., A.Z.-R. and V.J.; software, M.J.K.; validation, M.J.K.; formal analysis, M.J.K. and A.Z.-R.; investigation, M.J.K.; resources, A.D. and V.J.; writing—original draft preparation, M.J.K., A.Z.-R. and V.J.; writing—review and editing, M.J.K., A.Z.-R. and V.J.; visualization, M.J.K., A.Z.-R. and V.J.; supervision, V.J. and A.D.; project administration, A.Z.-R.; funding acquisition, V.J. and A.D. All authors have read and agreed to the published version of the manuscript.

Funding: This research was funded by the German Federal Ministry of Economy and Energy (BMWi) through the Forschungskreis der Ernährungsindustrie e. V.—FEI program (grant number: 20629N).

Institutional Review Board Statement: Not applicable.

Informed Consent Statement: Not applicable.

Data Availability Statement: Not applicable.

Acknowledgments: We acknowledge financial support from Deutsche Forschungsgemeinschaft and Friedrich-Alexander-Universität Erlangen-Nürnberg within the funding programme "Open Access

Publication Funding". Furthermore, we express our gratitude to the company Diener for support in the coupling of the plasma generation device and the treatment reactor.

Conflicts of Interest: The authors declare no conflict of interest. The founding sponsors had no role in the design of the study; in the collection, analyses or interpretation of data; in the writing of the manuscript or in the decision to publish the results.

References

1. McKevith, B. Nutritional aspects of cereals. *Nutr. Bull.* **2004**, *29*, 111–142. [CrossRef]
2. Laskowski, W.; Górska-Warsewicz, H.; Rejman, K.; Czeczotko, M.; Zwolińska, J. How important are cereals and cereal products in the average polish diet? *Nutrients* **2019**, *11*, 679. [CrossRef]
3. Shewry, P.R.; Hey, S.J. The contribution of wheat to human diet and health. *Food Energy Secur.* **2015**, *4*, 178–202. [CrossRef] [PubMed]
4. Scholtz, V.; Šerá, B.; Khun, J.; Šerý, M.; Julák, J. Effects of Nonthermal Plasma on Wheat Grains and Products. *J. Food Qual.* **2019**, *2019*, 1–10. [CrossRef]
5. Ahmed, J.; Mulla, M.Z.; Arfat, Y.A. Particle size, rheological and structural properties of whole wheat flour doughs as treated by high pressure. *Int. J. Food Prop.* **2017**, *20*, 1829–1842. [CrossRef]
6. Misra, N.N. Quality of Cold Plasma Treated Plant Foods. In *Cold Plasma in Food and Agriculture: Fundamentals and Applications*; Academic Press: Cambridge, MA, USA, 2016.
7. López, M.; Calvo, T.; Prieto, M.; Múgica-Vidal, R.; Muro-Fraguas, I.; Alba-Elías, F.; Alvarez-Ordóñez, A. A review on non-thermal atmospheric plasma for food preservation: Mode of action, determinants of effectiveness, and applications. *Front. Microbiol.* **2019**, *10*, 622. [CrossRef]
8. Fernández, A.; Shearer, N.; Wilson, D.R.; Thompson, A. Effect of microbial loading on the efficiency of cold atmospheric gas plasma inactivation of Salmonella enterica serovar Typhimurium. *Int. J. Food Microbiol.* **2012**, *152*, 175–180. [CrossRef]
9. Ziuzina, D.; Misra, N.N. Cold Plasma for Food Safety. In *Cold Plasma in Food and Agriculture: Fundamentals and Applications*; Elsevier: Amsterdam, The Netherlands, 2016; Chapter 9; pp. 223–252. [CrossRef]
10. Niemira, B.A. Cold plasma decontamination of foods. *Annu. Rev. Food Sci. Technol.* **2012**, *3*, 125–142. [CrossRef]
11. Jayasena, D.D.; Kim, H.J.; Yong, H.I.; Park, S.; Kim, K.; Choe, W.; Jo, C. Flexible thin-layer dielectric barrier discharge plasma treatment of pork butt and beef loin: Effects on pathogen inactivation and meat-quality attributes. *Food Microbiol.* **2015**, *46*, 51–55. [CrossRef]
12. Jay, J.M. *Food Preservation with Chemicals BT-Modern Food Microbiology*; Jay, J.M., Ed.; Springer: Boston, MA, USA, 1995; pp. 273–303.
13. Safefood. *Cleaning and Disinfection in Food Processing Operations*; Safefood 360 Inc., 2012; Available online: https://docplayer.net/23928366-Cleaning-and-disinfection-in-food-processing-operations.html (accessed on 30 March 2022).
14. Nath, S.; Chowdhury, S.; Dora, K.C.; Sarkar, S. Role Of Biopreservation In Improving Food Safety And Storage. *Int. J. Eng. Res. Appl.* **2014**, *4*, 26–32.
15. Poulsen, L.K. Thermal Processing of Food: Allergenicity. In *Thermal Processing of Food*; Wiley-VCH Verlag GmbH & Co. KgaA: Weinheim, Germany, 2007.
16. Chandrasekaran, S.; Ramanathan, S.; Basak, T. Microwave food processing-A review. *Food Res. Int.* **2013**, *52*, 243–261. [CrossRef]
17. Chemat, F.; Zill-E-Huma; Khan, M.K. Applications of ultrasound in food technology: Processing, preservation and extraction. *Ultrason. Sonochem.* **2011**, *18*, 813–835. [CrossRef] [PubMed]
18. Safefood 360. Whitepaper Water Activity (aw) in Foods. 2014. Available online: https://docplayer.net/20745103-Water-activity-a-w-in-foods-whitepaper-contents-summary.html. (accessed on 30 March 2022).
19. Koutchma, T.; Marcotte, M. High hydrostatic pressure processing of foods: Challenges for pasteurization and sterilization. In Proceedings of the 8th World Congress of Chemical Engineering, Montreal, QC, Canada, 23–27 August 2009.
20. Penchalaraju, M.; Shireesha, B. Preservation of Foods by High-pressure Processing-A Review. *Ind. J. Sci. Res. Tech.* **2013**, *1*, 30–38.
21. Food Processing and Packaging benefitting from Modern Vacuum Technology. *Food Marketing and Technology Magazine*, April 2016; 20–21.
22. Scholtz, V.; Pazlarova, J.; Souskova, H.; Khun, J.; Julak, J. Nonthermal plasma-A tool for decontamination and disinfection. *Biotechnol. Adv.* **2015**, *33*, 1108–1119. [CrossRef] [PubMed]
23. Gianibelli, M.C.; Larroque, O.R.; MacRitchie, F.; Wrigley, C.W. Biochemical, genetic, and molecular characterization of wheat glutenin and its component subunits. *Cereal Chem.* **2001**, *78*, 635–646. [CrossRef]
24. Lin, J.; Gu, Y.; Bian, K. Bulk and Surface Chemical Composition of Wheat Flour Particles of Different Sizes. *J. Chem.* **2019**, *2019*, 1–11. [CrossRef]
25. DSM Food Specialities. *How Adding BakeZyme ®AAA to Bread Reduces Ascorbic Acid Dosage While Maintaining Ideal Texture and Volume*; Technical Report; DSM Food Specialities B.V.: Delft, The Netherlands, July 2018.
26. Peighambardoust, S.H.; Dadpour, M.R.; Dokouhaki, M. Application of epifluorescence light microscopy (EFLM) to study the microstructure of wheat dough: A comparison with confocal scanning laser microscopy (CSLM) technique. *J. Cereal Sci.* **2010**, *51*, 21–27. [CrossRef]

27. Salmenkallio-Marttila, M.; Katina, K.; Autio, K. Effects of bran fermentation on quality and microstructure of high-fiber wheat bread. *Cereal Chem.* **2001**, *78*, 429–435. [CrossRef]
28. Chen, X.; Schofield, J.D. Effects of dough mixing and oxidising improvers on free reduced and free oxidised glutathione and protein-glutathione mixed disulphides of wheat flour. *Eur. Food Res. Technol.* **1996**, *203*, 255–261. [CrossRef]
29. Sandhu, H.P.S.; Manthey, F.A.; Simsek, S. Ozone gas affects physical and chemical properties of wheat (*Triticum aestivum* L.) starch. *Carbohydr. Polym.* **2012**, *87*, 1261–1268. [CrossRef]
30. Mei, J.; Liu, G.; Huang, X.; Ding, W. Effects of ozone treatment on medium hard wheat (*Triticum aestivum* L.) flour quality and performance in steamed bread making. *CYTA-J. Food* **2016**, *14*, 449–456. [CrossRef]
31. Naguib, K. Effect of ozonation of wheat grain on quality bread factory. *J. Agroaliment. Proc. Technol.* **2013**, *19*, 1–9.
32. Al-Dmoor, H.M. Cake Flour: Functionality and Quality (Review). *Eur. Sci. J.* **2013**, *9*, 166–180.
33. Afshari, R.; Hosseini, H. Non-thermal plasma as a new food preservation method, Its present and future prospect. *J. Paramed. Sci. Winter* **2014**, *5*, 2008–4978.
34. Bahrami, N.; Bayliss, D.; Chope, G.; Penson, S.; Perehinec, T.; Fisk, I.D. Cold plasma: A new technology to modify wheat flour functionality. *Food Chem.* **2016**, *202*, 247–253. [CrossRef]
35. Yiğit, E. *Introduction to Plasma BT-Atmospheric and Space Sciences: Ionospheres and Plasma Environments*; Yiğit, E., Ed.; Springer International Publishing: Cham, Switzerland, 2018; Volume 2, pp. 1–19.
36. Eliezer, S.; Eliezer, Y. *The Four State of Matter*; IOP Publishing Ltd.: Bristol, UK, 2001; p. 235.
37. Li, J.; Ma, C.; Zhu, S.; Yu, F.; Dai, B.; Yang, D. A review of recent advances of dielectric barrier discharge plasma in catalysis. *Nanomaterials* **2019**, *9*, 1428. [CrossRef]
38. Haertel, B.; von Woedtke, T.; Weltmann, K.D.; Lindequist, U. Non-thermal atmospheric-pressure plasma possible application in wound healing. *Biomol. Ther.* **2014**, *22*, 477–490. [CrossRef]
39. Heberlein, J.V.R. Generation of thermal and pseudo-thermal plasmas. *Pure Appl. Chem.* **1992**, *64*, 629–636. [CrossRef]
40. Li, X.; Wen, Y.; Zhang, J.; Ma, D.; Zhang, J.; An, Y.; Song, X.; Ren, X.; Zhang, W. Effects of non-thermal plasma treating wheat kernel on the physicochemical properties of wheat flour and the quality of fresh wet noodles. *Int. J. Food Sci. Technol.* **2022**, *57*, 1544–1553. [CrossRef]
41. Chaple, S.; Sarangapani, C.; Jones, J.; Carey, E.; Causeret, L.; Genson, A.; Duffy, B.; Bourke, P. Effect of atmospheric cold plasma on the functional properties of whole wheat (*Triticum aestivum* L.) grain and wheat flour. *Innov. Food Sci. Emerg. Technol.* **2020**, *66*, 102529. [CrossRef]
42. Lahijani, A.K.S.A.T.; Shahidi, F.; Habibian, M. Evaluation of the effect of non-thermal plasma on the physicochemical, technological and functional properties of wheat flour. *Iran. Food Sci. Technol. Res. J.* **2020**. Available online: https://ifstrj.um.ac.ir/article_39185.html?lang=en (accessed on 30 November 2020).
43. Montenegro, F.M.; Júnior, A.M.; Berteli, M.N.; Campelo, P.H.; Pedrosa, M.T.; Clerici, S. Effects of microwave-generated non-thermal plasma treatment applied to wheat flour and bran. *Soc. Dev.* **2021**, *2021*, 1–8. [CrossRef]
44. Shi, M.; Cheng, Y.; Wang, F.; Ji, X.; Liu, Y.; Yan, Y. Rheological Properties of Wheat Flour Modified by Plasma-Activated Water and Heat Moisture Treatment and in vitro Digestibility of Steamed Bread. *Front. Nutr.* **2022**, *9*, 1–8. [CrossRef] [PubMed]
45. Tang, Q.; Jiang, W.; Cheng, Y.; Lin, S.; Lim, T.M.; Xiong, J. Generation of reactive species by gas-phase dielectric barrier discharges. *Ind. Eng. Chem. Res.* **2011**, *50*, 9839–9846. [CrossRef]
46. Misra, N.N.; Kaur, S.; Tiwari, B.K.; Kaur, A.; Singh, N.; Cullen, P.J. Atmospheric pressure cold plasma (ACP) treatment of wheat flour. *Food Hydrocoll.* **2015**, *44*, 115–121. [CrossRef]
47. Arpagaus, C.; Sonnenfeld, A.; von Rohr, P.R. A downer reactor for short-time plasma surface modification of polymer powders. *Chem. Eng. Technol.* **2005**, *28*, 87–94. [CrossRef]
48. Diener, Diener Electronic GmbH. 2022. Available online: https://www.plasma.com/ (accessed on 30 March 2022).
49. Traynham, T.L.; Myers, D.J.; Carriquiry, A.L.; Johnson, L.A. Evaluation of water-holding capacity for wheat-soy flour blends. *JAOCS J. Am. Oil Chem. Soc.* **2007**, *84*, 151–155. [CrossRef]
50. Meerts, M.; Cardinaels, R.; Oosterlinck, F.; Courtin, C.M.; Moldenaers, P. The Impact of Water Content and Mixing Time on the Linear and Non-Linear Rheology of Wheat Flour Dough. *Food Biophys.* **2017**, *12*, 151–163. [CrossRef]
51. Paar, A. MCR 102e/302e/502e. 2022. Available online: https://www.anton-paar.com/corp-en/products/details/rheometer-mcr-102-302-502/ (accessed on 30 March 2022).
52. Jekle, M.; Becker, T. Wheat Dough Microstructure: The Relation Between Visual Structure and Mechanical Behavior. *Crit. Rev. Food Sci. Nutr.* **2014**, *55*, 369–382. [CrossRef]
53. Ahmed, J. Effect of barley β-glucan concentrate on oscillatory and creep behavior of composite wheat flour dough. *J. Food Eng.* **2015**, *152*, 85–94. [CrossRef]
54. Amemiya, J.I.; Menjivar, J.A. Comparison of small and large deformation measurements to characterize the rheology of wheat flour doughs. *J. Food Eng.* **1992**, *16*, 91–108. [CrossRef]
55. Morshed, M.N.; Behary, N.; Bouazizi, N.; Guan, J.; Chen, G.; Nierstrasz, V. Surface modification of polyester fabric using plasma-dendrimer for robust immobilization of glucose oxidase enzyme. *Sci. Rep.* **2019**, *9*, 1–16. [CrossRef] [PubMed]
56. Laukemper, R.; Becker, T.; Jekle, M. Surface Energy of Food Contact Materials and Its Relation to Wheat Dough Adhesion. *Food Bioprocess Technol.* **2021**, *14*, 1142–1154. [CrossRef]

57. Los, A.; Ziuzina, D.; Boehm, D.; Cullen, P.J.; Bourke, P. Investigation of mechanisms involved in germination enhancement of wheat (*Triticum aestivum*) by cold plasma: Effects on seed surface chemistry and characteristics. *Plasma Process. Polym.* **2019**, *16*, 1800148. [CrossRef]
58. Paar, A. Amplitude Sweeps. 2022. Available online: https://wiki.anton-paar.com/en/amplitude-sweeps/ (accessed on 16 May 2022).
59. Sawyer, S.F. Analysis of Variance: The Fundamental Concepts. *J. Man. Manip. Ther.* **2009**, *17*, 27E–38E. [CrossRef]
60. Chittrakorn, S. Use of Ozone As an Alternative to Chlorine for Treatment of Soft Wheat Flours. 2008. Available online: http://krex.k-state.edu/dspace/handle/2097/575 (accessed on 5 April 2022).
61. Estrada-Girón, Y.; Aguilar, J.; del Rio, J.A.M.; Botin, A.V.; Guerrero-Beltrán, J.; Martínez-Preciado, A.H.; Balleza, E.R.M.; Soltero, J.F.A.; Solorza-Feria, J. Effect of moisture content and temperature, on the rheological, microstructural and thermal properties of MASA (dough) from a hybrid corn (Zea Mays sp.) variety. *Rev. Mex. Ing. Quim.* **2014**, *13*, 429–446.
62. Opaliński, I.; Chutkowski, M.; Hassanpour, A. Rheology of moist food powders as affected by moisture content. *Powder Technol.* **2016**, *294*, 315–322. [CrossRef]
63. Bechtel, D.B.; Pomeranz, Y.; de Francisco, A. Breadmaking studied by light and transmission electron microscopy. *Cereal Chem.* **1978**, *55*, 392–401.
64. Indrani, D.; Prabhasankar, P.; Rajiv, J.; Rao, G.V. Scanning Electron Microscopy, Rheological Characteristics, and Bread-Baking Performance of Wheat-Flour Dough as Affected by Enzymes. *J. Food Sci.* **2003**, *68*, 2804–2809. [CrossRef]
65. Stoddard, F.L. Wheat Starch Granule Size. In *Woodhead Publishing Series in Food Science, Technology and Nutrition*; Cauvain, S., Salmon, S., Young, L., Eds.; Woodhead Publishing: Sawston, UK, 2005; pp. 461–465. [CrossRef]
66. Bajić, B.Ž.; Davidović, D.N.; Veličković, D.T.; Milosavljević, N.P.; Dodić, S.N.; Dodić, J.M. Effect of natural organic compounds on microstructure of wheat dough and bread quality. *Rom. Biotechnol. Lett.* **2017**, *22*, 12163.
67. Devahastin, S. *Food Microstructure and Its Relationship with Quality and Stability*; Woodhead Publishing: Sawston, UK, 2017.
68. Banerji, A.; Ananthanarayan, L.; Lele, S.S. *The Science and Technology of Chapatti and Other Indian Flatbreads*; CRC Press: Boca Raton, FL, USA, 2020.
69. Jukic, M.; Komlenić, D.; Mastanjević, K.; Mastanjević, K.; Lučan, M.; Popovici, C.; Nakov, G.; Lukinac, J. Influence of damaged starch on the quality parameters of wheat dough and bread. *Ukr. Food J.* **2019**, *8*, 512–521. [CrossRef]
70. Aqua-Calc. Density of Flour, Wheat (Material). 2022. Available online: https://www.aqua-calc.com/page/density-table/substance/flour-coma-and-blank-wheat (accessed on 24 June 2022).
71. Cauvain, S.P. Chapter 13-The use of redox agents in breadmaking. In *Woodhead Publishing Series in Food Science, Technology and Nutrition*; Cauvain, S.P., Ed.; Woodhead Publishing: Sawston, UK, 2020; pp. 391–413. [CrossRef]
72. Tozatti, P.; Fleitas, M.C.; Briggs, C.; Hucl, P.; Chibbar, R.N.; Nickerson, M.T. Effect of L-cysteine on the rheology and baking quality of doughs formulated with flour from five contrasting Canada spring wheat cultivars. *Cereal Chem.* **2020**, *97*, 235–247. [CrossRef]
73. Every, D.; Simmons, L.; Sutton, K.H.; Ross, M. Studies on the mechanism of the ascorbic acid improver effect on bread using flour fractionation and reconstitution methods. *J. Cereal Sci.* **1999**, *30*, 147–158. [CrossRef]
74. Wieser, H. *The Use of Redox Agents in Breadmaking*, 2nd ed.; Woodhead Publishing Limited: Sawston, UK, 2012.
75. Jia, F.; Ye, K.; Zhang, C.; Zhang, S.; Fu, M.; Liu, X.; Guo, R.; Yang, R.; Zhang, H.; Wang, J. Effects of vitamin C on the structural and functional characteristics of wheat gluten. *Grain Oil Sci. Technol.* **2022**, *5*, 79–86. [CrossRef]
76. Pauli, F.; Driendl, N.; Hameyer, K. Study on temperature dependence of partial discharge in low voltage traction drives. In Proceedings of the IEEE Workshop on Electrical Machines Design, Control and Diagnosis (WEMDCD), Athens, Greece, 22–23 April 2019; pp. 209–214. [CrossRef]
77. Nguyen, H.V.P.; Phung, B.T.; Blackburn, T. Effect of temperatures on very low frequency partial discharge diagnostics. In Proceedings of the IEEE 11th International Conference on the Properties and Applications of Dielectric Materials (ICPADM), Johor Bahru, Malaysia, 19–22 July 2015; pp. 272–275. [CrossRef]
78. Uhm, H.S.; Jung, S.J.; Kim, H.S. Influence of gas temperature on electrical breakdown in cylindrical electrodes. *J. Korean Phys. Soc.* **2003**, *42*, S989–S993.
79. de Podesta, M. *Understanding the Properties of Matter*; Taylor & Francis: New York, NY, USA, 2002.

applied sciences

MDPI

Article

SDBD Flexible Plasma Actuator with Ag-Ink Electrodes: Experimental Assessment

Viktoras Papadimas [1,†], Christos Doudesis [1,†], Panagiotis Svarnas [1,*], Polycarpos K. Papadopoulos [2], George P. Vafakos [2] and Panayiotis Vafeas [3]

1 High Voltage Laboratory, Department of Electrical & Computer Engineering, University of Patras, Rion, 26 504 Patras, Greece; up1047007@upnet.gr (V.P.); up1046893@upnet.gr (C.D.)
2 Department of Mechanical Engineering & Aeronautics, University of Patras, Rion, 26 504 Patras, Greece; p.papadopoulos@des.upatras.gr (P.K.P.); vafakos@upnet.gr (G.P.V.)
3 Department of Chemical Engineering, University of Patras, Rion, 26 504 Patras, Greece; vafeas@chemeng.upatras.gr
* Correspondence: svarnas@ece.upatras.gr
† Equal contribution.

Abstract: In the present work, a single dielectric barrier discharge (SDBD)-based actuator is developed and experimentally tested by means of various diagnostic techniques. Flexible dielectric barriers and conductive paint electrodes are used, making the design concept applicable to surfaces of different aerodynamic profiles. A technical drawing of the actuator is given in detail. The plasma is sustained by audio frequency sinusoidal high voltage, while it is probed electrically and optically. The consumed electric power is measured, and the optical emission spectrum is recorded in the ultraviolet–near infrared (UV–NIR) range. High-resolution spectroscopy provides molecular rotational distributions, which are treated appropriately to evaluate the gas temperature. The plasma-induced flow field is spatiotemporally surveyed with pitot-like tube and schlieren imaging. Briefly, the actuator consumes a mean power less than 10 W and shows a fair stability over one day, the average temperature of the gas above its surface is close to 400 K, and the fluid speed rises to 4.5 m s^{-1}. A long, thin layer (less than 1.5 mm) of laminar flow is unveiled on the actuator surface. This thin layer is interfaced with an outspread turbulent flow field, which occupies a centimeter-scale area. Molecular nitrogen-positive ions appear to be part of the charged heavy species in the generated filamentary discharge, which can transfer energy and momentum to the surrounding air molecules.

Keywords: atmospheric pressure plasma; DBD; actuator; pitot tube; schlieren imaging; UV–NIR OES

Citation: Papadimas, V.; Doudesis, C.; Svarnas, P.; Papadopoulos, P.K.; Vafakos, G.P.; Vafeas, P. SDBD Flexible Plasma Actuator with Ag-Ink Electrodes: Experimental Assessment. *Appl. Sci.* **2021**, *11*, 11930. https://doi.org/10.3390/app112411930

Academic Editor: Bogdan-George Rusu

Received: 25 November 2021
Accepted: 13 December 2021
Published: 15 December 2021

1. Introduction

When there is relative movement between a fluid and a solid surface, a boundary layer is formed. This is the layer of fluid in the immediate vicinity of the bounding surface where the effects of viscosity are significant, and it can be either laminar or turbulent. Simplified, the laminar boundary corresponds to a smooth flow, whereas the turbulent boundary layer contains eddies. At the same time, the solid surface experiences a force of resistance in the fluid due to frictional and pressure forces: the "drag force". Practically, this is the component of the surface force parallel to the flow direction (the other component of the surface force that is perpendicular to the oncoming flow direction is the "lift force"). A laminar boundary is associated with less skin friction than a turbulent one, but it tends to break down more suddenly. In the case of a full-size body (e.g., a wing surface), as the flow develops along its surface, the initial laminar boundary layer becomes thicker (and thus less stable) as the flow continues back from the leading edge, and at a certain distance, the laminar boundary layer breaks down and transitions into a turbulent one. It becomes apparent that any spatial delay of this transition is advantageous since the surface experiences lower drag. Furthermore, turbulent flow is a source of aerodynamic noise generated from the unsteady nature of this kind of flow. Finally, apart from the laminar-to-turbulent flow transition and the aerodynamic noise, a third important effect due to excessive momentum loss near the solid surface in a boundary layer trying to move downstream against increasing pressure (adverse pressure gradient) is the boundary layer detachment/separation from the surface (into a wake).

The tremendous technological and financial impact of the possibility of controlling the abovementioned flow field effects, e.g., in the aerospace industry and the aircraft market, has been recognized since decades and many methods for flow manipulation (e.g., lift enhancement and drag reduction) have been developed. Most of them refer to efficient mechanical devices, which however may be complicated, heavy, massive sources of noise and vibrations, or maintenance critical, thus partially offsetting the active airflow control value. As a counterweight, units based on atmospheric-pressure, low-temperature plasmas of electrical discharges have been devised for active airflow control. These are the plasma actuators. Two plausible principal physical mechanisms have been proposed on the operation of the plasma actuators. Either an electrohydrodynamic body force provokes collisions between ionic and neutral species, leading thus to the production of so-called electric or ionic wind [1,2], or electric energy is instantly transformed into heat energy, leading to the formation of moving blast waves responsible for large-scale flow field structures [3,4].

Excellent reviews on plasma actuators exist [5,6], gathering the fundamental concepts and the state-of-the-art in the field. We typically deal with surface electrical discharges exploiting unique features from the dielectric barrier discharge (DBD) [7]. This includes arc transition prevention due to the dielectric barrier, which in turn results in a low gas temperature, high engineerability, responsivity within the sub-microsecond time scale, absence of moving components, implicit conversion of electric power into a moving fluid, long background of studies and applications in various interdisciplinary scientific fields [7–9], etc. The great number of reports published over the last decade on the topic of plasma actuators and the ongoing research has a twofold meaning. First, it proves the importance and the potentiality of these devices, whereas second, it states that many issues have not yet been met and further challenges still exist (e.g., energy conversion efficiency factor enhancement). Numerous studies focus on the geometry-configuration optimization [10–12], the dielectric barrier specifications [12,13], the material endurance [13,14], the role of the driving voltage characteristics [12,15–17], the boundary layer separation control [18,19], the laminar-to-turbulent transition delay [20], etc., just to name a few.

As a contribution to the field, the present study is devoted to the implementation of a particular single dielectric barrier discharge (SDBD) [21] plasma actuator and its test under sinusoidal high voltage. Kapton® polyimide films are used as the dielectric barrier due to their ability to be mounted onto curved aerodynamic surfaces. On the other hand, silver (Ag) conductive paint is selected for the formation of the electrodes due to its provided feasibility to design electrodes of every shape with negligible thickness on a variety of surfaces. Both choices make the actuator fully flexible, and this is the main claim of the present communication. The actuator is probed by means of electrical and optical techniques. Electrical measurements are conducted to investigate the time evolution of the power consumption and the endurance of the actuator, over the time window of a day. High-resolution optical emission spectroscopy (OES) provides an insight into the emitting species of the plasma as well as an estimation of the temperature of the air above the actuator. Then, pitot-like tube and schlieren imaging give access to the induced fluid speed and the pattern of the relevant flow field, respectively. Eventually, the overall experimental results allow for a brief discussion on the physical mechanisms governing the aerodynamic specifications of this flexible plasma actuator.

2. Experimental Setup

Figure 1 shows the experimental setup, including the plasma actuator itself and the diagnostics employed in the present work. The actuator design is illustrated in detail in

Figure 2. It is an SDBD-based one, with the dielectric barrier to be a stack of Kapton® polyimide films. The patterns of the electrodes are formed on the polyimide films by means of silver ink (resistivity 100 μΩ cm) and stencils. The grounded electrode is encapsulated within a two-component epoxy resin.

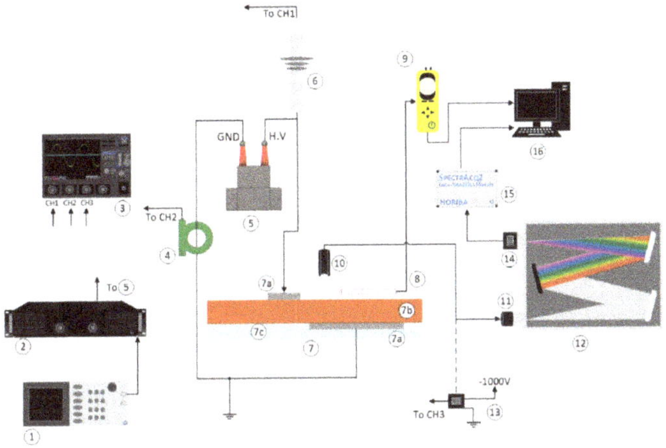

Figure 1. Conceptual diagram of the experimental setup. 1: signal generator; 2: audio power amplifier; 3: oscilloscope; 4: current monitor; 5: ferrite core, step up transformer; 6: high-voltage probe; 7: SDBD actuator; 7a: painted electrodes; 7b: flexible dielectric barrier; 7c: epoxy resin; 8: pitot-like tube on x–y–z, linear, micro-translation stage; 9: pitot-like tube hardware and interface; 10: optical fiber; 11: optical matcher; 12: monochromator; 13,14: photo-electron multiplier tube; 15: data acquisition unit; 16: personal computer.

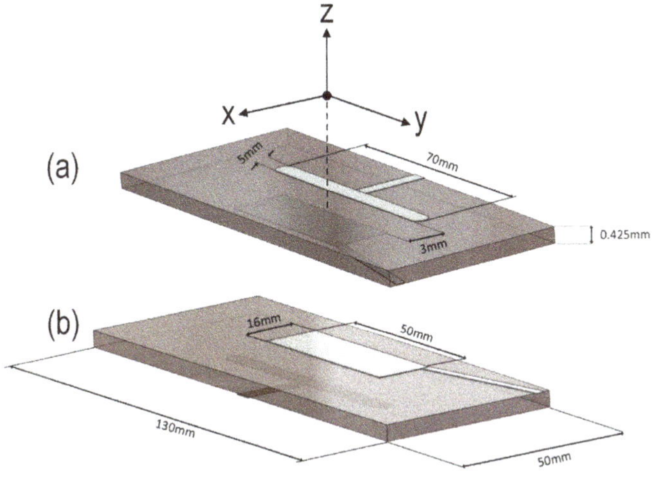

Figure 2. Design of the plasma actuator. (**a**) Top view depicting the high-voltage-driven electrode details. The inset defines the coordinate system that is used hereafter. The system origin coincides with the actuator surface (z = 0), the edge of the discharge gap toward the grounded electrode side (x = 0), and the middle of the grounded electrode length (y = 0). (**b**) Bottom view depicting the grounded electrode details. The stack of Kapton® polyimide films has a total thickness of 0.425 mm, whereas the epoxy resin (No_7c in Figure 1) is not shown for simplicity purposes.

The high voltage is generated by amplifying a reference sinusoidal signal (10 kHz) and supplying the primary winding of a specially designed, ferrite core, step-up transformer. The output high voltage, v(t), is permanently monitored with a passive probe (Tektronix; P6015; DC-75 MHz). The DBD current, i(t), is recorded with a wideband current transformer (Pearson Electronics; 6585; 400 Hz–200 MHz). The wavelength- and space-integrated light, emitted from the plasma, is collected with a high-grade fused silica optical fiber (Newport; 77576; 260–2200 nm), and then, it becomes time-resolved with a photo-electron multiplier tube (PMT; Hamamatsu R928; 185–900 nm). All waveforms are recorded by a four-channel, wideband, digital oscilloscope (LeCroy; WaveRunner 44Xi-A; 400 MHz; 5 GSamples s^{-1}).

The mean electric power consumed by the actuator is calculated by integrating the product [v(t:t + 5T) × i(t:t + 5T)] over five sequential voltage periods, i.e., 5T, and by dividing the result by this factor. The process is repeated for five independent [v(t:t + 5T) × i(t:t + 5T)] products. Two such measurement sets are realized on different dates. Hence, in total, 10 instantaneous power waveforms (5T duration each) are considered for extracting mean values and standard deviations (error bars in the graphs) of the electric power.

The time- and space-integrated light is guided by the abovementioned optical fiber to a monochromator (Jobin Yvon; THR 1000; 170–750 nm; 2400 grooves mm^{-1}) and the optical emission spectrum is thus identified. The wavelength calibration of this unit is carried out with an Hg (Ar) pencil-style lamp (Newport; 6035). Special attention is paid to calibrating the relative spectral efficiency of the entire optical system. This is accomplished with a quartz-tungsten-halogen lamp (Newport; 6334NS; 250 W) operated at 3400 K. The rotational temperature of principal excited molecular species is estimated by fitting their experimental rotational distributions to the corresponding theoretical ones, using a lab-built software [22]. In addition, a 0.25 m imaging spectrograph (Newport; MS260i) is used for exploring wider wavelength ranges. It is equipped with two motorized gratings: one holographic (2400 grooves mm^{-1}; blaze wavelength 250 nm; 180–700 nm) and one ruled (600 grooves mm^{-1}; blaze wavelength 400 nm; 250–1300 nm). The photodetector of this spectrograph is a linear CCD array (200–1100 nm). Optical matchers are used in both cases (monochromator and spectrograph) for optimal alignment of the fiber image.

The speed of the plasma-induced fluid is recorded in real time with a pitot-like tube (glass capillary tube; $\varnothing_{out}$ = 1.3 mm; $\varnothing_{in}$ = 0.8 mm) and appropriate hardware (Trotec; TA400). Precise, point-specific measurements are allowed due to the tube mounting on a x–y–z linear micro-translation stage.

Finally, flow field patterns are visualized by means of schlieren imaging. The main parts of the system are provided by Edmund Optics®. It contains a high-power green light emitting diode, two aluminized first surface spherical mirrors (152.4 mm in diameter, 1524 mm focal length and 1/8 wave surface accuracy) overcoated with silicon monoxide, and two Foucault knife edge testers mounted on separate micro-translator stages (one horizontal and one vertical). The components are arranged in a Z–type configuration. A camera (Nikon; D3300) is added to the system enabling photographic records. The camera is equipped with a zoom lens (Canon; FD 70–210 mm). The settings for the schlieren photos are ISO 400, exposure time 1/4000 s, and f-number 4. The settings for the conventional photos of the plasma are ISO 6400, f-number 5.6, and 1/30 s at 14 kV_{pp} and 1/40 s at 16 kV_{pp} ("kV_{pp}" stands for kV peak-to-peak).

3. Results and Discussion

Figure 3a–c provide representative oscillograms of the actuator driving voltage, DBD current, and plasma emission integrated over ultraviolet-near infrared (UV–NIR) wavelengths, respectively. Clearly, the main ionization and excitation processes are related to the rising part of the driving voltage, whereas much weaker current and emission are observed during the falling part. This fact has been mentioned and studied extensively in other DBD-based setups, showing that the propagation of cathode- and anode-directed streamers is involved [23].

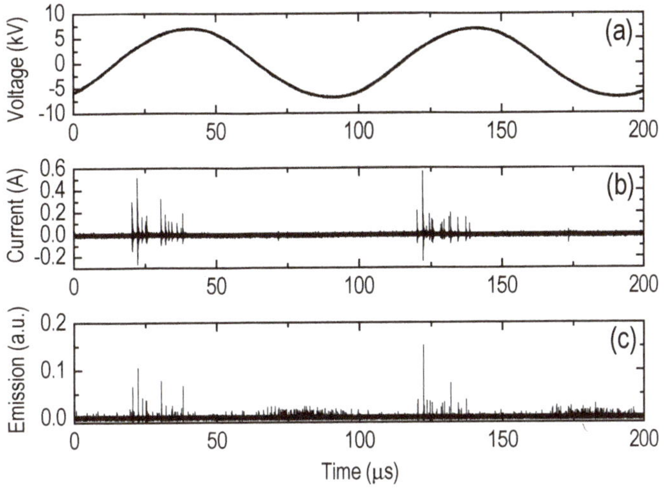

Figure 3. Representative waveforms of (**a**) the high voltage, (**b**) DBD current, and (**c**) wavelength-integrated optical emission over two periods. The projection of the optical fiber acceptance cone on the actuator surface corresponds to a circle of 12.5 mm in radius, centered on the point (x = 0, y = 0, z = 0).

During the rising part of the voltage, primary electrons propagate towards the anode, promoting ionization and excitation processes. The qualitative similarity between the current and emission impulses (Figure 3b,c) is underlined. At the same time, the resultant heavy positive ions are accelerated towards the dielectric-covered cathode, transferring momentum and energy to the surrounding air molecules, leading eventually to the flow field patterns that are illustrated below. On the other hand, during the falling part of the voltage, we probably deal with anode-directed streamers. According to this assumption, since the exposed electrode is now negatively driven, electrons are repealed towards the dielectric-covered electrode. They are following the field lines and diverging from each other giving a diffused and weaker excitation.

The impulsive form of the current (Figure 3b) and the optical emission (Figure 3c) are in accordance with the conventional photographs of the DBD pattern shown in Figure 4. The induced plasma is associated with filamentary DBDs. The number and the electron density of the filaments along the flat electrodes increase for higher voltage amplitude, but a homogeneous glow discharge is never reached with the voltage amplitudes used here. It is considered that the electric field is quite elevated due to the electrode design (thickness of a few micrometers only). Thus, important fluid perturbations are anticipated because of electrohydrodynamic forces [2,24–26]. Schlieren images are in line with this statement (discussed later).

Based on the above observations, it becomes apparent that the power is principally delivered to the actuator during the positive cycle of the driving voltage. Figure 5 shows that, under the present experimental conditions, the actuator consumes a mean power of less than 10 W. An increase at the voltage amplitude of just 2 kV_{pp} leads to power doubling (Figure 5a versus Figure 5b). However, the consumption remains practically unchanged over at least 24 h of operation (accumulative). The latter is an implication of a quite reliable actuator.

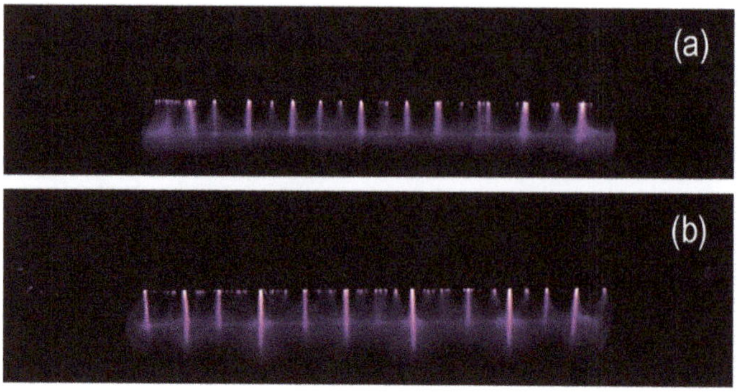

Figure 4. Representative conventional photographs of the DBD developed between the Ag-ink electrodes of the actuator. The filamentary nature of the discharge is manifested: (**a**) 14 kV_{pp}. (**b**) 16 kV_{pp}. The scale is the same in both photos (the plasma visible pattern has a length of about 50 mm).

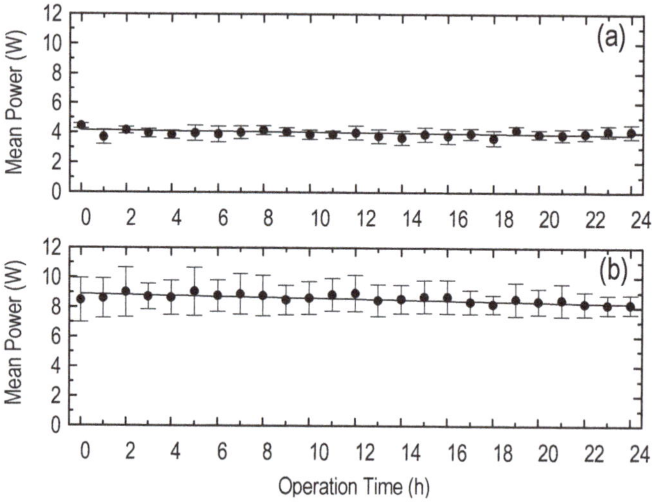

Figure 5. Electrical mean power consumed by a newly constructed actuator during the first 24 h of its operation (accumulative): (**a**) 14 kV_{pp} and (**b**) 16 kV_{pp}. Solid symbols: mean values following 10 sets of measurements (see Section 2 for details). Error bars: standard deviations derived from the 10 sets. Lines: linear fitting of the mean values.

However, despite the consistency of the actuator in terms of power consumption, both dielectric and electrode degradation are observed as the operation time accumulates. Figure 6 demonstrates this aging effect, as it is exhibited on the top surface of the actuator. The photo in Figure 6b refers to 24 h of accumulative operation and the worst-case stress scenario (i.e., 16 kV_{pp}). The actuator of Figure 6b remains functional, but the quantification of its material degradation and its possible efficiency deterioration might be the task of another study.

A better insight into the species contributing to the plasma-induced flow field may be gained by the OES spectrum of Figure 7a. Although a much wider wavelength range has been examined (see Section 2 for grating specifications), only N_2(SPS) and N_2^+(FNS), shown in Figure 7a, are detectable. The identification is organized in Table 1. Interestingly, with regard to ionic species, the nitrogen molecular ion is solely observable, and despite its weak relative spectral emission, its role in the flow field formation is emphasized. Otherwise, the spectrum is mainly populated by excited nitrogen molecules, whereas species such as NO_{γ}, OH, and N_2(FPS) are not detected.

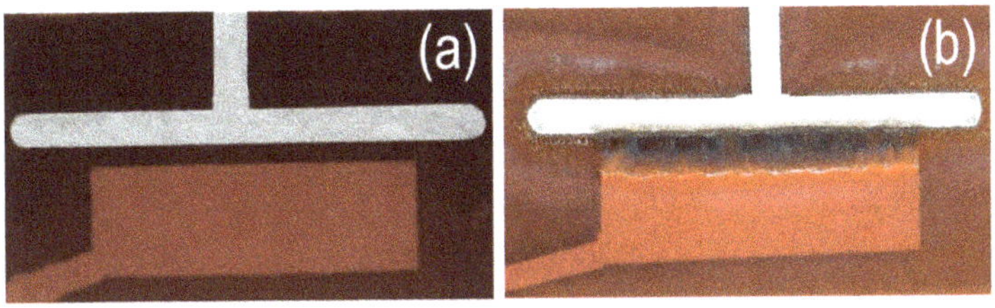

Figure 6. External top view of a newly constructed actuator (**a**) before and (**b**) after operation during 24 h (accumulative time) at 16 kV_{pp}.

Furthermore, high-resolution spectra can give the patterns of the rotational distributions of excited molecules, which thus serve as probe molecules for the gas temperature evaluation. In Figure 7b, the rotational distribution of the N_2 (SPS) species (337.13 nm in Table 1) is presented, being determined both experimentally and numerically. The numerical fitting of the latter to the former implies a gas temperature up to around 410 K at the maximum applied voltage (16 kV_{pp}). Further experiments have given values around 318 K at 12 kV_{pp} and 336 K at 14 kV_{pp}. Apart from the positive ions, the role of this rather elevated temperature in the flow field pattern should also be considered. This remark becomes more critical if one considers the local temperature, which is expected to be higher than the average one measured here. The term "local" means the temperature within specific elementary volumes of the plasma, contrary to the integrated emissive volume probed here (see the caption of Figure 7). In the frame of this work, the relative contribution of each factor, i.e., ions versus temperature, to the flow field modifications cannot be conclusive, but this topic remains challenging (see the further discussion below based on the schlieren imaging results).

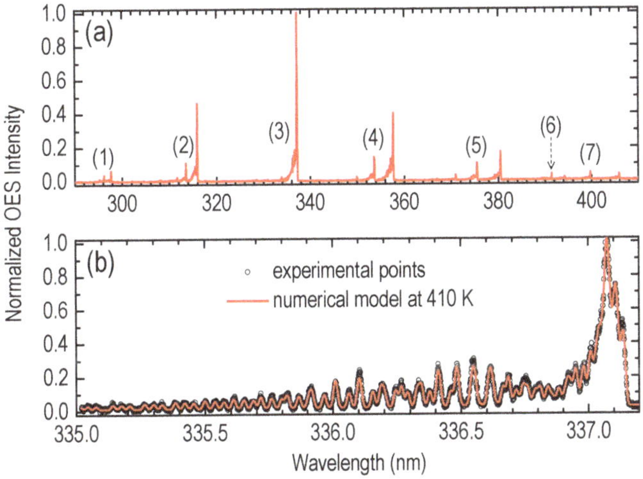

Figure 7. (**a**) Optical emission spectroscopy wide scan of the SDBD plasma (resolution 50 pm). For temporal evolution of the emission, see Figure 3c. (**b**) N_2(SPS; $v' = 0 - v'' = 0$) rotational distribution (resolution 1 pm). Solid symbols: experimental points. Line: theoretical rotational distribution, at 410 K, fitted to the experimental data. In both frames, the projection of the optical fiber acceptance cone on the actuator surface corresponds to a circle of 12.5 mm in radius, centered on the point (x = 0, y = 0, z = 0).

Table 1. Identification of the numbered bands of the spectrum given in Figure 7a.

Number/Label	Species	Vibrational Transition v′ − v″ (Δv)	Theoretical λ (nm)
(1)	N_2 (SPS): $C^3\Pi_u$–$B^3\Pi_g$	3−1 (+2)	296.2
	N_2 (SPS): $C^3\Pi_u$–$B^3\Pi_g$	2−0 (+2)	297.68
(2)	N_2 (SPS): $C^3\Pi_u$–$B^3\Pi_g$	3−2 (+1)	311.67
	N_2 (SPS): $C^3\Pi_u$–$B^3\Pi_g$	2−1 (+1)	313.6
	N_2 (SPS): $C^3\Pi_u$–$B^3\Pi_g$	1−0 (+1)	315.93
(3)	N_2 (SPS): $C^3\Pi_u$–$B^3\Pi_g$	1−1 (0)	333.89
	N_2 (SPS): $C^3\Pi_u$–$B^3\Pi_g$	0−0 (0)	337.13
(4)	N_2 (SPS): $C^3\Pi_u$–$B^3\Pi_g$	2−3 (−1)	350.05
	N_2 (SPS): $C^3\Pi_u$–$B^3\Pi_g$	1−2 (−1)	353.67
	N_2 (SPS): $C^3\Pi_u$–$B^3\Pi_g$	0−1 (−1)	357.69
(5)	N_2 (SPS): $C^3\Pi_u$–$B^3\Pi_g$	2−4 (−2)	371.05
	N_2 (SPS): $C^3\Pi_u$–$B^3\Pi_g$	1−3 (−2)	375.54
	N_2 (SPS): $C^3\Pi_u$–$B^3\Pi_g$	0−2 (−2)	380.49
(6)	N_2^+ (FNS) : $B^2\Sigma_u^+$–$X^2\Sigma_g^+$	0−0 (0)	391.44
(7)	N_2 (SPS): $C^3\Pi_u$–$B^3\Pi_g$	2−5 (−3)	394.3
	N_2 (SPS): $C^3\Pi_u$–$B^3\Pi_g$	1−4 (−3)	399.84
	N_2 (SPS): $C^3\Pi_u$–$B^3\Pi_g$	0−3 (−3)	405.94

Figure 8 presents the point-specific speed of the fluid over the actuator surface (z = 0.75 mm; y = 0 mm) at various positions far away from the discharge gap (x = 8, 18, and 24 mm) versus the time. These graphs unveil the variation in the speed that may take place as a function of the space coordinates and the time elapsed. Speed fluctuations are highly pronounced at longer distances from the discharge gap and they almost fade as the gap is approached (sequence Figure 8c → Figure 8b → Figure 8a). It is thus suggested that a transition from laminar to turbulent flow takes place along the x direction, even if we remain close to the surface of the actuator.

Based on time-resolved speed graphs such as those of Figure 8, the mean speed is calculated from each 300 s graph, and the 2D distribution (xz-plane) of the gas mean speed is mapped as in Figure 9 (y = 0). As regards the fluid speed close to the actuator surface (z = 0.75 mm; solid symbols in graphs), an increased speed is measured close to the discharge gap (x = 0 mm), whereas it decays monotonously along longer distances (up to x = 24 mm). This trend persists independently of the applied voltage amplitude. However, at 16 kV_{pp} (Figure 9b), a slightly higher speed is achieved compared with that at 14 kV_{pp} (Figure 9a). On the other hand, an abrupt decrease in the speed is observed at an almost double distance from the actuator surface (z = 1.4 mm; open symbols in graphs), and this is more noticeable when the actuator is driven by a lower voltage (Figure 9a). Another remarkable fact is the increased values of the standard deviations (error bars) calculated in the case of z = 1.4 mm compared with those found for the measurements closer to the surface (z = 0.75 mm). This fact should not be attributed to experimental uncertainties but, as it is mentioned above, it is rather related to the transition from a laminar flow layer to a turbulent phase. The subtleties of this assumption are considered below along with the schlieren imaging results.

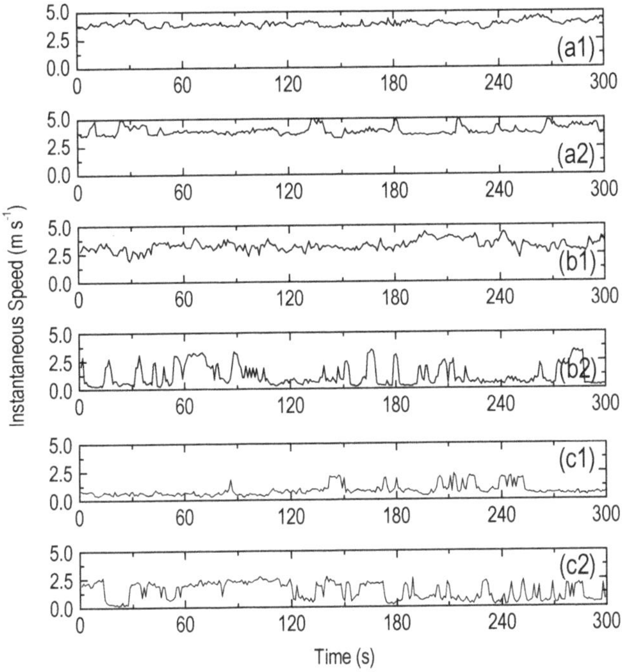

Figure 8. Real-time recordings of the point-specific, "instantaneous" speed (integration time 1 s) over 300 s time intervals. Two independent sets are obtained at x = 8 mm, y = 0 mm, z = 0.75 mm (**a1**,**a2**); x = 18 mm, y = 0 mm, z = 0.75 mm (**b1**,**b2**); and x = 24 mm, y = 0 mm, z = 0.75 mm (**c1**,**c2**). A newly constructed actuator is used for each set (first set: **a1**–**c1**; second set: **a2**–**c2**).

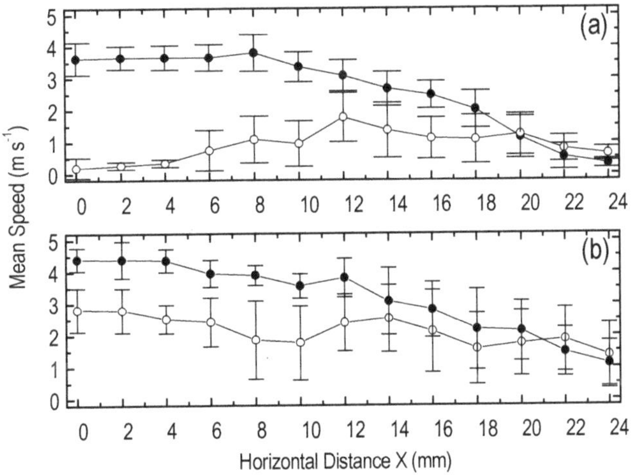

Figure 9. Mean speed along the *x*-axis at two different positions over the actuator surface. Solid symbols: y = 0 mm and z = 0.75 mm. Open symbols: y = 0 mm and z = 1.4 mm. Driving voltage: (**a**) 14 kV_{pp} and (**b**) 16 kV_{pp}. Mean values and standard deviations are derived from two sets of measurements. Four newly constructed actuators are used (first and second: 14 kV_{pp}/z = 0.75 mm/z = 1.4 mm; third and fourth: 16 kV_{pp}/z = 0.75 mm/z = 1.4 mm).

The vertical (i.e., along the z-axis) variation in the mean speed for two representative positions behind the discharge gap is plotted in Figure 10. In both cases, i.e., x = 4 mm and x = 12 mm, as the actuator surface is approached, the fluid speed increases constantly, whereas it becomes negligible at a vertical distance z = 1.5–2 mm. Comparing Figure 10a,b, the turbulent nature of the flow as we move behind the discharge gap is mirrored in the increasing standard deviation values, similarly to what is implied by the data in Figure 8.

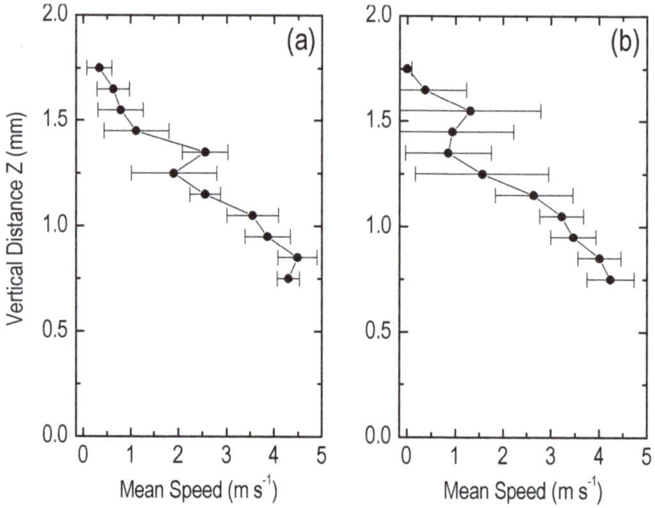

Figure 10. Mean speed along the z-axis at two different positions behind the discharge gap. (**a**) x = 4 mm and y = 0 mm; (**b**) x = 12 mm and y = 0 mm. Mean values and standard deviations are derived from two sets of measurements. Two newly constructed actuators are used (first: 16 kV_{pp}/x = 4 mm/x = 12 mm; second: 16 kV_{pp}/x = 4 mm/x = 12 mm).

A direct comparison of the above measured parameters with the corresponding values appearing in the bibliography does not make sense since an identical plasma actuator operating at the same conditions has not been evaluated earlier. Nevertheless, we can appose indicative information from experiments on SDBD plasma actuators in terms of fluid speed, electrical features, electrode dimensions, etc. For an actuator with both electrodes exposed (Al tapes of 200 mm length, 5 mm width, and 0.1 mm thickness), a 2 mm PMMA barrier, an electrode gap equal to 5 mm, and a sinusoidal (700 Hz) driving voltage at 40 kV_{pp}, a maximum speed of about 4.5 m s^{-1} has been noted [27]. In the same work, an electrode width of 20 mm, an electrode gap of 0 mm, a frequency of 1.5 kHz, and a voltage of 40 kV_{pp} led to a maximum speed of about 6.5 m s^{-1}. In another case [4], where a 300 mm long actuator consisting of 0.1 mm thickness Kapton® barrier, 12.7 mm wide covered grounded electrode, and 6.35 mm wide exposed high-voltage electrode were used, the time-averaged consumed power was reported to be less than 0.3 W mm^{-1} when the actuator was driven by short nanosecond pulses at frequencies less than 3 kHz and typical peak voltage at 16 kV. The velocity field generated in still air gave ensemble-averaged speed values up to 0.5 m s^{-1}, 20 mm downstream of the discharge for repetition frequency 2 kHz. In a last instance [28], a 0.15 mm thick Kapton® barrier, a 0.025 mm thick copper foil, and a 12.7 mm wide exposed electrode were employed. For a 24 mm wide insulated lower electrode and 16 kV_{pp} triangular (5 kHz) high voltage, a maximum fluid speed between 2.5 and 3 m s^{-1} was recorded.

Regarding the present actuator, the above speed plots provide a reasonable picture of the flow field pattern within the 2D space. This picture is validated by the schlieren images of Figure 11. It is noticed that schlieren images, unavoidably, correspond to side-on snapshots (xz-plane). This may point to an integration of optical events along the Y direction and their projection onto the xz-plane. However, following this angle, three different regions and regimes of flow field are readily distinguished. The first region (1) refers to the area above the high-voltage-driven electrode. This area is associated with an eddy-like flow field, which appears concentrated on the electrode edge adjacent to the discharge gap. The second region (2) is the interelectrode one, i.e., the gap itself, where a laminar flow well bounded onto the actuator surface is established. The thickness of this layer is approximately 1 mm. The third region (3) is the extended area above the grounded electrode, where the boundary laminar layer continues to propagate onto the surface. Nonetheless, it becomes progressively thicker along the *x*-axis, and a clear transition to intense perturbated (turbulent) flow field is observed along the *z*-axis. In addition, it tends to bend upwards as it approaches the end of the grounded electrode, resembling the separation effect. The perturbated field occupies more and more space as the distance along the *x*- or/and *z*-axis increases. This result is reflected in the speed and standard deviation values discussed above. The distinction of the three areas holds true for both voltage amplitudes in Figure 11. Nevertheless, the 16 kV_{pp} case promotes more intense perturbations.

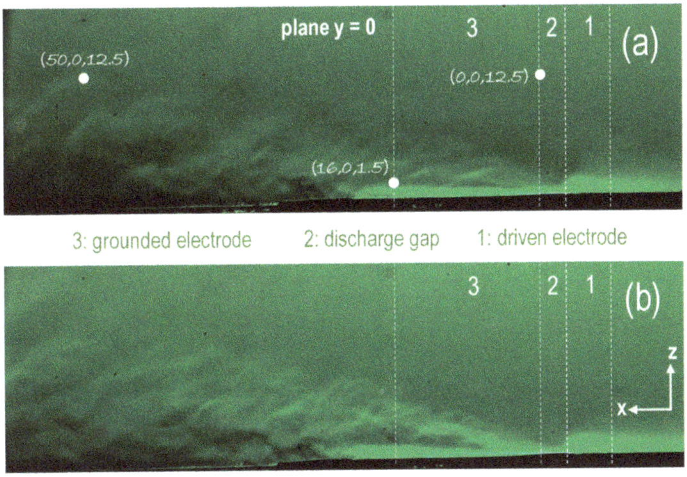

Figure 11. Representative flow field patterns recorded by means of schlieren imaging for two different voltage amplitudes: (**a**) 14 kV_{pp} and (**b**) 16 kV_{pp}. A newly constructed reactor is used. The three white bullets (insets) refer to indicative coordinates (x, y, z) in millimeters, common to (**a**,**b**). They mark off the image scale and facilitate the discussion in the text. The coordinates are given with respect to the Cartesian system defined in Figure 2.

Lastly, the flow field perturbations induced by the actuator propagate to long distances, even behind the grounded electrode. The snapshots of Figure 11 unveil perturbations far away from (i) the grounded electrode left edge (up to about 60 mm on the *x*-axis) and (ii) the electrode plane (up to about 20 mm on the *z*-axis). Such an intense directed motion of neutrals should be attributed to collisions with ions drifting into high local electric fields. The extremely thin electrodes were painted on the dielectric point to electric field enhancement as a dominant factor determining the effectiveness of momentum coupling into the surrounding air [28]. The role of temperature remains ambiguous even after the present results. However, similar electrohydrodynamic and thermal effects have been extensively studied by our group numerically [24–26,29], and the adaptation of the available numerical models to the present actuator case is in progress.

4. Conclusions

An SDBD-based plasma actuator having flexible a dielectric barrier and electrodes made of conductive ink was implemented and tested. Being driven by sinusoidal high voltage at 10 kHz, the actuator consumed up to 10 W of electric power and yielded a fluid mean speed of up to 4.5 m s^{-1}. Molecular nitrogen ions were produced during the rising part of the driving voltage, originating from air ionization due to the propagation of cathode-directed streamers. These ionic species were considered potential agents for the flow field establishment. This consisted of (i) a thin laminar flow layer, better developed closer to the actuator surface and the discharge gap, and (ii) an extended turbulent structure, which prevailed as being moved away from the surface and the gap. The average temperature of the neutral species over the actuator was found to be around 410 K at the maximum power level. Consequently, although the fluid directed speeds were presumably accredited to an ionic wind effect, the role of the temperature in the flow field formation remained debatable.

Author Contributions: V.P. and C.D. contributed equally: conceptualization; investigation; methodology; software; data curation; writing—original draft preparation; writing—review and editing; formal analysis; validation; visualization. P.S.: project administration; funding acquisition; supervision; resources; writing—original draft preparation; writing—review and editing; validation. P.K.P.: resources; validation; writing—review and editing. G.P.V.: resources; investigation. P.V.: validation; writing—review and editing. All authors have read and agreed to the published version of the manuscript.

Funding: This research received no external funding.

Data Availability Statement: The data presented in this study are available from the corresponding author upon request. The data are not publicly available due to privacy.

Conflicts of Interest: The authors declare no conflict of interest.

References

1. Sato, S.; Furukawa, H.; Komuro, A.; Takahashi, M.; Ohnishi, N. Successively accelerated ionic wind with integrated dielectric-barrier-discharge plasma actuator for low-voltage operation. *Sci. Rep.* **2019**, *9*, 5813. [CrossRef]
2. Boeuf, J.P.; Lagmich, Y.; Unfer, T.; Callegari, T.; Pitchford, L.C. Electrohydrodynamic force in dielectric barrier discharge plasma actuators. *J. Phys. D Appl. Phys.* **2007**, *40*, 652–662. [CrossRef]
3. Mursenkova, I.V.; Znamenskaya, I.A.; Lutsky, A.E. Influence of shock waves from plasma actuators on transonic and supersonic airflow. *J. Phys. D Appl. Phys.* **2018**, *51*, 105201. [CrossRef]
4. Little, J.; Takashima, K.; Nishihara, M.; Adamovich, I.; Samimy, M. Separation control with nanosecond-pulse-driven dielectric barrier discharge plasma actuators. *AIAA J.* **2012**, *50*, 350–365. [CrossRef]
5. Moreau, E. Airflow control by non-thermal plasma actuators. *J. Phys. D Appl. Phys.* **2007**, *40*, 605–636. [CrossRef]
6. Corke, T.C.; Enloe, C.L.; Wilkinson, S.P. Dielectric barrier discharge plasma actuators for flow control. *Annu. Rev. Fluid Mech.* **2010**, *42*, 505–529. [CrossRef]
7. Kogelschatz, U. Dielectric-barrier Discharges: Their History, Discharge Physics, and Industrial Applications. *Plasma Chem. Plasma Process.* **2003**, *23*, 1–46. [CrossRef]
8. Svarnas, P.; Giannakopoulos, E.; Kalavrouziotis, I.; Krontiras, C.; Georga, S.; Pasolari, R.S.; Papadopoulos, P.K.; Apostolou, I.; Chrysochoou, D. Sanitary effect of FE-DBD cold plasma in ambient air on sewage biosolids. *Sci. Total Environ.* **2020**, *705*, 135940. [CrossRef]
9. Svarnas, P.; Asimakoulas, L.; Katsafadou, M.; Pachis, K.; Kostazos, N.; Antimisiaris, S.G. Liposomal membrane disruption by means of miniaturized dielectric-barrier discharge in air: Liposome characterization. *J. Phys. D Appl. Phys.* **2017**, *50*, 345403. [CrossRef]
10. Ndong, A.C.A.; Zouzou, N.; Benard, N.; Moreau, E. Geometrical optimization of a surface DBD powered by a nanosecond pulsed high voltage. *J. Electrostat.* **2013**, *71*, 246–253. [CrossRef]
11. Gao, G.; Dong, L.; Peng, K.; Wei, W.; Li, C.; Wu, G. Comparison of the surface dielectric barrier discharge characteristics under different electrode gaps. *Phys. Plasmas* **2017**, *24*, 013510. [CrossRef]
12. Thomas, F.O.; Corke, T.C.; Iqbal, M.; Kozlov, A.; Schatzman, D. Optimization of dielectric barrier discharge plasma actuators for active aerodynamic flow control. *AIAA J.* **2009**, *47*, 2169–2178. [CrossRef]
13. Bian, D.; Wu, Y.; Long, C.; Lin, B. Effects of material degradation on electrical and optical characteristics of surface dielectric barrier discharge. *J. Appl. Phys.* **2018**, *124*, 183301. [CrossRef]

14. Hanson, R.E.; Houser, N.M.; Lavoie, P. Dielectric material degradation monitoring of dielectric barrier discharge plasma actuators. *J. Appl. Phys.* **2014**, *115*, 043301. [CrossRef]
15. Kong, F.; Wang, Y.; Zhang, C.; Che, X.; Yan, P.; Shao, T. Electrical and optical characteristics of surface plasma actuator based on a three-electrode geometry excited by nanosecond-pulse and DC sources. *Phys. Plasmas* **2017**, *24*, 123503.
16. Dawson, R.A.; Little, J. Effects of pulse polarity on nanosecond pulse driven dielectric barrier discharge plasma actuators. *J. Appl. Phys.* **2014**, *115*, 043306. [CrossRef]
17. Benard, N.; Moreau, E. Role of the electric waveform supplying a dielectric barrier discharge plasma actuator. *Appl. Phys. Lett.* **2012**, *100*, 193503. [CrossRef]
18. Roupassov, D.V.; Nikipelov, A.A.; Nudnova, M.M.; Starikovskii, A.Y. Flow separation control by plasma actuator with nanosecond pulse periodic discharge. *AIAA J.* **2009**, *47*, 168–185. [CrossRef]
19. Labergue, A.; Moreau, E.; Zouzou, N.; Touchard, G. Separation control using plasma actuators: Application to a free turbulent jet. *J. Phys. D Appl. Phys.* **2007**, *40*, 674–684. [CrossRef]
20. Grundmann, S.; Tropea, C. Experimental transition delay using glow-discharge plasma actuators. *Exp. Fluids* **2007**, *42*, 653–657. [CrossRef]
21. Corke, T.C.; Post, M.L.; Orlov, D.M. SDBD plasma enhanced aerodynamics: Concepts, optimization and applications. *Prog. Aerosp. Sci.* **2007**, *43*, 193–217. [CrossRef]
22. Cardoso, R.P.; Belmonte, Y.; Keravec, P.; Kosior, F.; Henrion, G. Influence of impurities on the temperature of an atmospheric helium plasma in microwave resonant cavity. *J. Phys. D Appl. Phys.* **2007**, *40*, 1394. [CrossRef]
23. Gazeli, K.; Svarnas, P.; Vafeas, P.; Papadopoulos, P.K.; Gkelios, A.; Clément, F. Investigation on streamers propagating into a helium jet in air at atmospheric pressure: Electrical and optical emission analysis. *J. Appl. Phys.* **2013**, *114*, 103304. [CrossRef]
24. Logothetis, D.K.; Papadopoulos, P.K.; Svarnas, P.; Vafeas, P. Numerical simulation of the interaction between helium jet flow and an atmospheric-pressure "plasma jet". *Comput. Fluids* **2016**, *140*, 11–18. [CrossRef]
25. Papadopoulos, P.K.; Vafeas, P.; Svarnas, P.; Gazeli, K.; Hatzikonstantinou, P.M.; Gkelios, A.; Clément, F. Interpretation of the gas flow field modification induced by guided streamer ('plasma bullet') propagation. *J. Phys. D Appl. Phys.* **2014**, *47*, 425203. [CrossRef]
26. Papadopoulos, P.K.; Athanasopoulos, D.; Sklias, K.; Svarnas, P.; Mourousias, N.; Vratsinis, K.; Vafeas, P. Generic residual charge based model for the interpretation of the electrohydrodynamic effects in cold atmospheric pressure plasmas. *Plasma Sources Sci. Technol.* **2019**, *28*, 065005. [CrossRef]
27. Forte, M.; Jolibois, J.; Pons, J.; Moreau, E.; Touchard, G.; Cazalens, M. Optimization of a dielectric barrier discharge actuator by stationary and non-stationary measurements of the induced flow velocity: Application to airflow control. *Exp. Fluids* **2007**, *43*, 917–928. [CrossRef]
28. Enloe, C.L.; McLaughlin, T.E.; VanDyken, R.D.; Kachner, K.D.; Jumper, E.J.; Corke, T.C.; Haddad, O. Mechanisms and Responses of a Single Dielectric Barrier Plasma Actuator: Geometric Effects. *AIAA J.* **2004**, *42*, 595–604. [CrossRef]
29. Svarnas, P.; Papadopoulos, P.; Athanasopoulos, D.; Sklias, K.; Gazeli, K.; Vafeas, P. Parametric study of thermal effects in a capillary dielectric-barrier discharge related to plasma jet production: Experiments and numerical modelling. *J. Appl. Phys.* **2018**, *124*, 064902. [CrossRef]

applied sciences

MDPI

Article

Plasma Gas Temperature Control Performance of Metal 3D-Printed Multi-Gas Temperature-Controllable Plasma Jet

Yuma Suenaga [1], Toshihiro Takamatsu [2,3,*], Toshiki Aizawa [1], Shohei Moriya [1], Yuriko Matsumura [4], Atsuo Iwasawa [4] and Akitoshi Okino [1]

1 Laboratory for Future Interdisciplinary Research of Science and Technology, Institute of Innovative Research, Tokyo Institute of Technology, J2-32, 4259 Nagatsuta, Midori-ku, Yokohama 226-8502, Japan; suenaga@plasma.es.titech.ac.jp (Y.S.); atoshiki@plasma.es.titech.ac.jp (T.A.); moriya@plasma.es.titech.ac.jp (S.M.); aokino@es.titech.ac.jp (A.O.)

2 Research Institute for Biomedical Sciences, Tokyo University of Science, 2669 Yamazaki, Noda 278-0022, Japan

3 Exploratory Oncology Research & Clinical Trial Center, National Cancer Center, 6-5-1 Kashiwanoha, Kashiwa 277-8577, Japan

4 Division of Infection Prevention and Control, Tokyo Healthcare University, 4-1-17 Higashi-Gotanda, Shinagawa-ku, Tokyo 141-8648, Japan; y-matsumura@thcu.ac.jp (Y.M.); a-iwasawa@thcu.ac.jp (A.I.)

* Correspondence: totakama@east.ncc.go.jp

Abstract: The aim of the study was to design and build a multi-gas temperature-controllable plasma jet that can control the gas temperature of plasmas with various gas species, and evaluated its temperature control performance. In this device, a fluid at an arbitrary controlled temperature is circulated through the plasma jet body. The gas exchanges heat with the plasma jet body to control the plasma temperature. Based on this concept, a complex-shaped plasma jet with two channels in the plasma jet body, a temperature control fluid (TCF) channel, and a gas channel was designed. The temperature control performance of nitrogen gas was evaluated using computational fluid dynamics analysis, which found that the gas temperature changed proportionally to the TCF temperature. The designed plasma jet body was fabricated using metal 3D-printer technology. Using the fabricated plasma jet body, stable plasmas of argon, oxygen, carbon dioxide, and nitrogen were generated. By varying the plasma jet body temperature from −30 °C to 90 °C, the gas temperature was successfully controlled linearly in the range of 29–85 °C for all plasma gas species. This is expected to further expand the range of applications of atmospheric low temperature plasma and to improve the plasma treatment effect.

Keywords: atmospheric plasma; metal 3D printing; temperature-controllable plasma gas

Citation: Suenaga, Y.; Takamatsu, T.; Aizawa, T.; Moriya, S.; Matsumura, Y.; Iwasawa, A.; Okino, A. Plasma Gas Temperature Control Performance of Metal 3D-Printed Multi-Gas Temperature-Controllable Plasma Jet. *Appl. Sci.* **2021**, *11*, 11686. https://doi.org/10.3390/app112411686

Academic Editor: Bogdan-George Rusu

Received: 15 November 2021
Accepted: 6 December 2021
Published: 9 December 2021

1. Introduction

Plasma has been actively applied in industrial fields, such as semiconductor manufacturing and fluorescent lighting. For example, in the field of surface treatment, plasma is used to harden the surface of materials [1] and surface modification [2]. These surface treatments are techniques that change the properties of solid surfaces using the action of the ions and electrons generated by plasma, for which low-pressure plasma has been used. Low-pressure plasmas are generated at low pressures of 1/1000 atm or less, which enables uniform surface treatment; however, this has limitations in terms of the types of treatment objects and throughput.

In recent years, it has become possible to stably generate low-temperature plasmas under atmospheric pressure; therefore, these plasmas have been applied in various fields such as medicine, industry, and chemical analysis. For example, in the medical field, they are used for disinfection [3–5], hemostasis [6], and wound healing [7], and they are used for surface modification in the industrial field [8]. In the field of chemical analysis, they have been utilized for surface adhesion analysis [9] and on-site analysis [10]. To increase the processing effectiveness of atmospheric low-temperature plasma, the energy applied to a unit volume can be increased by means such as discharge [11]. For materials that are resistant to thermal damage, an increase in temperature promotes the reaction with the reactive species, improving the treatment effect. Ohkubo et al. reported the adhesion of PTFE using atmospheric pressure plasma controlled at 260 °C [12]. A high adhesion effect and radical density were observed in the high temperature plasma by increasing the input power. However, this temperature increase is a problem for heat-sensitive materials, such as biological samples. To solve this problem, cryo-microplasma, in which He gas is cooled by liquid nitrogen before the plasma is generated, was developed [13,14]. Oshita et al. developed a temperature-controllable atmospheric plasma source as an advanced plasma jet [15]. They succeeded in controlling the gas temperature of He plasma in the range of −54–160 °C by cooling with liquid nitrogen and heating with a heater. Another way to increase the treatment effect of atmospheric low-temperature plasma is to change the gas species of the plasma. Takamatsu et al. evaluated the effect of plasma gas species on the surface treatment effect of polyimide films and found that carbon dioxide plasma was the most effective treatment [16]. Thus, to obtain a high treatment effect without thermal damage to the target in atmospheric low-temperature plasma application, it is necessary to control the gas temperature of the plasma and generate plasmas of various gas species.

We developed a multi-gas temperature-controllable plasma jet that can easily control the gas temperature of plasmas of various gas species over a wide range of temperatures. In this study, because the temperature of gases other than He can be controlled, the excessive cooling using liquid nitrogen in the previous study must be avoided. In this study, to control the gas temperature in the plasma, the gas was stagnated in the plasma jet body before plasma generation, and heat exchange was performed. To achieve a wide temperature control range, a plasma jet body was designed and analyzed using computational fluid dynamics (CFD) to improve the temperature control performance. To fabricate a plasma jet body with a complex shape, a metal 3D printer was used. 3D-printing technology has attracted increasing attention in manufacturing, including its use in plasma systems, due to its low cost and high flexibility [17–19]. Recently, a plasma jet for an endoscope with a diameter of approximately 3 mm produced by a metal 3D printer has been reported [20]. Nitrogen, carbon dioxide, oxygen, and argon plasmas were generated using a multi-gas temperature-controllable plasma jet fabricated using a metal 3D printer. The gas temperature control performance of each plasma sample was evaluated.

2. Materials and Methods

2.1. Concept of Multi-Gas Temperature-Controllable Plasma Jet

The concept of a multi-gas temperature-controllable plasma jet is shown in Figure 1. The gas temperature before the plasma generation was controlled in the multi-gas temperature-controllable plasma jet. To achieve this, the plasma jet body was designed with a mechanism to change the gas temperature before plasma generation through heat exchange with the body. In the plasma jet body, there are two channels: a temperature control fluid (TCF) flow channel and a gas channel used to generate the plasma. The TCF flow channel spiraled around the gas channel. The plasma jet body was maintained at a constant temperature by flowing TCF through the TCF channel. The gas introduced into the plasma jet body reaches the hot and ground electrodes while conducting heat exchange with the plasma jet body. Plasma is generated by an inter-electrode discharge, and the afterglow of the plasma flows out of the plasma jet body.

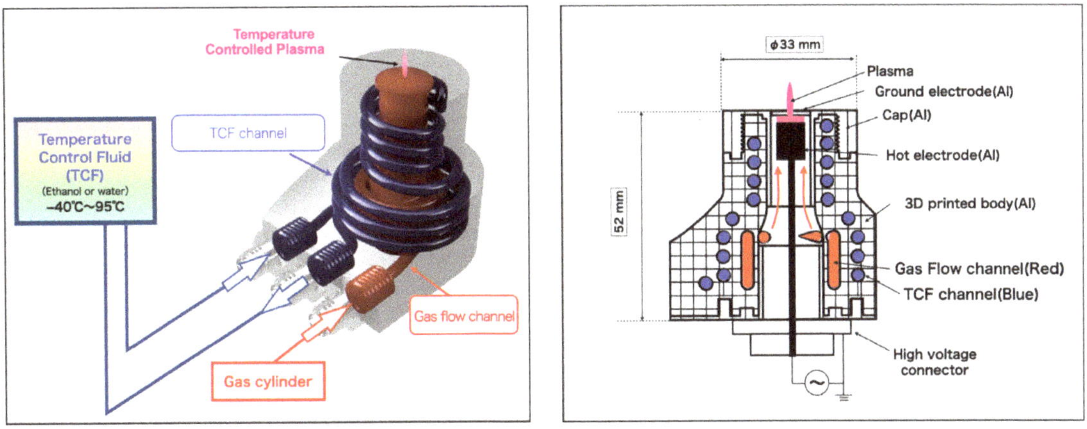

(a) (b)

Figure 1. Concept of multi-gas temperature-controllable plasma jet: (**a**) concept of flow channel; (**b**) cross-sectional view.

2.2. Evaluation of Temperature Control Performance Using CFD Analysis

CFD analysis is used in the design of plasma devices to understand fluid dynamics and heat transfer [21]. In this study, CFD analysis using Autodesk CFD (Autodesk Inc., San Rafael, CA, USA) was performed to design the flow channels of the plasma jet. To analyze the heat transfer and gas flow, the continuity, Navier-Stokes, and energy equations are discretized and calculated by the finite element method. The respective equations for incompressible fluids are shown below. The continuity equation is

$$\rho(\nabla \cdot \boldsymbol{U}) = 0 \tag{1}$$

where ρ is the density and $\boldsymbol{U}$ is the velocity vector. The Navier-Stokes equation is

$$\rho\frac{\partial \boldsymbol{U}}{\partial t} + \rho(\nabla \cdot \boldsymbol{U})\boldsymbol{U} = \rho \boldsymbol{g} - \nabla P + \mu\nabla^2\boldsymbol{U} \tag{2}$$

where $\boldsymbol{g}$ are the gravitational acceleration vector, P is pressure, and μ is viscosity. The energy equation is

$$\frac{\partial \rho C_p T}{\partial t} + \nabla \cdot (\rho C_p T \boldsymbol{U}) = \nabla^2 kT \tag{3}$$

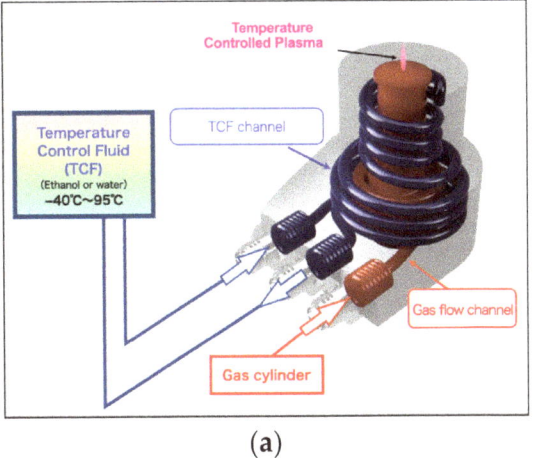

where C_p is the constant pressure specific heat, T is the temperature, and k is the thermal conductivity. For turbulence analysis, these equations were time-averaged. The Reynolds stress terms generated by this averaging were approximated using the turbulence model k-ε. A modified Petrov–Galerkin method was used for calculation of the convection term in the Navier-Stokes equations. In the simplified model shown in Figure 2, the joints and screws of the parts that did not have a significant effect on the CFD were omitted. The mesh size of the model was set to "Automatic", and the parameters are resolution factor: 1.000, edge growth rate: 1.100, minimum points on edge: 2, points on longest edge: 10, surface limiting aspect: 20. The total number of nodes is 236,971 (fluid nodes: 169,458, solid nodes: 67,513), and the total number of elements is 1,008,496 (fluid elements: 532,224, solid elements: 476,272). In the analysis of the low-temperature side (−30–0 °C), 80 wt% ethanol was used as the TCF and supplied to the TCF channel at a rate of 0.5 L/min. For the analysis of the high-temperature side (0–90 °C), water was used as the TCF and supplied to the TCF flow channel at a rate of 0.5 L/min. The TCF was supplied to the plasma jet body using an insulated silicon rubber tube. The pressure at the outlet surface of the TCF flow channel was set to 0 Pa, and there was no pressure loss in the temperature-controlled fluid flow. Dry nitrogen gas at 3 L/min and 24 °C was used as the gas for plasma generation. The plasma jet body was made of aluminum and surrounded by a 5 mm-thick porous ethylene propylene diene rubber insulation material. The thermal conductivity of the insulation material was set to 0.032 W/m·k. However, no insulation was placed on the surface where the plasma outlet was placed and on the upper surface because these surfaces are impediments to plasma processing in practical use. To analyze the heat transfer to the external gas, the plasma jet was placed in a nitrogen external fluid. Nitrogen at a temperature of 24 °C and humidity of 60% was used as the external fluid to match the operating environment. The surface of the external fluid was analyzed assuming no pressure loss. To clarify the effect of the temperature of the TCF on the gas before plasma generation, the temperature of the plasma jet body and gas temperature were calculated by varying the TCF from −30 to 90 °C. The temperature at the 2 mm point of the plasma outlet was calculated. A component analysis was performed on the plasma jet body, and the average temperature was calculated. It should be noted that the plasma was not considered in the CFD in this study.

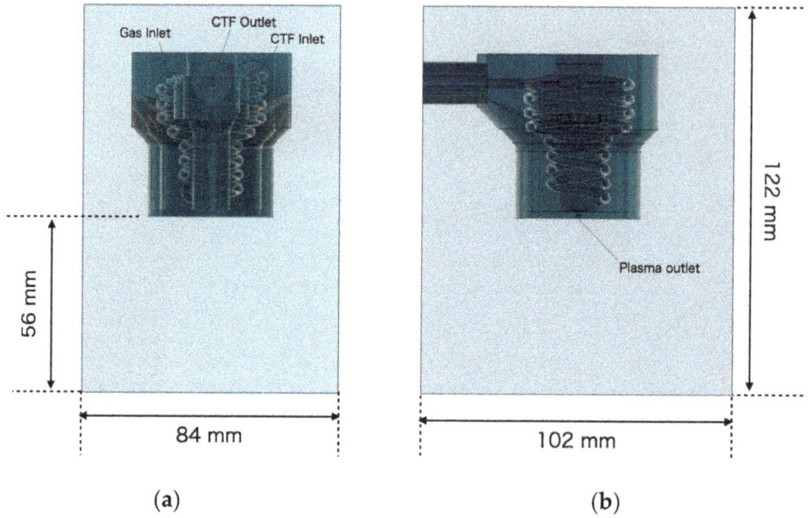

Figure 2. Geometry of multi-gas temperature-controllable plasma jet for computational fluid dynamics (CFD) analysis: (**a**) front view; (**b**) side view.

2.3. Temperature Control Performance of Multi-Gas Temperature-Controllable Plasma Jet

The temperature control performance of the multi-gas temperature-controllable plasma jet was evaluated. The designed plasma jet produced 3 L/min (standard) plasmas of carbon dioxide, argon, nitrogen, and oxygen. The plasma jet body temperature was varied from −30 to 90 °C, and the change in the plasma gas temperature was measured. For the TCF, an 80 wt% ethanol solution and water were used for the plasma jet body temperature range of −30–0 and 10–90 °C, respectively. The temperature of the TCF was controlled using a low-temperature thermostatic bath (NCB-2410B, TOKYO RIKAKIKAI CO, LTD., Tokyo, Japan) and a thermostatic bath (NCB-1210B, TOKYO RIKAKIKAI CO, LTD., Tokyo, Japan) at −30–0 °C and 10–90 °C, respectively.

The temperature of the plasma jet body was measured using a K-type thermocouple attached to the side of the body and a logger (RX-450K, AS ONE CORPORATION, Osaka, Japan). The TCF temperature was measured using a K-type thermocouple in the TCF channel immediately before the plasma jet body. The plasma gas temperature was measured using a K-type thermocouple at a distance of 2 mm from the plasma outlet 120 s after the plasma was generated. The temperature at each gas irradiation without the plasma generation was also measured under the same conditions. The ambient temperature and humidity were 22 °C and 60%, respectively. The plasma jet body was covered with insulation material to reduce the influence of the surrounding environment.

3. Results and Discussion

3.1. Evaluation of Temperature Control Performance Using CFD Analysis

CFD analysis was performed to design the flow path of the multi-gas temperature-controllable plasma jet. Figure 3a,b show the temperature distribution in the cross-section of the plasma jet when a TCF of −30 °C and 90 °C flows in the TCF channel, respectively. When a TCF of −30 °C was supplied, the average temperature of the plasma jet body decreased to −29.1 °C. The gas temperature 2 mm from the plasma outlet was −23.0 °C. When a TCF of 90 °C was supplied, the temperature of the plasma body was 89.5 °C. The gas temperature at 2 mm from the plasma outlet was 82.1 °C. In each case, it was shown that the gas temperature approached the room temperature of 24 °C as the distance from the plasma outlet increased.

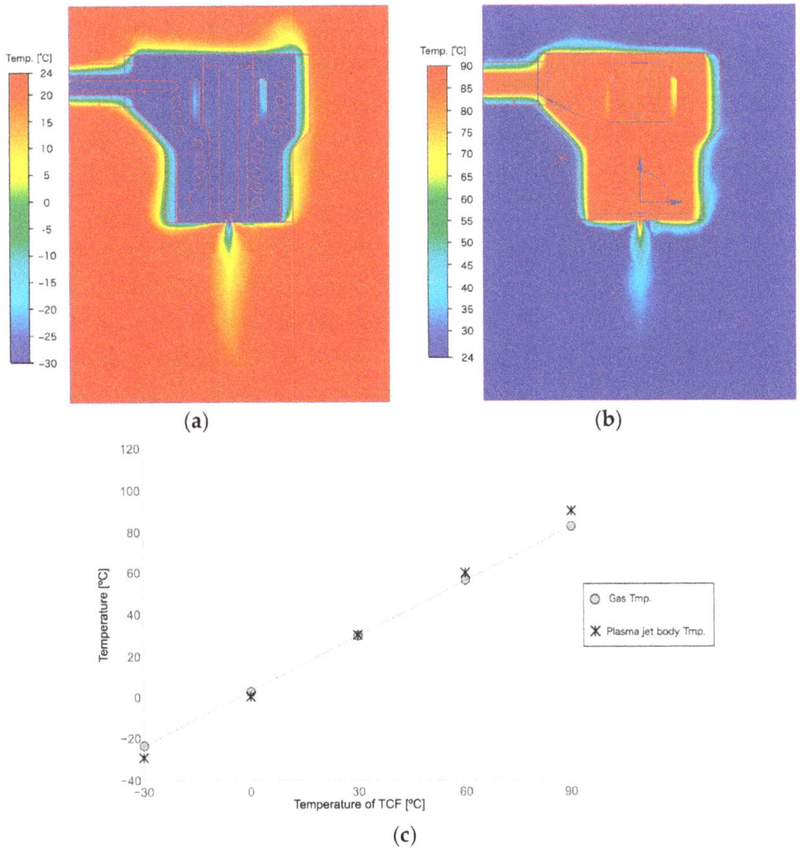

Figure 3. Evaluation of plasma jet body using CFD analysis: (**a**) temperature distribution at temperature control fluid (TCF) of −30 °C; (**b**) temperature distribution at TCF of 90 °C; (**c**) gas temperature at a distance of 2 mm from the plasma outlet calculated by CFD.

Figure 3c shows the relationship between the TCF temperature and gas temperature at a distance of 2 mm from the plasma outlet. As the TCF temperature increased, the gas temperature increased proportionally. The CFD analysis shows that the gas temperature before the plasma generation can be easily changed using a plasma jet body containing a TCF channel. It has been reported that the gas temperature of the plasma can be changed by varying the gas temperature before the plasma generation [15]. The gas temperature of the plasma can also be controlled by varying the TCF temperature used in the designed plasma jet.

3.2. Fabrication of Multi-Gas Temperature-Controllable Plasma Jet

The CFD analysis showed that the gas temperature could be controlled by the TCF temperature. Therefore, a multi-gas temperature-controllable plasma jet containing a TCF channel and a gas channel was fabricated. This device is difficult to fabricate by general machining due to the complex flow channels inside the plasma jet body. The plasma jet body was fabricated using a direct metal-printing 3D printer (Prox300 from 3DSystems Inc., San Diego, CA, USA) that sintered the metal powder with a laser. The plasma jet body was fabricated by SOLIZE Corporation, Tokyo, Japan. The metal powder used was aluminum–silicon alloy (AlSi12), which has excellent thermal conductivity. In the particle size distribution of metal powder, D10, D50, D90 were 9 μm, 20 μm, and 36 μm, respectively. When the metal powder is reused, it is sieved to remove foreign matter. The parameters of the 3D printer are 40 μm thickness per layer. The standard tolerance of the built object is ±0.3 mm. The parts that required high precision, such as screws and parts that needed to be airtight, were fabricated using machine tools. The fabricated plasma jet is shown in Figure 4a. The plasma was generated by applying a sinusoidal wave of 9 kV and 16 kHz to the hot electrode of the fabricated plasma jet. Figure 4b shows the generated plasmas of carbon dioxide, argon, nitrogen, and oxygen. Stable plasma generation was observed in the plasma jet body with multiple channels formed by a metal 3D printer.

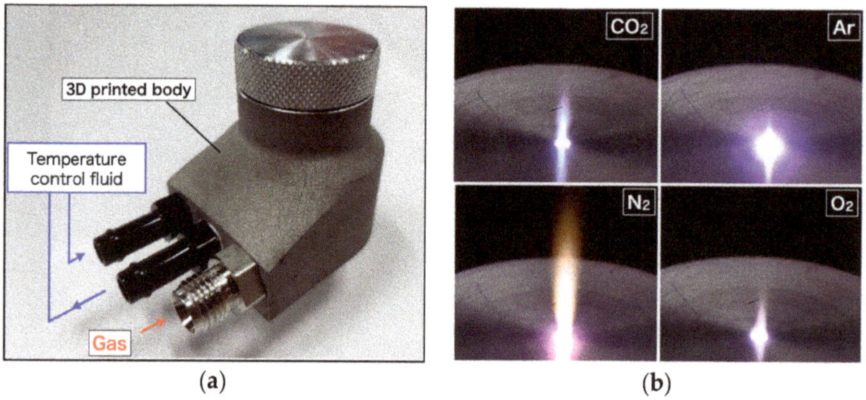

Figure 4. Metal 3D-printed multi-gas temperature-controllable plasma jet: (**a**) outside view; (**b**) plasma generation for various gas species.

3.3. Temperature Control Performance of Multi-Gas Temperature-Controllable Plasma Jet

Figure 5 shows the relationship between the TCF temperature, the plasma jet body temperature, and the gas temperature before and after the plasma generation. The results of the CFD analysis are also plotted in the N_2 result. The gas and plasma gas temperatures of carbon dioxide, argon, nitrogen, and oxygen were varied in the ranges of −17–77 and 29–108, −18–74.5 and 3–85, −20–78 and 28–108, and −21–78 and 17–106 °C, respectively, by varying the plasma jet body temperature from −30 °C to 90 °C. Assuming that the plasma jet body temperature affects the plasma gas temperature, a single regression analysis was performed. The coefficients of determination for each approximation line are listed in Table 1. In the case of gas irradiation, the coefficients of determination for the R^2 values were greater than 0.99 for all gas species. The gas temperatures of the plasmas had a coefficient of determination for the R^2 values greater than 0.98 for all gas species. These results show that the approximation line fits effectively and that the plasma jet body temperature, gas temperature, and plasma gas temperature vary proportionally. The gas temperature of the plasma was indirectly controlled by controlling the temperature of the plasma jet body. The instability of the plasma gas temperature was observed when the plasma jet body temperature was between −10 °C and 20 °C because of the water droplets that condensed on the plasma jet body near the plasma outlet. These water droplets were caught in the gas flow of the plasma, causing instability in the plasma temperature. When the measured nitrogen gas temperature was compared with the CFD temperature control performance, a decrease in the temperature control performance of approximately 3 °C and 5 °C was observed at a plasma jet body temperature of −30 and 90 °C, respectively. The CFD results and actual measurements were not in perfect agreement. This may be due to the fact that the CFD does not reproduce external disturbances such as the air flow around the plasma jet.

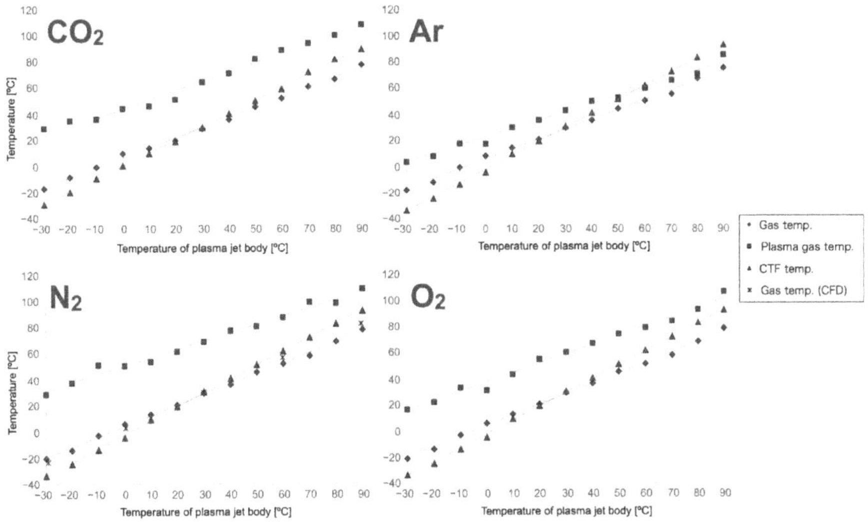

Figure 5. Relationship between plasma gas temperature and plasma jet body temperature.

Table 1. Coefficient of determination between plasma jet body temperature and gas temperature for each gas species.

	CO_2	Ar	N_2	O_2
Gas	0.9975	0.9967	0.9981	0.9996
Plasma	0.9828	0.9898	0.9861	0.9893

For all gas species, a temperature increase was observed when the plasma was generated. The ranges of the temperature increase for carbon dioxide, argon, nitrogen, and oxygen at the plasma jet body temperature of −30 °C were 46, 22, 49, and 37 °C, respectively. The range of temperature increase for carbon dioxide, argon, nitrogen, and oxygen at the plasma jet body temperature of 20 °C, which was close to the room temperature, was 31, 15, 41, and 34 °C, respectively. The temperature increase for carbon dioxide, argon, nitrogen, and oxygen at the plasma jet body temperature of 90 °C was 31, 10, 31, and 28 °C, respectively. For all gas species of plasma, the range of temperature increase due to plasma generation decreased as the gas temperature increased. One of the reasons for this phenomenon may be the influence of the room temperature through mixing with the ambient air. To achieve lower or higher plasma gas temperatures, it is necessary to vary the temperature of the TCF significantly.

By lowering the temperature of the plasma jet body to −30 °C, a plasma gas temperature of less than 30 °C can be achieved, and irradiation of heat-sensitive processing materials such as plants is possible. Gas temperatures up to 108 °C can be achieved in carbon dioxide and nitrogen plasmas, which is useful for studying the conditions for improving the treatment effect. In the future, the developed multi-gas temperature-controllable plasma jet will be applied in medical and agriculture applications. Additionally, it is necessary to clarify the gas species and gas temperature of the plasma to maximize the treatment effect.

4. Conclusions

In this study, we developed a multi-gas temperature-controllable plasma jet that can generate plasma of various gas species at an arbitrary controlled temperature. A multi-gas temperature-controllable plasma jet was designed using CFD analysis with a TCF channel spiraled around the gas channel. The designed plasma jet was fabricated using metal 3D-printer technology. In the multi-gas temperature-controllable plasma jet, the stable generation of the plasma of nitrogen, oxygen, carbon dioxide, and argon was successfully achieved. The temperature of the plasma gas can be easily changed by controlling the temperature of the supplied TCF. Additionally, the gas temperature after plasma generation changed linearly by changing the TCF temperature. The gas temperature of the plasma was controlled between a minimum of 3 °C and a maximum of 108 °C by varying the plasma jet body temperature from −30 to 90 °C. The gas temperature was increased by the plasma generation. The range of the temperature increase obtained for carbon dioxide, argon, nitrogen, and oxygen was 31, 15, 41, and 34 °C, respectively, when the plasma jet body temperature was 20 °C. These results indicate that the gas temperature control characteristics of plasma vary significantly depending on the gas species.

It was shown that it is possible to design and fabricate plasma jets with a higher level of flexibility. A multi-gas temperature-controllable plasma jet of any shape can be fabricated for plasma applications in medicine, agriculture, and material processing. The use of multi-gas temperature-controllable plasma jets is expected to control the gas temperature of the plasma of various gas species and achieve stable treatment effects without damaging the treated object. In the future, we will study the gas species and temperature of the plasma for various applications such as hemostasis, disinfection, surface treatment, and plant genome editing.

Author Contributions: Conceptualization, S.M., T.T., Y.M., A.I., A.O.; methodology, Y.S., T.T., T.A., S.M., A.O.; validation, Y.S., T.A.; formal analysis, Y.S.; investigation, Y.S., S.M., T.A.; resources, Y.S., T.A., S.M.; data curation, Y.S., T.A., S.M., T.T.; writing—original draft preparation, Y.S.; writing—review and editing, S.M., T.T., Y.M., A.I., A.O.; Visualization, Y.S., T.A., S.M.; supervision, T.T., Y.M., A.I., A.O.; project administration, Y.M., A.I., A.O.; funding acquisition, A.I., A.O. All authors have read and agreed to the published version of the manuscript.

Funding: This study was supported by JSPS KAKENHI (Grant Number: 20K07039) and the Cooperative Research Project of the Research Center for Biomedical Engineering, National Cancer Center Research and Development Fund (Grant Number: 31-A-11), TERUMO LIFE SCIENCE FOUNDATION (Grant Number: 18-II106).

Institutional Review Board Statement: Not applicable.

Informed Consent Statement: Not applicable.

Data Availability Statement: Data is contained within the article.

Acknowledgments: The authors would like to thank Norihiko Yamamoto at the Design and Manufacturing Division, Open Facility Center, Tokyo Institute of Technology, for preparing the plasma jet parts. The authors would like to thank Syosaku Ota at the Kobe Design University, for useful discussions on plasma jet fabrication.

Conflicts of Interest: The authors declare no conflict of interest.

References

1. Kashapov, N.F.; Sharifullin, S.N. Hardening of the Surface Plasma Jet High- Frequency Induction Discharge of Low Pressure. *Mater. Sci. Eng. Pap.* **2015**, *86*, 012021. [CrossRef]
2. Wilson, D.J.; Williams, R.L.; Pond, R.C. Plasma Modification of PTFE Surfaces. *Surf. Interface Anal.* **2001**, *31*, 385–396. [CrossRef]
3. Pan, J.; Li, Y.L.; Liu, C.M.; Tian, Y.; Yu, S.; Wang, K.L.; Zhang, J.; Fang, J. Investigation of cold atmospheric plasma-activated water for the dental unit waterline system contamination and safety evaluation in vitro. *Plasma Chem. Plasma Process.* **2017**, *37*, 1091–1103. [CrossRef]
4. Maisch, T.; Shimizu, T.; Li, Y.F.; Heinlin, J.; Karrer, S.; Morfill, G.; Zimmermann, J.L. Decolonisation of MRSA, *S. Aureus* and *E. Coli* by Cold-Atmospheric Plasma Using a Porcine Skin Model In Vitro. *PLoS ONE* **2012**, *7*, e34610. [CrossRef]
5. Abonti, T.R.; Kaku, M.; Kojima, S.; Sumi, H.; Kojima, S.; Yamamoto, T.; Yashima, Y.; Miyahara, H.; Okino, A.; Kawata, T.; et al. Irradiation Effects of Low Temperature Multi Gas Plasma Jet on Oral Bacteria. *Dent. Mater. J.* **2016**, *35*, 822–828. [CrossRef] [PubMed]
6. Fridman, G.; Peddinghaus, M.; Ayan, H.; Fridman, A.; Balasubramanian, M.; Gutsol, A.; Brooks, A.; Friedman, G. Blood Coagulation and Living Tissue Sterilization by Floating-Electrode Dielectric Barrier Discharge in Air. *Plasma Chem. Plasma Process.* **2006**, *26*, 425–442. [CrossRef]
7. Shimatani, A.; Toyoda, H.; Orita, K.; Hirakawa, Y.; Aoki, K.; Oh, J.; Shirafuji, T.; Nakamura, H. In Vivo Study on the Healing of Bone Defect Treated with Non-Thermal Atmospheric Pressure Gas Discharge Plasma. *PLoS ONE* **2021**, *16*, e0255861. [CrossRef]
8. Čerňáková, L.; Kováčik, D.; Zahoranová, A.; Černák, M.; Mazúr, M. Surface Modification of Polypropylene Non-Woven Fabrics by Atmospheric-Pressure Plasma Activation Followed by Acrylic Acid Grafting. *Plasma Chem. Plasma Process.* **2005**, *25*, 427–437. [CrossRef]
9. Aida, M.; Iwai, T.; Okamoto, Y.; Kohno, S.; Kakegawa, K.; Miyahara, H.; Seto, Y.; Okino, A. Development of a Dual Plasma Desorption/Ionization System for the Noncontact and Highly Sensitive Analysis of Surface Adhesive Compounds. *Mass Spectrom.* **2017**, *6*, S0075. [CrossRef] [PubMed]
10. Iwai, T.; Kakegawa, K.; Aida, M.; Nagashima, H.; Nagoya, T.; Kanamori-kataoka, M.; Miyahara, H.; Seto, Y.; Okino, A. Development of a Gas-Cylinder-Free Plasma Desorption/Ionization System for On-Site Detection of Chemical Warfare Agents. *Anal. Chem.* **2015**, *87*, 5707–5715. [CrossRef] [PubMed]
11. Van Deynse, A.; Cools, P.; Leys, C.; De Geyter, N.; Morent, R. Surface Activation of Polyethylene with an Argon Atmospheric Pressure Plasma Jet: Influence of Applied Power and Flow Rate. *Appl. Surf. Sci.* **2015**, *328*, 269–278. [CrossRef]
12. Ohkubo, Y.; Ishihara, K.; Shibahara, M.; Nagatani, A.; Honda, K.; Endo, K.; Yamamura, K. Drastic Improvement in Adhesion Property of Polytetrafluoroethylene (PTFE) via Heat-Assisted Plasma Treatment Using a Heater. *Sci. Rep.* **2017**, *7*, 9476. [CrossRef] [PubMed]
13. Noma, Y.; Choi, J.H.; Tomai, T.; Terashima, K. Gas-Temperature-Dependent Generation of Cryoplasma Jet under Atmospheric Pressure. *Appl. Phys. Lett.* **2008**, *93*, 101503. [CrossRef]
14. Ishihara, D.; Noma, Y.; Stauss, S.; Sai, M.; Tomai, T.; Terashima, K. Development of a Dielectric Barrier Discharge (DBD) Cryo-Microplasma: Generation and diagnostics. *Plasma Sources Sci. Technol. Dev.* **2008**, *17*, 035008. [CrossRef]
15. Oshita, T.; Kawano, H.; Takamatsu, T.; Miyahara, H.; Okino, A. Temperature Controllable Atmospheric Plasma Source. *IEEE Trans. Plasma Sci.* **2015**, *43*, 1987–1992. [CrossRef]
16. Takamatsu, T.; Hirai, H.; Sasaki, R.; Miyahara, H.; Okino, A. Surface Hydrophilization of Polyimide Films Using Atmospheric Damage-Free Multigas Plasma Jet Source. *Kagaku Kogaku Ronbunshu* **2013**, *39*, 372–377. [CrossRef]
17. Martínez-Jarquín, S.; Moreno-Pedraza, A.; Guillén-Alonso, H.; Winkler, R. Template for 3D Printing a Low-Temperature Plasma Probe. *Anal. Chem.* **2016**, *88*, 6976–6980. [CrossRef] [PubMed]
18. Barillas, L.; Makhneva, E.; An, S.; Fricke, K. Functional Thin Films Synthesized from Liquid Precursors by Combining Mist Chambers and Atmospheric-Pressure Plasma Polymerization. *Coatings* **2021**, *11*, 1336. [CrossRef]
19. Takamatsu, T.; Kawano, H.; Miyahara, H.; Azuma, T.; Okino, A. Atmospheric Nonequilibrium Mini-Plasma Jet Created by a 3D Printer. *AIP Adv.* **2015**, *5*, 077184. [CrossRef]
20. Kurosawa, M.; Takamatsu, T.; Kawano, H.; Hayashi, Y.; Miyahara, H.; Ota, S.; Okino, A.; Yoshida, M. Endoscopic Hemostasis in Porcine Gastrointestinal Tract Using CO_2 Low-Temperature Plasma Jet. *J. Surg. Res.* **2018**, *234*, 334–342. [CrossRef] [PubMed]
21. Onyshchenko, I.; De Geyter, N.; Morent, R. Improvement of the Plasma Treatment Effect on PET with a Newly Designed Atmospheric Pressure Plasma Jet. *Plasma Process. Polym.* **2017**, *14*, 1600200. [CrossRef]

applied sciences

MDPI

Article

Influence of Controlling Plasma Gas Species and Temperature on Reactive Species and Bactericidal Effect of the Plasma

Yuma Suenaga [1], Toshihiro Takamatsu [2,3,*], Toshiki Aizawa [1], Shohei Moriya [1], Yuriko Matsumura [4], Atsuo Iwasawa [4] and Akitoshi Okino [1]

1 Laboratory for Future Interdisciplinary Research of Science and Technology, Institute of Innovative Research, Tokyo Institute of Technology, J2-32, 4259 Nagatsuta, Midori-ku, Yokohama 226-8502, Japan; suenaga@plasma.es.titech.ac.jp (Y.S.); atoshiki@plasma.es.titech.ac.jp (T.A.); moriya@plasma.es.titech.ac.jp (S.M.); aokino@es.titech.ac.jp (A.O.)
2 Research Institute for Biomedical Sciences, Tokyo University of Science, 2669 Yamazaki, Noda 278-0022, Japan
3 Exploratory Oncology Research & Clinical Trial Center, National Cancer Center, 6-5-1 Kashiwanoha, Kashiwa 277-8577, Japan
4 Division of Infection Prevention and Control, Tokyo Healthcare University, 4-1-17 Higashi-Gotanda, Shinagawa-ku, Tokyo 141-8648, Japan; y-matsumura@thcu.ac.jp (Y.M.); a-iwasawa@thcu.ac.jp (A.I.)
* Correspondence: totakama@east.ncc.go.jp

Abstract: In this study, plasma gas species and temperature were varied to evaluate the reactive species produced and the bactericidal effect of plasma. Nitrogen, carbon dioxide, oxygen, and argon were used as the gas species, and the gas temperature of each plasma was varied from 30 to 90 °C. Singlet oxygen, OH radicals, hydrogen peroxide, and ozone generated by the plasma were trapped in a liquid, and then measured. Nitrogen plasma produced up to 172 μM of the OH radical, which was higher than that of the other plasmas. In carbon dioxide plasma, the concentration of singlet oxygen increased from 77 to 812 μM, as the plasma gas temperature increased from 30 to 90 °C. The bactericidal effect of carbon dioxide and nitrogen plasma was evaluated using bactericidal ability, which indicated the log reduction per minute. In carbon dioxide plasma, the bactericidal ability increased from 5.6 to 38.8, as the temperature of the plasma gas increased from 30 to 90 °C. Conversely, nitrogen plasma did not exhibit a high bactericidal effect. These results demonstrate that the plasma gas type and temperature have a significant influence on the reactive species produced and the bactericidal effect of plasma.

Keywords: atmospheric low-temperature plasma; reactive species; plasma disinfection

Citation: Suenaga, Y.; Takamatsu, T.; Aizawa, T.; Moriya, S.; Matsumura, Y.; Iwasawa, A.; Okino, A. Influence of Controlling Plasma Gas Species and Temperature on Reactive Species and Bactericidal Effect of the Plasma. *Appl. Sci.* **2021**, *11*, 11674. https://doi.org/10.3390/app112411674

Academic Editor: Bogdan-George Rusu

Received: 1 November 2021
Accepted: 6 December 2021
Published: 9 December 2021

1. Introduction

In the conventional plasma applications, high-temperature (several thousand degrees Celsius or higher) atmospheric plasma and low-pressure (1/10,000 atm) nonthermal plasma have been used for analysis [1] and semiconductor manufacturing [2]. Recently, the stable generation of low-temperature plasma at approximately 50–100 °C under atmospheric pressure has become possible. This has significantly expanded the range of plasma applications. Applications of plasma, such as in disinfection [3] and hemostasis [4], wound healing [5], analysis of surface-adhesive compounds [6], and mobile on-site analytical devices [7], are examples that take advantage of the characteristics of atmospheric pressure and low-temperature generation of plasma. A simple technique to improve the effectiveness of plasma treatment, such as surface treatment, involves increasing the energy input during plasma generation [8]. In atmospheric low-temperature plasmas, the gas temperature of the plasma is inevitably higher than room temperature (15–25 °C), because energy is supplied to the gas at room temperature through discharge to generate the plasma [9]. Therefore, for the treatment of plants and other particularly heat-sensitive processing targets, it is necessary to design a system that allows processing to be performed at a temperature that is close to room temperature. Ishihara et al. generated helium plasmas cooled with liquid nitrogen, and showed that it is possible to generate plasmas from cryogenic temperature to room temperature [10]. In addition, Oshita et al. reported a method to generate plasma at an arbitrary temperature by heating helium gas that is cooled by liquid nitrogen using a heater [11]. Although there are advantages to controlling plasma at low or room temperature to expand the range of applications, low- or room-temperature plasmas are not ideal for achieving certain processing effects. Kawano et al. investigated the influence of the gas temperature of helium plasma with oxygen on the bactericidal effect of plasma, and reported that it was enhanced by increasing the gas temperature of the plasma [12].

It has also been reported that the selection of the gas species in plasma is important for improving the treatment effect. Different plasma gas species produce different surface treatments and bactericidal effects, which affects the type and number of reactive species produced [13–15]. Yanagawa et al. reported the introduction of proteins into tobacco leaves via plasma treatment with various gas species, such as argon, nitrogen, oxygen, and carbon dioxide. In this process, liquid nitrogen is used to cool the gas temperature of the plasma, to avoid thermal damage to the plant [16]. Thus, the gas species and temperature of the plasma have a significant influence on the plasma treatment effect. Therefore, if the gas species and temperature of the plasma can be arbitrarily controlled, it is expected that the range of applications will expand, and the conditions of plasma treatment can be optimized to maximize the effect.

We have developed a multi-gas temperature-controllable plasma jet that can generate stable plasma with various gas species and control the gas temperature of the plasma. In this system, the plasmas can be generated with argon, helium, nitrogen, oxygen, carbon dioxide, or a mixture of these gases, and the gas temperature can be controlled in the range of 30–90 °C. In this study, the liquid was treated with plasma, and the reactive species generated by each plasma gas species were evaluated. In addition, the effects of plasma gas species and temperature on the bactericidal effects of carbon dioxide and nitrogen plasmas were evaluated.

2. Materials and Methods

2.1. Multi-Gas Temperature-Controllable Plasma Jet

The developed multi-gas, temperature-controllable plasma jet can generate plasma with various gas species, such as carbon dioxide, argon, nitrogen, oxygen, and their mixtures, and the gas temperature of each plasma can be changed in the range of 30–90 °C. The plasma jet has two channels in its metal body: one for the temperature-control fluid, and the other for the plasma gas. The temperature of the metal body can be changed by flowing liquid at any temperature through the temperature-control fluid channel. The plasma gas temperature can be changed through heat exchange with the metal body. In this study, ethylene glycol, or 80 wt.% ethanol, was used as the temperature-control fluid for −30 to 20 °C, and tap water was used as the temperature-control fluid for 20–90 °C. The temperature of the fluid was controlled using a thermostatic bath (NCB-1210B, TOKYO RIKAKIKAI CO, LTD., Tokyo Japan). In the plasma generation section, a voltage of 9 kV and 16 kHz was applied between the two electrodes to generate the plasma. The generated plasma flowed through a hole with a diameter of 1 mm.

2.2. Measurement of the Generated Reactive Species

The concentration of the reactive species in the solution after plasma treatment was measured to determine the influence of the plasma gas species on reactive species' generation. In this experiment, OH radicals, singlet oxygen, ozone, and hydrogen peroxide were measured. The concentrations of OH radicals and singlet oxygen were measured using electron spin resonance (ESR; JES-FA100, JEOL Ltd., Tokyo, Japan). The concentrations of ozone and hydrogen peroxide were measured via a colorimetric method using a pocket ozonometer (DR300, Hach Company, Loveland, CO, USA) and double-beam spectrophotometer (U-2900, Hitachi High-Tech Science Corporation, Tokyo, Japan). An overview of the plasma treatment is shown in Figure 1. Nitrogen, carbon dioxide, oxygen, and argon plasma at 3 L/min (standard) were used. The gas temperature of each plasma was controlled at 30, 45, 60, 75, and 90 °C at a distance of 2 mm from the plasma outlet. Thereafter, 200 μL of the solution was dispensed in a 10.3 mm diameter well, and treated from a height of 16.5 mm above the liquid surface for 15 s.

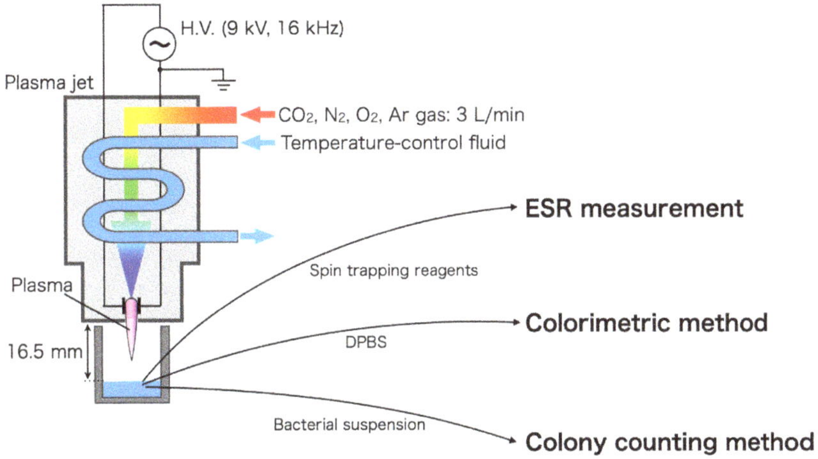

Figure 1. Overview of the plasma treatment.

The spin-trapping reagents for the OH radical and singlet oxygen were 5,5-dimethyl-1-pyrroline-N-oxide (DMPO) [17] and 2,2,5,5-tetramethyl-3-pyrroline-3-carboxamide (TPC) [18]. These reagents were dissolved in Dulbecco's phosphate-buffered saline (DPBS) solution, and the concentrations of DMPO and TPC were fixed at 200 and 75 mM, respectively. Each 150 μL of plasma-treated spin-trapping reagent was measured using ESR within 30 s. The ESR measurement was set to a microwave frequency of 9.425 GHz, modulation frequency of 100 kHz, sweep time of 2 min, magnetic field of 335.5 ± 5 mT, and modulation width of 0.1 mT.

The colorimetric method with ozone reagent (AccuVac® Mid-Range 0–0.75 mg/L, Hach Company, Loveland, CO, USA) was used to measure the ozone. Plasma-treated 120 μL of DPBS was immediately mixed with the ozone reagent, and the ozone concentration was determined using a pocket ozonometer. The hydrogen peroxide was also measured using the colorimetric method based on the reaction of Fe^{3+} with xylenol orange [19]. Fe^{3+} is a product formed by the reaction between Fe^{2+} and hydrogen peroxide. Plasma-treated 120 μL of DPBS and 120 μL of colorimetric reagent (200 μM xylenol orange, 500 μM ammonium ferrous sulfate, 50 mM sulfuric acid, and 200 mM sorbitol) were mixed. After 40 min of mixing, the hydrogen peroxide was quantified by measuring the absorbance at 586 nm.

2.3. *Influence of Plasma Gas Temperature on Bactericidal Effect*

Disinfection using plasma, such as direct treatment and with plasma-activated liquids, has been reported [20,21]. In this study, we treated bacterial suspensions with temperature-controlled plasma, and evaluated their bactericidal effects. *Staphylococcus aureus* ATCC6538, the target of disinfection, was transferred to Luria-Broth agar medium on the day before the experiment, and incubated overnight at 36 °C. The bacterial suspensions were prepared by suspending *Staphylococcus aureus* in the DPBS solution to 10^8 CFU/mL. Carbon dioxide and nitrogen at 3 L/min (standard) were used as the plasma gases. The plasma gas temperature was controlled at 30, 45, 60, 75, and 90 °C, at 2 mm from the plasma outlet. The bacterial suspension (500 μL) was dispensed into a 24-well plate (MS-8024R, Sumitomo Bakelite Co., Ltd., Tokyo, Japan), and the plasma was treated from 16.5 mm above the liquid surface.

Subsequently, 100 μL of the bacterial suspension was collected and diluted, and the number of surviving bacteria was evaluated using the colony counting method. For comparison, the bacterial suspension was treated with carbon dioxide and nitrogen gas at 90 °C, and the number of surviving bacteria was evaluated. In this case, temperature control using a chiller could not achieve 90 °C gas without generating plasma. Therefore, the plasma jet body was directly heated using a ribbon heater, and the gas at 90 °C was generated by adjusting the voltage applied to the heater.

To quantitatively evaluate the bactericidal effect, we used the bactericidal activity (*BA*) value, which can be calculated using Equation (1) [12]:

$$BA = \frac{\log_{10}(N1/N2)}{T2 - T1} \quad (1)$$

The *BA* value indicates the number of bacteria inactivated per minute. It has been shown that plasma disinfection takes time after treatment, until the disinfection effect is achieved [22]. In this study, we evaluated the disinfection effect by calculating the *BA* value from the time when the number of surviving bacteria decreased by more than one log reduction from the initial number to the time just before the number of bacteria decreased below the detection limit. Here, *T1* is the time at the measurement point just before the number of surviving bacteria decreased by more than one digit from the initial number, and *T2* is the time at the measuring point just before the number of surviving bacteria fell below the detection limit. The numbers of surviving bacteria at *T1* and *T2* are denoted as *N1* and *N2*, respectively.

3. Results

3.1. Measurement of Generated Reactive Species

The relationship between the gas temperature of the plasma and the number of reactive species produced for each gas species is shown in Figure 2. The concentration of OH radicals was highest at approximately 130 μM or more in the nitrogen plasma and at 20–40 μM in the carbon dioxide and argon plasmas. The lowest concentration was detected in oxygen plasma at 10 μM or less. In the nitrogen plasma, the concentration of OH radicals increased from 146 to 172 μM with a change in the plasma gas temperature from 30 to 45 °C, showed an insignificant change from 45 to 75 °C, and decreased to 131 μM with a change in temperature from 75 to 90 °C. In the carbon dioxide plasma, the concentration increased from 26 to 39 μM with a change in the plasma gas temperature from 30 to 90 °C. In the argon plasma, the concentration increased from 28 to 34 μM with a change in the plasma gas temperature from 30 to 45 °C. There was almost no change in concentration when the plasma gas temperature increased from 45 to 75 °C, and the concentration decreased to 27 μM with a change in the plasma gas temperature from 75 to 90 °C. In the oxygen plasma, the concentration increased from 5.7 to 10 μM with a change in the plasma gas temperature from 30 to 90 °C.

The concentration of the singlet oxygen was higher in each plasma variant in the order of oxygen, carbon dioxide, nitrogen, and argon when the plasma gas temperature was 30 °C. A significant increase in concentration was observed in the carbon dioxide plasma above 45 °C. The concentration of the singlet oxygen in the carbon dioxide plasma increased from 77 to 459 μM, as the plasma gas temperature changed from 30 to 45 °C. From 45 to 60 °C, there was almost no change in the concentration, and from 60 to 90 °C, there was an increase in the concentration from 435 to 812 μM. In the oxygen plasma, the concentration increased from 96 to 208 μM with a change in the plasma gas temperature from 30 to 90 °C. In the nitrogen plasma, the amount produced increased from 56 to 115 μM with a change in the plasma gas temperature from 30 to 90 °C. In the case of argon plasma, the amount produced increased from 16 to 24 μM with a temperature change from 30 to 75 °C, and decreased to 13 μM at 90 °C.

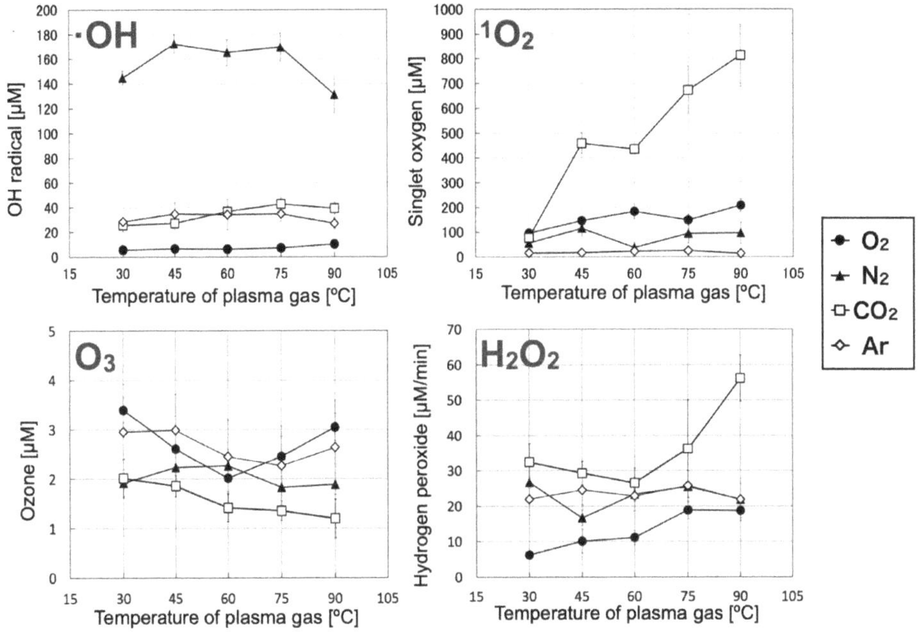

Figure 2. Influence of gas species and gas temperature of plasma on the generation of reactive species.

In the oxygen plasma, the concentration of ozone was 3.4 µM at 30 °C, reached a minimum of 2.0 µM at 60 °C, and increased to 3.1 µM as the temperature increased to 90 °C. In the argon plasma, the concentration decreased slowly between 30 and 75 °C from 3.0 to 2.3 µM, and then increased to 2.6 µM at 90 °C. In the nitrogen plasma, the concentration was not significantly affected by the plasma gas temperature, and was 2.0 ± 0.2 µM between 30 and 90 °C. In the carbon dioxide plasma, the concentration decreased slowly from 2.0 to 1.2 µM with a change in temperature from 30 to 90 °C.

The concentration of hydrogen peroxide was higher in the carbon dioxide plasma, similar to the argon and nitrogen plasmas, and lower in the oxygen plasma. In the carbon dioxide plasma, the concentration decreased from 32 to 26 µM between 30 and 60 °C, and increased significantly to 56 µM as the gas temperature increased to 90 °C. In the nitrogen plasma, the concentration was almost constant between 30 and 90 °C, but decreased to 17 µM only at 45 °C. In the argon plasma, the change in the plasma gas temperature had an insignificant effect on the concentration, which remained constant at 21 µM. In the oxygen plasma, the concentration increased slowly from 6 to 19 µM between 30 and 90 °C.

3.2. *Influence of Plasma Gas Temperature on Bactericidal Effect*

Figure 3 shows the relationship between the gas temperature and bactericidal effects of the carbon dioxide and nitrogen plasmas. At a gas temperature of 30 °C, the carbon dioxide plasma showed a bactericidal effect of more than a 4-log reduction in the number of surviving bacteria in 60 s. At a gas temperature of 45 °C, the carbon dioxide plasma demonstrated a bactericidal effect of more than a 6-log reduction in the number of surviving bacteria in 60 s. At gas temperatures of 60 and 75 °C, the carbon dioxide plasma showed a bactericidal effect of more than a 6-log reduction in the number of surviving bacteria in 15 s. At a gas temperature of 90 °C, the carbon dioxide plasma showed a bactericidal effect of more than a 6-log reduction in the number of surviving bacteria in 10 s. The increase in the gas temperature of the plasma significantly increased its bactericidal effect. In the case of the carbon dioxide gas treatment at 90 °C, the number of surviving bacteria did not decrease by 1-log even after 60 s of treatment. The maximum bactericidal effect of the nitrogen plasma was only approximately a 1-log reduction after 60 s of treatment, showing a significant difference from the bactericidal effect of the carbon dioxide plasma. No difference in its bactericidal effect was observed when the plasma gas temperature was varied from 30 to 75 °C. In the case of the nitrogen gas treatment at 90 °C, the number of surviving bacteria did not decrease by 1-log even after 60 s of treatment.

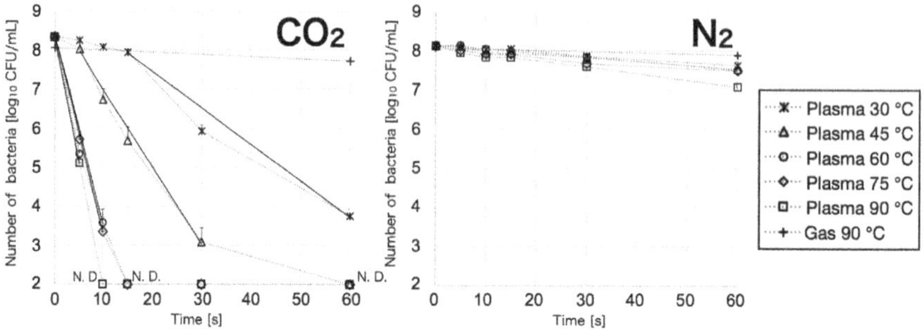

Figure 3. Relationship between the gas temperature and bactericidal effect of carbon dioxide and nitrogen plasma. In the left graph of the carbon dioxide treatment result, the solid black line shows the result used to calculate the *BA* value. The slope represents the *BA* value.

The *BA* values that were calculated for the carbon dioxide plasma showed a significant bactericidal effect. The results are shown in Table 1. The *BA* value in the carbon dioxide plasma treatment increased with an increase in the plasma gas temperature. In the case of the plasma treatment at 90 °C, the *BA* value increased by approximately seven times, compared to that at 30 °C.

Table 1. Relationship between the plasma gas temperature and *BA* value.

Plasma Temp. (°C)	30	45	60	75	90
BA value (min^{-1})	5.6	11.9	28.6	29.9	38.8

3.3. Relationship between Bactericidal Effect and Reactive Species in Carbon Dioxide Plasma

The correlation coefficients between the bactericidal effect and number of reactive species produced in the carbon dioxide plasma were calculated. Figure 4 shows the relationship between the bactericidal effect and the number of reactive species produced. Table 2 shows the correlation coefficients for the bactericidal effects and reactive species. The amount of OH radicals produced was strongly and positively correlated with the bactericidal effect, with a correlation coefficient (R) of 0.914. The singlet oxygen production showed a strong positive correlation with the bactericidal effect, with an R value of 0.885. The amount of ozone produced had a strong negative correlation with the bactericidal effect, with an R value of −0.997. The amount of hydrogen peroxide produced was positively correlated with the bactericidal effect, with an R value of 0.623.

Table 2. Correlation coefficient value (R) of *BA* values and reactive species.

	Correlation Coefficient Value, R			
	OH Radical	**Singlet Oxygen**	**Ozone**	**Hydrogen Peroxide**
BA value	0.914	0.885	−0.997	0.623

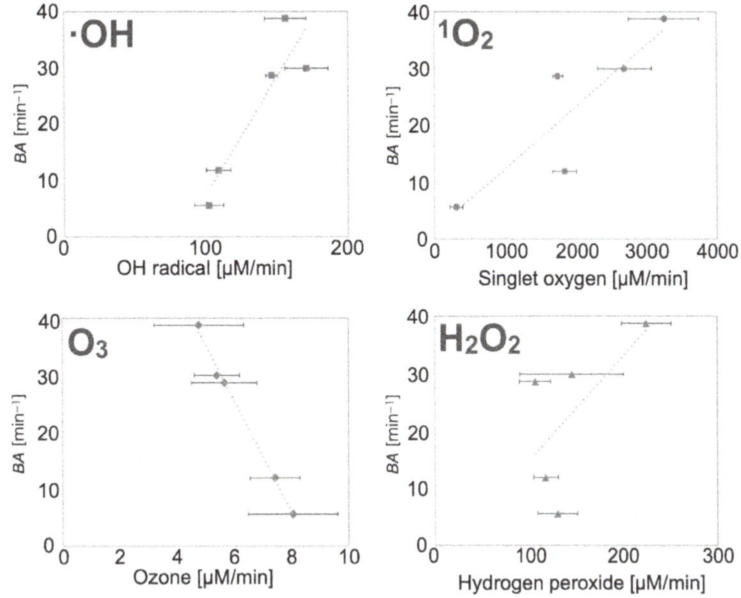

Figure 4. Correlation between bactericidal effect and reactive species in carbon dioxide plasma.

4. Discussion

As shown in Figure 2, the reactive species produced by the plasma were affected by varying the gas species and temperature. The OH radicals are produced largely from the nitrogen plasma. In the nitrogen plasma generated in the atmosphere, spectroscopic measurements have indicated the existence of nitrogen atoms [13]. The metastable atomic states of nitrogen $2^2D_{5/2}$, argon 4^3P_2, and oxygen 2^1D_2 have lifetimes of 6.1×10^4 s [23], 56 s [24], and 1.0×10^2 s [23], respectively. It is thought that metastable nitrogen, which has a longer lifetime than other metastable atoms, remained active and contacted water or water droplets in the air, producing OH radicals at the gas–liquid interface [25]. In a previous study, we reported that more OH radicals were produced from nitrogen plasmas than from any other gas species [15]. Singlet oxygen was produced more in the higher-temperature carbon dioxide plasma than in the oxygen plasma. This may be because, in the oxygen plasma, the atomic oxygen that produces singlet oxygen reacts with the ambient triplet oxygen, which is abundant, and quickly turns into ozone [26]. In fact, the amount of ozone produced by the oxygen plasma was higher than that produced by the carbon dioxide plasma.

In the oxygen and carbon dioxide plasmas, the production of OH radicals, singlet oxygen, and hydrogen peroxide tended to increase as the gas temperature increased. This is similar to the report by Kawano et al. on the increase in the production of the same reactive species when the gas temperature of the helium–oxygen mixture is increased [12]. In other words, the above-mentioned reactive species are considered to increase with increasing temperature in gas species that contain oxygen elements.

There was a significant difference in the bactericidal effect of the nitrogen and carbon dioxide plasmas, as shown in Figure 3, depending on the gas species. The nitrogen plasma showed only a weak bactericidal effect of less than 1-log reduction after 60 s of treatment. These results were different from our previous results, which confirmed the high bactericidal effect of nitrogen gas [14]. In the formation of reactive species in the nitrogen plasma, mixing with air is important because the gas does not contain oxygen. Therefore, it is considered that the difference in treatment conditions, such as gas flow rate and treatment distance, had a considerable influence. In contrast, the carbon dioxide plasma at 90 °C showed a high bactericidal effect of 6-log reduction after 10 s of treatment. In the treatment with the carbon dioxide gas at 90 °C, the number of surviving bacteria did not decrease by 1-log even after 60 s of treatment. Therefore, these results indicate that the improvement in the bactericidal effect is not due to the gas temperature, but due to the introduction of reactive species generated by the plasma. In the carbon dioxide plasma, the production of reactive species, such as singlet oxygen and OH radicals, changed significantly as the plasma gas temperature increased, suggesting that these reactive species contribute to the bactericidal effect.

As shown in Table 2, the bactericidal effect of the carbon dioxide plasma exhibited a strong negative correlation with the ozone and a strong positive correlation with the OH radicals and singlet oxygen. Ozone is also used for disinfection, and Lezcano et al. reported 90% disinfection of *Escherichia coli* by 0.94 mg/L (19.6 μM) of ozone in 0.41 min [27]. In our study, the highest ozone concentration in the carbon dioxide plasma was 2.0 μM, which is an insufficient concentration for disinfection. If the OH radical is assumed to be the reactive species contributing to its bactericidal effect, the observation is inconsistent with the fact that no bactericidal effect was observed in the nitrogen plasma. In our previous study, we investigated the bactericidal factor in the plasma treatment of carbon dioxide using a radical scavenger [14]. This study also suggested the contribution of singlet oxygen to the bactericidal effect, which is consistent with the results of the present study. These results suggest that the bactericidal effect of the carbon dioxide plasma is mainly due to the singlet oxygen. The bactericidal effect was improved by increasing the temperature, because the amount of singlet oxygen produced by the plasma increased with an increase in temperature, and the amount of singlet oxygen that contributed to the bactericidal effect in the liquid increased. However, in the disinfection of atmospheric low-temperature plasma, it has been reported that there are complex effects of reactive species, UV, and charged particles on microorganisms [28]; thus, singlet oxygen is not the only factor contributing to the bactericidal effect. In the future, other bactericidal factors should be investigated, such as reactive nitrogen species and UV, to clarify their contribution to the bactericidal effect.

5. Conclusions

In this study, plasma gas species and temperature were varied to evaluate the reactive species produced and the bactericidal effect of plasma. The reactive species produced by the plasma vary greatly depending on the gas species. It was found that a considerable amount of OH radicals were produced in the nitrogen plasma. Varying the plasma gas temperature resulted in a change in the concentration of the generated reactive species. In carbon dioxide plasma, the amount of singlet oxygen produced increased significantly with increasing temperature, and the amount of singlet oxygen produced was more than eight times greater at 90 than at 30 °C. The bactericidal effects of nitrogen and carbon dioxide plasmas on *Staphylococcus aureus* in liquids were compared. The bactericidal effect of nitrogen plasma was not significantly affected by the temperature of the plasma gas. In the case of carbon dioxide plasma, the bactericidal effect was significantly improved by increasing the plasma gas temperature. The contribution of the singlet oxygen to the bactericidal effect of carbon dioxide was expected, based on the results of the bactericidal effect and reactive species produced.

It was also found that the effectiveness of the disinfection process could be improved by properly selecting the plasma gas species and temperature. This result can be attributed to the changes in the type and number of reactive species. Therefore, it is expected that the treatment effect can be improved by changing the plasma gas species and temperature in treatments other than disinfection, such as hemostasis, treatment of plants, and surface treatment. In the case of plasma treatment in air, mixing with ambient air is considered to have a significant effect on the generation of reactive species. To realize a more stable treatment, it is necessary to control the air mixing or to construct a treatment method that does not depend on air. To effectively control plasma gas species and temperature, it is necessary to understand the reactive species that contribute to the effect, and to study the conditions according to the purpose of each treatment. In the future, we will study other plasma applications, such as hemostasis and surface treatments, to improve the treatment effect and clarify the effect mechanism using changes in the plasma gas species and temperature.

Author Contributions: Conceptualization, S.M., T.T. and A.O.; methodology, Y.S., T.A., S.M., Y.M. and A.I.; validation, Y.S. and T.A.; formal analysis, Y.S.; investigation, Y.S., S.M., T.A., T.T. and Y.M.; resources, S.M., Y.M. and A.I.; data curation, Y.S., S.M., T.T. and Y.M.; writing—original draft preparation, Y.S.; writing—review and editing, S.M., T.T., Y.M., A.I. and A.O.; visualization, Y.S. and T.A.; supervision, T.T. and Y.M.; project administration, Y.M., A.I. and A.O.; funding acquisition, A.I. and A.O. All authors have read and agreed to the published version of the manuscript.

Funding: This study was supported by JSPS KAKENHI (Grant Number: 20K07039) and the Cooperative Research Project of the Research Center for Biomedical Engineering, National Cancer Center Research and Development Fund (Grant Number: 31-A-11), TERUMO LIFE SCIENCE FOUNDATION (Grant Number: 18-II106).

Institutional Review Board Statement: Not applicable.

Informed Consent Statement: Not applicable.

Data Availability Statement: The data that support the findings of this study are available from the corresponding author, T.T., upon reasonable request.

Acknowledgments: The authors would like to thank Ikuo Nakanishi at Quantum RedOx Chemistry Group, Institute for Quantum Life Science, Quantum Life and Medical Science Directorate, National Institutes for Quantum Science and Technology, for providing the measurement equipment for the electron spin resonance method. The authors would like to thank Norihiko Yamamoto at the Design and Manufacturing Division, Open Facility Center, Tokyo Institute of Technology, for preparing the plasma jet parts.

Conflicts of Interest: The authors declare no conflict of interest.

References

1. Taylor, H.E. *Inductively Coupled Plasma-Mass Spectrometry: Practices and Techniques*; Academic Press: Cambridge, MA, USA, 2000; pp. 1–5.
2. Kortshagen, U. Nonthermal plasma synthesis of semiconductor nanocrystals. *J. Phys. D Appl. Phys.* **2009**, *42*, 113001. [CrossRef]
3. Maisch, T.; Shimizu, T.; Li, Y.F.; Heinlin, J.; Karrer, S.; Morfill, G.; Zimmermann, J.L. Decolonisation of MRSA, *S. Aureus* and *E. Coli* by cold-atmospheric plasma using a porcine skin model in vitro. *PLoS ONE* **2012**, *7*, e34610. [CrossRef] [PubMed]
4. Nomura, Y.; Takamatsu, T.; Kawano, H.; Miyahara, H.; Okino, A.; Masaru, Y.; Takeshi, A. Investigation of blood coagulation effect of nonthermal multigas plasma jet in vitro and in vivo. *J. Surg. Res.* **2017**, *219*, 302–309. [CrossRef] [PubMed]
5. Shimatani, A.; Toyoda, H.; Orita, K.; Hirakawa, Y.; Aoki, K.; Oh, J.; Shirafuji, T.; Nakamura, H. In vivo study on the healing of bone defect treated with non-thermal atmospheric pressure gas discharge plasma. *PLoS ONE* **2021**, *16*, e0255861. [CrossRef] [PubMed]
6. Aida, M.; Iwai, T.; Okamoto, Y.; Miyahara, H.; Seto, Y.; Okino, A. Development of an ionization method using hydrogenated plasma for mass analysis of surface. *J. Anal. At. Spectrom.* **2018**, *33*, 578–584. [CrossRef]
7. Iwai, T.; Kakegawa, K.; Aida, M.; Nagashima, H.; Nagoya, T.; Kanamori-kataoka, M.; Miyahara, H.; Seto, Y.; Okino, A. Development of a gas-cylinder-free plasma desorption/ionization system for on-site detection of chemical warfare agents. *Anal. Chem.* **2015**, *87*, 5707–5715. [CrossRef]
8. Van Deynse, A.; Cools, P.; Leys, C.; De Geyter, N.; Morent, R. Surface activation of polyethylene with an argon atmospheric pressure plasma jet: Influence of applied power and flow rate. *Appl. Surf. Sci.* **2015**, *328*, 269–278. [CrossRef]
9. Yoshimura, S.; Aramaki, M.; Otsubo, Y.; Yamashita, A.; Koga, K. Controlling feeding gas temperature of plasma jet with Peltier device for experiments with fission yeast. *Jpn. J. Appl. Phys.* **2019**, *58*, SEEG03. [CrossRef]
10. Ishihara, D.; Noma, Y.; Stauss, S.; Sai, M.; Tomai, T.; Terashima, K. Development of a dielectric barrier discharge (DBD) cryo-microplasma. *Plasma Sources Sci. Technol. Dev.* **2008**, *17*, 035008. [CrossRef]
11. Oshita, T.; Kawano, H.; Takamatsu, T.; Miyahara, H.; Okino, A. Temperature controllable atmospheric plasma source. *IEEE Trans. Plasma Sci.* **2015**, *43*, 1987–1992. [CrossRef]
12. Kawano, H.; Takamatsu, T.; Matsumura, Y.; Miyahara, H.; Iwasawa, A.; Okino, A. Influence of gas temperature in atmospheric non-equilibrium plasma on bactericidal effect. *Biocontrol Sci.* **2018**, *23*, 167–175. [CrossRef] [PubMed]
13. Takamatsu, T.; Hirai, H.; Sasaki, R.; Miyahara, H.; Okino, A. Surface hydrophilization of polyimide films using atmospheric damage-free multigas plasma jet source. *Kagaku Kogaku Ronbunshu* **2013**, *39*, 372–377. [CrossRef]

14. Takamatsu, T.; Uehara, K.; Sasaki, Y.; Hidekazu, M.; Matsumura, Y.; Iwasawa, A.; Ito, N.; Kohno, M.; Azuma, T.; Okino, A. Microbial inactivation in the liquid phase induced by multigas plasma jet. *PLoS ONE* **2015**, *10*, e0132381. [CrossRef]
15. Takamatsu, T.; Uehara, K.; Sasaki, Y.; Miyahara, H.; Matsumura, Y.; Iwasawa, A.; Ito, N.; Azuma, T.; Kohno, M.; Okino, A. Investigation of reactive species using various gas plasmas. *RSC Adv.* **2014**, *4*, 39901–39905. [CrossRef]
16. Yanagawa, Y.; Kawano, H.; Kobayashi, T.; Miyahara, H.; Okino, A.; Mitsuhara, I. Direct protein introduction into plant cells using a multi-gas plasma jet. *PLoS ONE* **2017**, *12*, e0171942. [CrossRef] [PubMed]
17. Kohno, M.; Yamada, M.; Mitsuta, K.; Mizuta, Y.; Yoshikawa, T. Spin-trapping studies on the reaction of iron complexes with peroxides and the effects of water-soluble antioxidants. *Bull. Chem. Soc. Jpn.* **1991**, *64*, 1447–1453. [CrossRef]
18. Matsumura, Y.; Iwasawa, A.; Kobayashi, T.; Kamachi, T.; Ozawa, T.; Kohno, M. Detection of high-frequency ultrasound-induced singlet oxygen by the ESR spin-trapping method. *Chem. Lett.* **2013**, *42*, 1291–1293. [CrossRef]
19. Ikai, H.; Nakamura, K.; Kanno, T.; Shirato, M.; Meirelles, L.; Sasaki, K.; Niwano, Y. Synergistic effect of proanthocyanidin on the bactericidal action of the photolysis of H_2O_2. *Biocontrol Sci.* **2013**, *18*, 137–141. [CrossRef] [PubMed]
20. Abonti, T.R.; Kaku, M.; Kojima, S.; Sumi, H.; Kojima, S.; Yamamoto, T.; Yashima, Y.; Miyahara, H.; Okino, A.; Kawata, T.; et al. Irradiation effects of low temperature multi gas plasma jet on oral bacteria. *Dent. Mater. J.* **2016**, *35*, 822–828. [CrossRef]
21. Pan, J.; Li, Y.L.; Liu, C.M.; Tian, Y.; Yu, S.; Wang, K.L.; Zhang, J.; Fang, J. Investigation of cold atmospheric plasma-activated water for the dental unit waterline system contamination and safety evaluation in vitro. *Plasma Chem. Plasma Process.* **2017**, *37*, 1091–1103. [CrossRef]
22. Lee, M.H.; Park, B.J.; Jin, S.C.; Kim, D.; Han, I.; Kim, J.; Hyun, S.O.; Chung, K.H.; Park, J.C. Removal and sterilization of biofilms and planktonic bacteria by microwave-induced argon plasma at atmospheric pressure. *New J. Phys.* **2009**, *11*, 115022. [CrossRef]
23. Smirnov, B.M. Excited Atoms. In *Physics of Atoms and Ions*, 1st ed.; Springer: New York, NY, USA, 2003; p. 148.
24. Small-Warren, N.E.; Chiu, L.-Y.C. Lifetime of the metastable $3P_2$ anti $^3P_0$ states of rare-gas atoms. *Phys. Rev. A* **1975**, *11*, 1777–1783. [CrossRef]
25. Herron, J.T.; Green, D.S. Chemical kinetics database and predictive schemes for nonthermal humid air plasma chemistry. Part II. Neutral species reactions. *Plasma Chem. Plasma Process.* **2001**, *21*, 459–481. [CrossRef]
26. Laroussi, M.; Leipold, F. Evaluation of the roles of reactive species, heat, and UV radiation in the inactivation of bacterial cells by air plasmas at atmospheric pressure. *Int. J. Mass Spectrom.* **2004**, *233*, 81–86. [CrossRef]
27. Lezcano, I.; Rey, R.P.; Baluja, C.; Sánchez, E. Ozone inactivation of Pseudomonas Aeruginosa, Escherichia Coli, Shigella Sonnei and Salmonella Typhimurium in water. *Ozone Sci. Eng.* **1999**, *12*, 293–300. [CrossRef]
28. Guo, J.; Huang, K.; Wang, J. Bactericidal effect of various non-thermal plasma agents and the influence of experimental conditions in microbial inactivation: A review. *Food Control* **2015**, *50*, 482–490. [CrossRef]

applied sciences

MDPI

Article

Modelling of a Non-Transferred Plasma Torch Used for Nano-Silica Powders Production

Ibrahim A. AlShunaifi [1], Samira Elaissi [2], Imed Ghiloufi [3,4,*], Seham S. Alterary [5] and Ahmed A. Alharbi [1]

1 Energy and Water Research Institute, King Abdulaziz City for Science and Technology (KACST), Riyadh 11442, Saudi Arabia; ialshunaifi@kacst.edu.sa (I.A.A.); ahalharbi@kacst.edu.sa (A.A.A.)
2 Department of Physics, College of Sciences, Princess Nourah Bint Abdulrahman University, Riyadh 11671, Saudi Arabia; samira_aissi@yahoo.fr
3 Department of Physics, College of Sciences, Imam Mohammad Ibn Saud Islamic University (IMSIU), Riyadh 11623, Saudi Arabia
4 Laboratory of Physics of Materials and Nanomaterials Applied at Environment (LaPhyMNE), Faculty of Sciences in Gabes, Gabes University, Gabes 6072, Tunisia
5 Chemistry Department, College of Science, King Saud University, Riyadh 11451, Saudi Arabia; salterary@ksu.edu.sa
* Correspondence: ghiloufimed@yahoo.fr

Abstract: In this study, a two-dimensional numerical model was developed to simulate operation conditions in the non-transferred plasma torch, used to synthesis nanosilica powder. The turbulent magnetohydrodynamic model was presented to predict the nitrogen plasma flow and heat transfer characteristics inside and outside the plasma torch. The continuity, momentum, energy, current continuity equations, and the turbulence model were expressed in cylindrical coordinates and numerically solved by COMSOL Multiphysics software with a finite element method. The operation conditions of the mass flow rate of ionized gas ranging from 78 sccm to 240 sccm and the current varying between 50 A to 200 A were systematically analyzed. The variation in the electrothermal efficiency with the gas flow rate, the plasma current, and the enthalpy was also reported. The results revealed that the increase in working current lead to a raise in the effective electric power and then an increase in the distribution of plasma velocity and temperature. The efficiency of the torch was found to be between 36% and 75%. The plasma jet exited the nozzle torch with a larger fast and hot core diameter with increasing current. The numerical results showed good correlation and good trends with the experimental measurement. This study allowed us to obtain more efficient control of the process conditions and a better optimization of this process in terms of the production rate and primary particle size. X-ray diffraction (XRD) and transmission electron microscopy (TEM) were used to characterize the primary nanosilica powder that was experimentally collected. The arc plasma method enabled us to produce a spherical silicon ultra-fine powder of about 20 nm in diameter.

Keywords: plasma torch; nano silica; numerical simulation; experimental measurement

Citation: AlShunaifi, I.A.; Elaissi, S.; Ghiloufi, I.; Alterary, S.S.; Alharbi, A.A. Modelling of a Non-Transferred Plasma Torch Used for Nano-Silica Powders Production. *Appl. Sci.* **2021**, *11*, 9842. https://doi.org/10.3390/app11219842

Academic Editor: Bogdan-George Rusu

Received: 19 September 2021
Accepted: 11 October 2021
Published: 21 October 2021

1. Introduction

Plasma technology has in the last years evolved to be a promising technique for the efficient manufacture of nano-sized materials, which are in increasing demand by recent technological advancement for diverse applications such as industrial, biomedical, and environmental purification processes [1–7]. For example, Ananth and Mok [8] revealed that the nanomaterials prepared by atmospheric plasma exhibit high crystallinity and good thermal resistivity. Additionally, Post et al. [9] describe that the plasma-manufactured nanoparticles are the best technique to obtain homogenized coating on metal nanoparticles and to control their outer surface properties. Another important aspect of plasma-based nanomaterials is the possibility to adjust the thermal efficiency of the solar cells and the use of atmospheric pressure plasma in order to generate silver and gold nanoparticles on tin oxide solar cells [10]. By virtue of these characteristics, plasma nanofabrication has grown into an interesting new field, which exhibits many advantages for the synthesis of nanoparticles and the deposition of nanostructured films and coatings, in a more cost-effective and ecologically friendly manner.

The present invention has attracted intense and increasing industrial interest as a novel mass-production method, using a variety of thermal plasma sources, such as alternating current at radiofrequency (RF plasma) and direct current (DC plasma), which can be operated in transferred and non-transferred arc-modes. Nano-metal powders have been broadly generated by transferred DC plasma torches [11,12]. However, in this kind of plasma torch the manufacturing process often becomes non-continuous because target metals, used as electrodes, should be replaced after each batch of metal nano-powder by reason of their non-resistance to the elevated temperature generated in the plasma torch. Alternative technologies, non-transferred DC, or RF plasma torches have been used to offer a continuous production system of nano-sized powders.

In non-transferred DC plasma torches, the electrodes are exclusively utilized for maintaining the arc plasma formation, and the targeted materials are introduced into the flame of thermal plasma as a precursor powder [13,14]. In comparison with RF plasma jets [15,16], there are multiple advantages of using non-transferred DC plasma torches in nanomanufacturing. The DC plasma torch has a narrow diameter that confines the plasma jet, resulting in an increase in the temperature and the velocity of the plasma flow at the torch axis. In addition, DC plasma jets are commonly turbulent, which reinforces mixing of the precursors injected. Generally, a DC plasma torch can attain 90% thermal efficiency, while RF plasma only attains 75% [17,18].

To synthesize nanosilica particles, a non-transferred arc system is run on nitrogen plasma gas, followed by a short mixing section of silicon tetrachloride ($SiCl4$) and carrier mixing gas (nitrogen and hydrogen) heated to about 1373.15 K and injected in the plasma tail flame.

The process starts with vaporization of precursor materials owing to the high enthalpy of the plasma, and then the temperature of the material vapor transported by the nitrogen tail flame decreases drastically; the vapor is highly supersaturated due to this quenching, which results in a rapid production of numerous nanoparticles via homogeneous nucleation, heterogeneous condensation, and coagulation between nanoparticles themselves.

Nowadays, the manufacturing processes of nanoparticles by a thermal plasma process is experimentally achieved. However, the understanding of the growth mechanism of the nanoparticles and the control of the size and the composition of the particle remains insufficient. In most cases, it is impossible to measure different aspects of the process, and only the characteristics of the final products are evaluated because there is a complex interaction between the thermo-fluid field, the induced electromagnetic field, and the particle concentration field [19].

Numerical modelling can be a powerful approach, allowing a better understanding of the growth mechanism of nanoparticles and improving torch designs and plasma processes at relatively low prices. Several research efforts have been dedicated to modelling the plasma flow and heat transfer coupled with the electromagnetic field inside and outside the plasma torch. Simulation of the arc inside a DC torch was first developed by Li and Chen [20] and Trelles [21]. In these models, the arc breakdown and reattachment operations in the plasma torch are accurately evaluated. A transient simulation of a DC plasma torch has been performed later by Selvan [22] to evaluate the substrate temperature with heating time and to estimate different precursor effects on the thermal flux to the substrate. Subsequently, Guo [23] and Modirkhazeni [24] employed new models with the large eddy simulation technique to simulate the turbulent plasma flow inside a DC non-transferred arc plasma torch and the effect of particle injection. For nanopowder production, the nanoparticles are generated not in the high-temperature plasma core but in the interfacial regions between the plasma and the cold gas at low to intermediate temperature. Lower-temperature regions tend to be more turbulent with multiscale eddies. These eddies strongly affect the transport processes of nanoparticles.

Moreover, a combined plasma torch including a plasma jet of the DC arc plasma torch fed to the inlet of the RF-ICP plasma torch and used for nano-powder production has been presented by Frolov [25] in order to reduce the power of the RF discharge in the plasma torch. Recently, a numerical model applied to a triple DC plasma torch used to synthesize nanoparticles was performed by Kim [26]. The results of the simulation presented an analysis of the thermal environment inside the reactor to control the condensation process of the nanoparticles.

In the present study, a two-dimensional axisymmetric turbulent model of a DC non-transferred plasma torch used for the synthesis of nano-silica was developed. Moreover, the effect of different plasma parameters such as the current and the gas flow rate were investigated, and discussion about the efficiency of the torch for different cases was realized. Furthermore, in this work, a DC non-transferred plasma torch was used to synthesis silica nanoparticles. In this study, the principal objective was the optimization of the circumstances of this process in terms of the production rate and the primary particle size. Numerical results were compared with the experimental measurements.

2. Numerical Model

2.1. Basic Assumptions

To simulate the heat transfer and the gas flow of the plasma, the following assumptions were used:

- The plasma is optically thin (when the optical depth approaches to zero, radiation has a small effect on the overall heat transfer process within the plasma, and the opacity can be neglected).
- Turbulence thermal plasma flow is considered (turbulence offers a strong mixing of plasma flow, and its eddies affects the transport processes of nanoparticles).
- The flow is treated as being weakly compressible when the Mach number (the ratio of the speed of the flow to the speed of sound) is smaller than 0.3 (Ma < 0.3), and the density change due to velocity is about 5% in that case.
- High collision frequencies among constituents in thermal plasma leads to a state close to local thermodynamic equilibrium (LTE), in which all plasma components (electrons, ions, and neutrons) have the same temperature.
- The gravity effects are negligible due to a high Froude number ($\approx 3 \times 10^6$).
- The arc is assumed to be steady and rotationally symmetric.
- Thermodynamic and transport properties of gas plasma expressed as a function of the local temperature and pressure are obtained from the literature provided by Boulos et al. study [27].

2.2. Control Equations

Based on the model assumptions cited above, the conservation equations of mass, momentum, and energy, as well as the electric potential and magnetic vector potential, are given by the following equations, respectively:

$$\nabla \cdot \left(\rho \vec{u}\right) = 0 \tag{1}$$

$$\nabla \cdot \left(\rho \vec{u}\vec{u}\right) = -\nabla P + \nabla \cdot \left(\overline{\overline{\tau}}\right) + \vec{J} \times \vec{B} \tag{2}$$

$$\nabla \cdot \left(\rho h \vec{u}\right) = \nabla \left(\frac{\lambda}{c_p} \nabla h\right) + \vec{J} \cdot \vec{E} - 4\pi\varepsilon_r \tag{3}$$

$$\nabla \cdot \vec{J} = \nabla \cdot (\sigma(-\nabla \cdot \varnothing)) = 0 \tag{4}$$

$$\nabla^2 \cdot \vec{A} = -\mu_0 \cdot \vec{J} \tag{5}$$

where $\vec{u}$, ∇P, $\bar{\bar{\tau}}$, $\vec{J}$, $\vec{B}$, $\vec{E}$, h, $\varnothing$ and $\vec{A}$ are the gas velocity, pressure work, stress tensor, current density, magnetic field, electric field, plasma enthalpy, electric potential, and magnetic vector potential, respectively. The terms ρ, λ, c_p, σ, μ_0 and ε_r are the gas density, thermal conductivity, specific heat, electric conductivity, permeability of free space, and the effective net emission coefficient, respectively, whereas $\left(\vec{J} \times \vec{B}\right)$, $\left(\vec{J} \cdot \vec{E}\right)$, and $4\pi\varepsilon_r$ are the electromagnetic force (Lorentz force), the Joule heating, and the volumetric radiation loss, respectively.

The stress tensor can be written as:

$$\bar{\bar{\tau}} = \mu\left[\left(\nabla\vec{u} + \nabla\vec{u}^{T}\right) - \frac{2}{3}\nabla\cdot\vec{u}\delta\right] \tag{6}$$

where μ is the dynamic viscosity, the superscript "T" indicates the transpose of matrix $\vec{u}$, and δ is the unit tensor.

To obtain the electromagnetic field within the plasma torch, it is necessary to combine Equations (4) and (5) with the following equations:

$$\vec{E} = -\nabla\varnothing \tag{7}$$

$$\vec{J} = \sigma\vec{E} \tag{8}$$

$$\vec{B} = \vec{\nabla} \times \vec{A} \tag{9}$$

The use of turbulence models in thermal plasma flows simulation is significantly requested due to their inherent characteristics (reactivity, large variation, and the electromagnetic effect). Hence, the standard $(K - \varepsilon)$ turbulence model developed by Launder and Splalding [28] was implemented in our model, where K stands for the turbulent kinetic energy, and ε is the turbulent kinetic energy dissipation rate.

$$\nabla\cdot\left(\rho K\vec{u}\right) = \nabla\cdot\left[\left(\mu + \frac{\mu_t}{\sigma_K}\right)\cdot\nabla K\right] + G_K - \rho\varepsilon + Y_M \tag{10}$$

$$\nabla\cdot\left(\rho\varepsilon\vec{u}\right) = \nabla\cdot\left[\left(\mu + \frac{\mu_t}{\sigma_\varepsilon}\right)\cdot\nabla\varepsilon\right] + \frac{\varepsilon}{K}\left(C_{1\varepsilon}G_K - C_{2\varepsilon}\rho\varepsilon\right) \tag{11}$$

Y_M represents the contribution of fluctuating dilatation. The turbulent viscosity μ_t, and the turbulent generation term G_K are defined as:

$$\mu_t = \rho C_\mu\left(\frac{K^2}{\varepsilon}\right) \tag{12}$$

$$G_K = \mu_t\left(\frac{\partial u_i}{\partial x_j} + \frac{\partial u_j}{\partial x_i}\right) \tag{13}$$

where $\frac{\partial u_i}{\partial x_j}$ is the production of turbulence kinetic energy. The turbulent model constants $C_{1\varepsilon}$, $C_{2\varepsilon}$, C_μ, σ_K, and σ_ε were identified as 1.44, 1.92, 0.09, 1.0, and 1.3, respectively.

2.3. Calculation Domain and Boundary Conditions

The geometry of the DC plasma torch consists typically of a tungsten tip rod-type cathode and a copper anode. The nitrogen gas was input through a nozzle with a diameter of 8.2 mm on either side of the cathode. The length of the anode nozzle channel and the exit diameter were 225 mm and 17.2 mm, respectively (Figure 1). The nozzle at the end of the torch was used to spread out the heated gas in the form of a plasma jet.

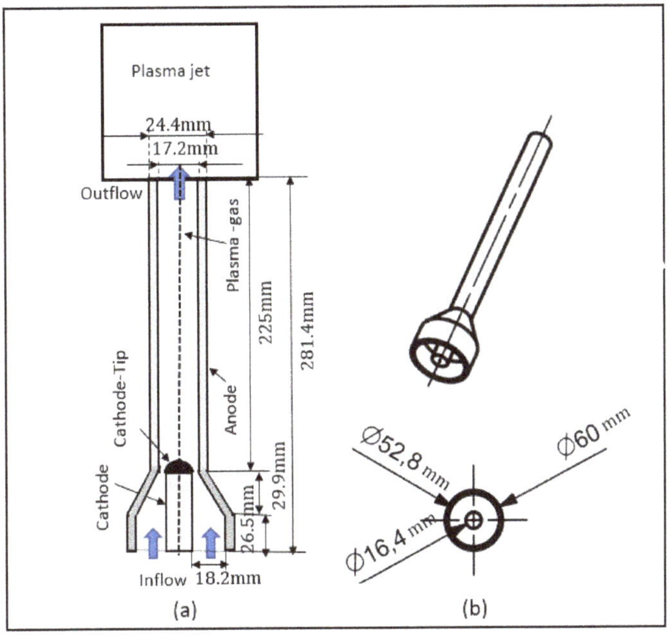

Figure 1. (**a**) The geometry of the plasma torch. (**b**) Revolution of the 3D geometry of the torch. All dimensions are in mm.

The axisymmetric boundary conditions performed in this study are mentioned in Table 1. Inflow boundary conditions are typically specified by imposing values of known properties of the gas injection, typically velocity and temperature. At the torch inlet, the gas was injected at 300 K, with a uniform axial (u_{zin}) and zero radial velocity component (u_{rin}). A swirl flow was required to enhance gas mixing, and an inflow tangential velocity component $(u_{\theta in})$ was introduced. In addition, the turbulent inlet parameter of the kinetic turbulent energy, $(K = 0.005 \times u_{in}^2)$, and its rate of dissipation $(\varepsilon = 0.1 \times K^2)$ were considered. The inflow mass flow rate of the plasma gas can be obtained by integrating the axial velocity at the surface of the torch inlet, namely:

$$Q_{in} = \int_{S_{inlet}} u_{zin}\, ds = u_{zin} S_{inlet} \vec{z} \tag{14}$$

where S_{inlet} is the inlet surface and $\vec{z}$ is the unit vector along the torch axis.

Table 1. Boundary conditions of the numerical model.

Boundary	P	$\vec{u}$	T	$\varnothing$	$\vec{A}$
Inlet	$P = P_{in}$	u_{in}	$T_{in} = 300$ K	$\partial_n \varnothing = 0$	$\partial_n \vec{A} = 0$
Cathode	$\partial_n P = 0$	$\vec{u} = 0$	$T = T_{cath}(r)$	$-\rho \partial_n \varnothing = J_{cath}(r)$	$\partial_n \vec{A} = 0$
Anode	$\partial_n P = 0$	$\vec{u} = 0$	$-k\partial_n T = h_w(T - T_w)$	$\varnothing = 0$	$\partial_n \vec{A} = 0$
Torch wall	$\partial_n P = 0$	$\vec{u} = 0$	$\partial_n T = 0$	$\partial_n \varnothing = 0$	$\partial_n \vec{A} = 0$
Outlet	$P = P_{out}$	$\partial_n \vec{u} = 0$	$\partial_n T = 0$	$\partial_n \varnothing = 0$	$\vec{A} = 0$

The temperature and the current density implemented on the cathode surface of the torch can be estimated by Gaussian profiles:

$$T_{cath}(r) = 500 + 3000\exp\left[-\left(\frac{r}{2R_{cath}}\right)^{n_{cath}}\right] \quad (15)$$

$$J_{cath}(r) = J_{max}\exp\left[-\left(\frac{r}{R_{cath}}\right)^{n_{cath}}\right] \quad (16)$$

where r is the radial distance from the torch axis, and n_{cath}, J_{max}, and R_{cath} are parameters that satisfy the distribution of the working current and temperature profiles over the cathode surface. The values of shape parameters for three cases are given in Table 2.

Table 2. Parameters of current density profiles.

Current (A)	J_{max} (A/m^2)	n_{cath}	R_{cath} (m)
100	0.17×10^7	4	8.2×10^{-3}
150	0.26×10^7	4	8.6×10^{-3}
200	0.35×10^7	4	8.9×10^{-3}

In non-transferred arc torches, an overall convective heat transfer is used for the modelling of heat transfer of the regions of the anode far from arc attachment, namely:

$$-k\partial_n T = h_w(T - T_w) \quad (17)$$

The term ($\partial_n \equiv n\cdot\nabla$), denotes the derivative in the direction of the outer normal to the surface, where n represents the outer normal to the surface boundary. $h_w = 1 \times 10^4$ W/(m^{2}K) is the convective heat transfer coefficient at the anode surface, and $T_w = 500$ K is the temperature of cooling water. At the torch exit, P_{out} was set equal to the atmospheric pressure.

To solve the Maxwell equations in terms of the potentials ∅ and A as indicated in Table 1, we defined a normal current density $J_{cathode}$ in the range of 10^6 A/m^2.

There was electric insulation, i.e., $n\cdot J = 0$, on the remaining surface of the cathode and a grounded anode ($\varnothing = 0$) on the anode's outer surface and magnetic insulation in all boundaries, with the magnetic potential $n \times A = 0$ and a gauge fixing $\Psi_0 = 1$ A/m.

According to the LTE hypothesis, the current is not able to pass through the plasma electrode interface. For this reason, an artificially high electrical conductivity (8×10^3 S/m) was set in a thin layer close to the electrodes, allowing the formation of a new arc attachment, even when the arc fringe gets near to the anode surface.

Then, we specified the physical values for the electrodes of the plasma torch in the equilibrium discharge interface. Both the cathode tip and the copper anode wall were modeled as boundary plasma heat sources mapping the electromagnetic surface losses as heat sources on the boundary. In this case, a surface work function of 4.15 V was the default value for copper electrodes in COMSOL Multiphysics®.

The numerical model of the DC non-transferred plasma torch was implemented in COMSOL Multiphysics® 5.4 software [29–32] using the physics of CFD (turbulent flow), heat transfer (heat transfer in fluid/solid), AC/DC (electric currents, magnetic fields), and plasma (equilibrium discharge interface). The steady state equations of conservation of fluid mechanics, heat transfer, and electromagnetics were developed by using the Multiphysics couplings options available in the software.

The thermodynamic and transport properties of gas plasma (ρ, λ, c_p, σ, μ_0, and ε_r) obtained from literature and expressed as a function of the local temperature and pressure were implemented in the COMSOL Multiphysics using a piecewise cubic interpolation method and a linear extrapolation method to preserve the shape of the data and to respect monitoring.

The partial differential equations used in this stationary model were numerically solved by the finite element method, where a SIMPLE-Type algorithm was adopted to decouple velocity components and pressure. Triangular instructed grids were generated with refinement close to the torch wall, gas inlet, cathode, and the symmetric axis in order to resolve the strong variation in flow properties within these regions. The computational domain included the inside and the outside of the plasma torch region, which was discretized using 105,600 mesh points. Averaged values of the physical quantities at the grid points in the mesh were calculated. Temperature and velocity distributions results were generated directly with COMSOL Multiphysics.

3. Equipment and Operating Conditions

Figure 2 shows the plasma system used to synthesis nano-silica. A non-transferred DC torch was used to create extremely reactive gas species at a high temperature for the reaction of gas precursors and for the synthesis of nanoparticles. The torch was operated with nitrogen gas followed by a short mixing section where a $SiCl_4$ and carrier gas mixture (nitrogen and hydrogen) were introduced and heated in the plasma tail flame to about 1100 °C. This torch used a (10–30 kW) power supply at a pressure slightly above one atmosphere (4 atm). The electric arc was initially generated by applying a voltage varied between 80 and 200 V, and gases were flown around the arc column for heating via conductive, convective, and radiative heat exchanges. A typical non-transferred DC torch with a rod-type cathode produced a plasma jet with temperature in the interval of (2400–4800 °C) and few hundreds of m/s velocity at the torch exit. The temperature or velocity jet conditions were largely determined by the nozzle design and thus can be adjusted for an efficient manufacturing of nanomaterials. Table 3 summarizes the optimum operation conditions used to synthesis the silica nanoparticles.

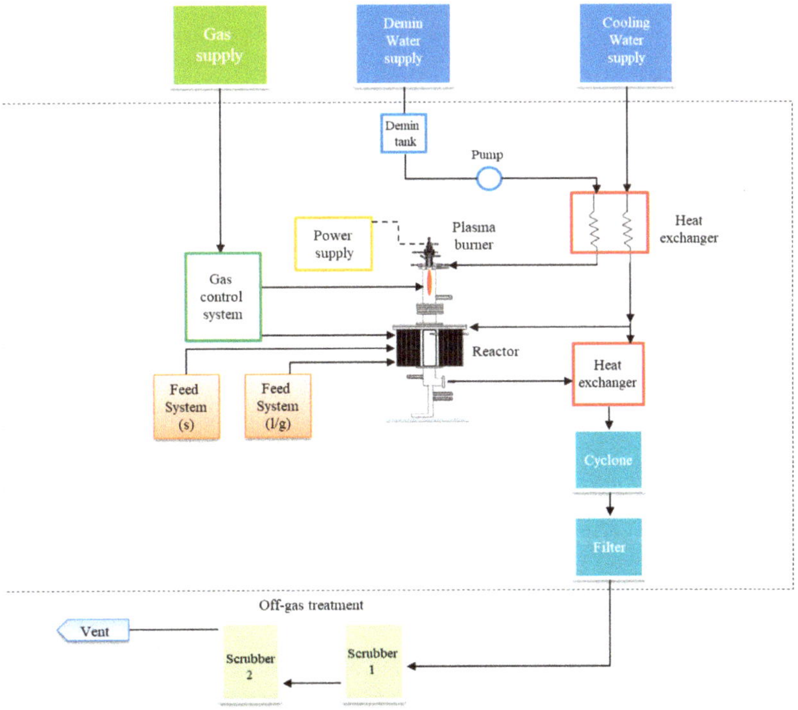

Figure 2. Plasma pilot for the synthesis of nano-silica.

Table 3. Operation conditions used to synthesis nano-silica.

Item	Description
Working gas	Nitrogen
Reactor pressure	400 kPa
Nitrogen flow rate	(78–240) sccm
Power range	10–30 kW
Current plasma	100–200 A
Plasma voltage	80–200 V
Cathode material	Thoriated tungsten
Anode material	High-purity copper
Interelectrode gap	1.8–2 mm
Overall length	250 mm
Outlet electrode diameter	17.2 mm
Temperature of exit gas	2400–4800 °C

Different technics were used to characterize the silica nanopowder prepared by the thermal plasma. These techniques were X-ray diffraction (XRD) and transmission electron microscopy (TEM). The XRD patterns of silica nanopowder were determined with a Bruker D5005 diffractometer and using CuKα radiation (λ = 1.78901 Å). In the TEM characterization, the synthesized products were placed in EtOH, then the samples were immersed for 15 min in an ultrasonic bath, and in the last step a few drops of the resulting suspension containing the synthesized materials were placed onto a TEM grid.

4. Results and Discussion

In this section, the simulation results of the DC non-transferred arc plasma torch used for the synthesis of nano-silica are presented. Furthermore, the influence of the working current on the plasma distribution fields is analyzed, and the efficiency of the torch is discussed for different cases based on comparisons with experimental results. At the nozzle exit, the distributions of temperature and velocity plasma jet are represented. Moreover, the nanosilica particles elaborated in the experimental device were characterized by X-ray diffraction and transmission electron microscopy. For all representative results, the operating gas introduced in the torch was nitrogen gas with flow rates varying in the range (78–240) sccm and current varying in the range (100–200 A).

4.1. Flow of Plasma in the Torch

In Figure 3, the distribution of plasma temperature is presented in the torch under the fixed gas flow rate $Q_{in} = 78$ sccm and for different current values. When the cold plasma forming gas passes through the anode column, it will be strongly heated and accelerated, so there is a fast increase in the temperature and velocity. Indeed, when the current rose from 100 A to 200 A the maximum temperature was increased from 5200 K to 5500 K.

To show with greater clarity the effect of increasing current on plasma temperature changes, the temperature distributions, in front of the cathode tip, are represented in Figure 4. It can be clearly seen that the region area of the plasma temperature higher than 5000 K expands when the current increases. This can be explicated by the effect of the Joule heat produced, namely:

$$Q_{joule} = \vec{J} \cdot \vec{E} = \frac{\left|\vec{J}\right|^2}{\sigma} \quad (18)$$

Indeed, the rising of the current leads to an increase in the current density responsible for Joule heating. Although the electric conductivity of nitrogen gas presents a slow raise as the temperature increases, its influence remains insignificant compared to the current density. Then, the plasma temperature increases with increasing current.

A small temperature variation was observed at the torch exit (from 5200 K to 5500 K), when the current rose from 100 A to 200 A. This was because the energy benefit of joule heating that contributed to the current growth was practically offset by the energy loss due to the length reduction in the electric arc. This effect consequently leads to a trivial dependance of the arc current on the average temperature at the torch exit [33].

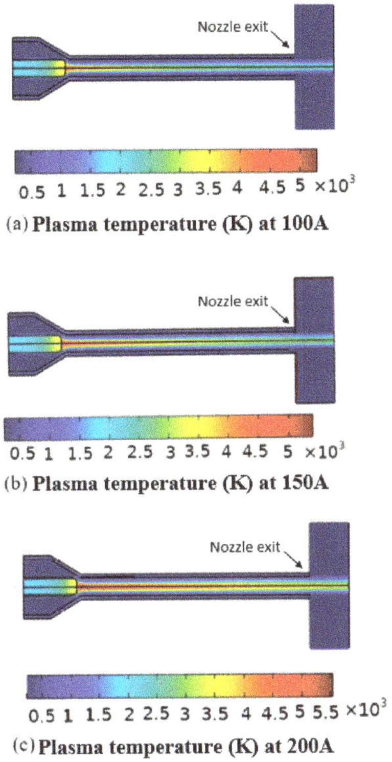

Figure 3. Distribution of plasma temperature for different current values ((**a**) 100 A, (**b**) 150 A, (**c**) 200 A) in the torch.

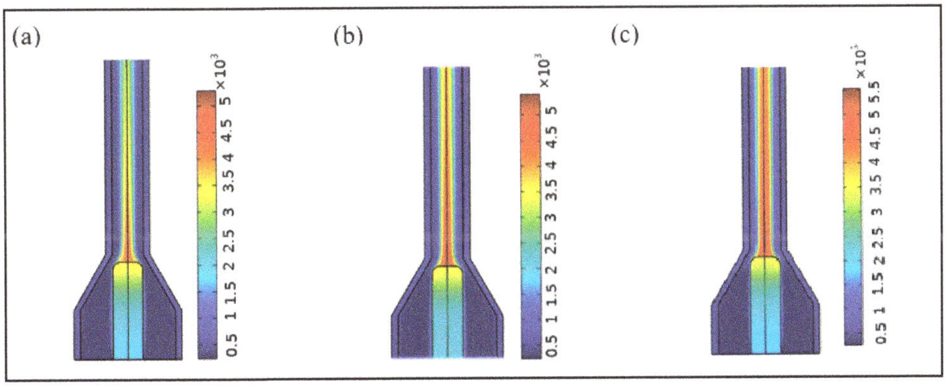

Figure 4. Distribution of the temperature of plasma at the nozzle exit for different current value ((**a**) 100 A, (**b**) 150 A, (**c**) 200 A).

A temperature above 3000 K was observed at the electrode tip, indicating that a melt could occur at the electrode tip. This high temperature was generally compensated by the cooling water of the cathode that causes thermal power loss through it, which can be calculated by:

$$Cathode_{loss} = \frac{Q_{cathode}}{I \cdot V_{arc}} \quad (19)$$

where $Cathode_{loss}$ represents the thermal power loss through cathode cooling water. However, sometimes after several hours we could observe erosion in the cathode tip [34]. This indicates that cooling of the cathode was not sufficient in this case.

In Figure 5, the distribution of the velocity magnitude field is presented in the torch under the fixed gas flow rate $Q_{in} = 78$ sccm and for different current values. The results show that the highest plasma velocities within the torch were approximately 90, 110, and 150 m/s for current values of 150, 200, and 200 A, respectively. The augmentation of working current led to the increase in velocity magnitude.

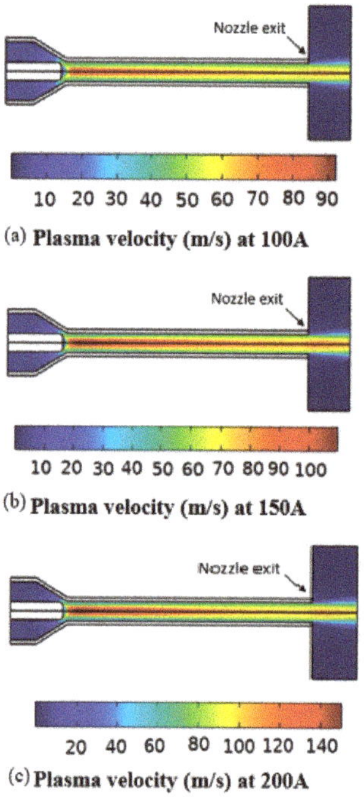

Figure 5. Distribution of plasma velocity for different current values ((**a**) 100 A, (**b**) 150 A, (**c**) 200 A) in the torch.

This axial acceleration of plasma flow was simultaneously influenced by the Lorentz force and by the rise in temperature driven by the joule heating effect [35], which reduces the gas density and reinforces the expansion of the plasma.

Figure 6 shows the variation in plasma voltage versus current at different nitrogen mass flow rates (Q). An increase in the current led to an increase in the voltage of the plasma arc, which reinforced the electric power of the plasma. This linear variation in plasma voltage with plasma current shows that the plasma closely obeys Ohm's law. Moreover, it can be clearly seen that the voltage increased with the increasing nitrogen flow rate, and the plasma was stable when the current and the nitrogen flow rate varied.

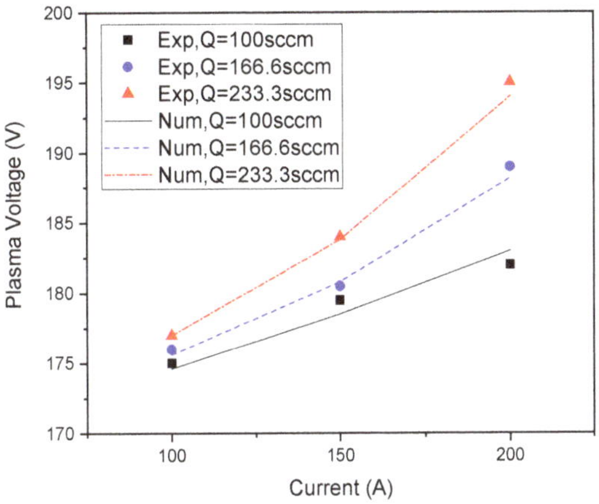

Figure 6. Plasma voltage as a function of current.

To study the efficiency of the plasma torch, we must consider that a portion of the input electric power was transferred to the plasma arc, and the rest of energy was extracted by the cooling water. The energy balance for the plasma torch is written as:

$$E_{exp} = U_{exp}I - Q_{lost} \tag{20}$$

where E_{exp} is the effective power transferred to the plasma arc, $U_{exp}I$ is the electric power supplied by the DC generator, and Q_{lost} represents the energy lost by the cooling water.

$$Q_{lost} = 4.18 \times C_{pw} \times \dot{m}_w(T_{out} - T_{in}) \tag{21}$$

where C_{pw} is the specific heat capacity of water (1 cal/cm^3), 4.18 is the conversion factor for converting cal/s into watts, $\dot{m}_w$ is the amount of cooling water flow rate (sccm), and T_{out} and T_{in} are the outlet and inlet temperatures, respectively.

However, for numerical simulation, the energy of the plasma leaving the torch can be calculated by integrating the plasma enthalpy at the surface of the torch output:

$$E_{cal} = \oiint \dot{m}_g h ds \tag{22}$$

The electrothermal efficiency can be obtained by dividing the energy transferred to the plasma gas by the electric power, mainly:

$$\eta = \frac{E_{exp}}{U_{exp}I} = \frac{E_{cal}}{U_{cal}\ I} \tag{23}$$

Figure 7 illustrates the numerical results and experimental measurements of electrothermal efficiency of the plasma torch for different working currents and at different mass flow rates. At lower mass flow rates, the increase in current led to an increase in the degree of ionization, which increased the plasma pressure inside the torch; then, the plasma velocity increased, and more plasma came out from the nozzle exit of the torch. Thus, the efficiency increased with current. However, at a higher gas flow rate, the amount of plasma coming out from the torch did not increase significantly because the increase in the plasma pressure inside the torch due to the increase in the current caused a higher collision of the plasma particles with the anode wall (limitation of the velocity) and led to more heat loss from the plasma to the walls, decreasing the total efficiency of the torch [36].

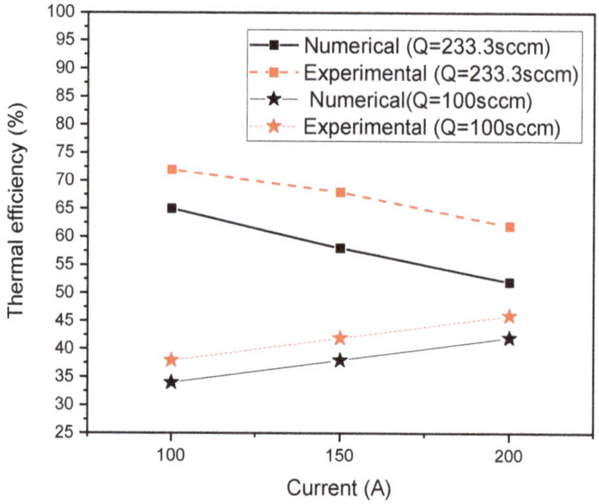

Figure 7. Numerical and experimental variation of thermal efficiency with working current (100 A, 150 A, 200 A) for different gas flow rates (Q = 233.3 sccm and Q = 100 sccm).

Furthermore, in Figure 8, experimental measurements and numerical predictions of electrothermal efficiency display that the plasma efficiency decreased linearly when the enthalpy increased.

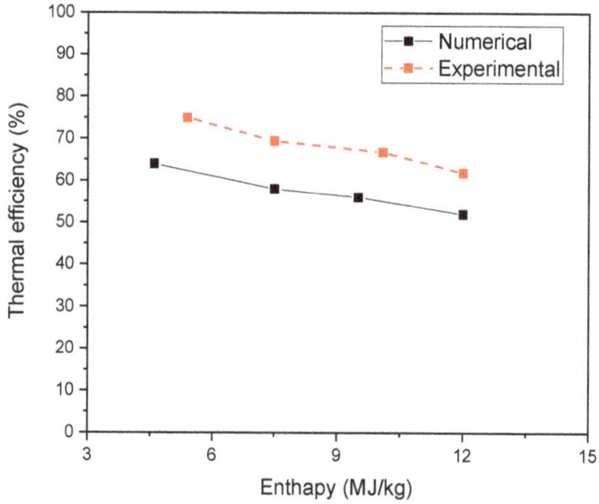

Figure 8. Numerical and experimental variation in thermal efficiency as a function of enthalpy with a gas flow rate Q = 233.3 sccm.

The comparison between the value of numerical results and the measured one showed the same variation tendency of the efficiency, but the values of the numerical model were less than those of experimental measurements. Indeed, the measured value of total energy included both the energy transferred to the plasma arc and the heat dissipated by cooled water. Experimentally, the energy extracted by the cooling water was under-evaluated because a part of heat dissipated into the environment. In this case, the effective thermal efficiency was overestimated.

In addition, Figure 9 shows that the specific enthalpy of nitrogen gas increased rapidly as temperature increased, which led to greater electrical energy needed.

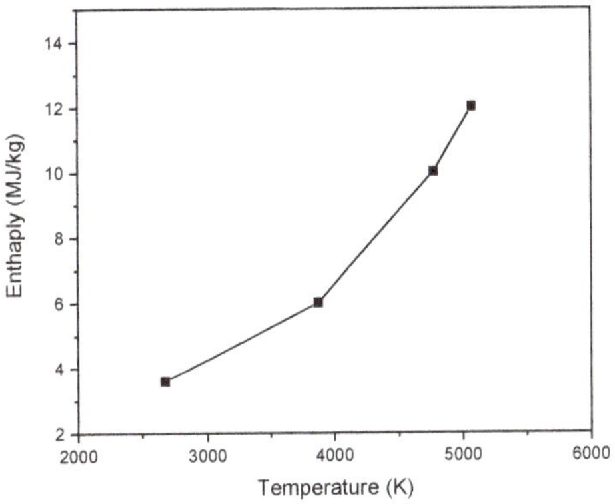

Figure 9. Enthalpy of plasma gas (N_2) as a function of temperature.

Another effect of current on the plasma characteristics, at the torch exit, can be intuitively shown in Figure 10. As the current increased from 100 to 200 A, the plasma temperature and velocity distributions were plotted in the ranges of 0–4000 K and 0–150 m/s scales, respectively. Figure 10a exhibits that the area of the high temperature (>2800 K) was progressively increased. Simultaneously, as shown in Figure 10b, the plasma velocity had the same variation tendency. This occurrence suggests that the increment in working current forced the plasma jet to exit the nozzle torch with a faster and larger hot core diameter.

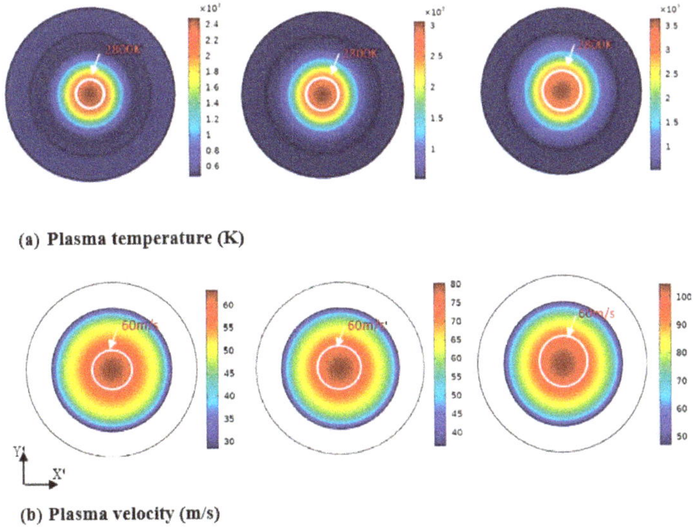

Figure 10. Distributions of plasma temperature (**a**) and velocity (**b**) at the torch exit at different current 100 A, 150 A, and 200 A.

Figure 11 represents the radial profiles of the temperature and velocity plasma jet at the torch exit for different values of working current. The increase in current had a greater effect on the plasma velocity (Figure 11a) compared to the temperature. Indeed, the maximum temperature had only risen by about 600 K when the current varied from 100 A to 200 A (Figure 11b). This was due to the dissipation of electrical energy by the cooling water. This effect can be confirmed by the decrease in the thermal efficiency versus current, presented in Figure 7.

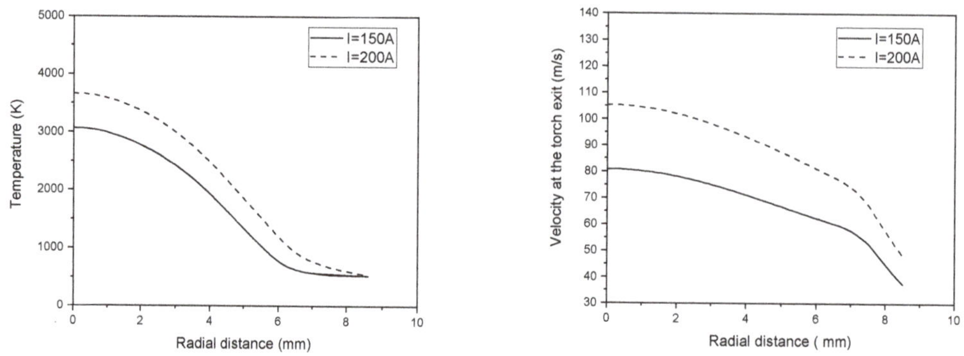

(a) (b)

Figure 11. The radial profiles of the temperature (**a**) and velocity (**b**) plasma jet at the torch exit for different values of working current.

4.2. Plasma Jet Outside the Torch

Figure 12a shows the velocity distribution inside and outside the torch. When leaving the torch exit, the velocity displayed a high downward tendency, which was mainly due to the expansion process of the plasma jet outside the torch. This expansion process was due to the absence of a constrained effect and to the entrainment of cold ambient air. Indeed, the considerable increase in driven cold air resulting from the fluctuated plasma jet led to a significant decrease in plasma temperature and velocity.

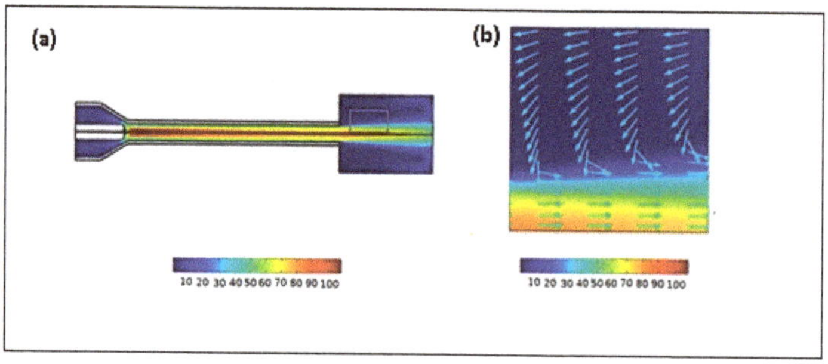

Figure 12. Velocity field distribution (**a**) and the corresponding velocity vector (**b**) in the grey rectangle.

The local enlarged picture of velocity vector in the grey rectangle (Figure 12a) is shown in Figure 12b. These arrows pointing in the opposite side to the flow of the plasma jet signal that a vortex roll-up formed, which displayed obvious evidence of the cold air driven into the plasma jet. Indeed, the velocity vector distribution presents alternating forward and backward stripes of the velocity vector direction, where forward velocity vectors show the blowing of the plasma jet outside the nozzle exit of the torch, and backward velocity vectors show the effect of the cold air outside the jet.

Both radial profiles of plasma temperature (Figure 13a) and velocity (Figure 13b) at 80 mm from the nozzle torch exit are shown in Figure 13. If we compare these radial profiles with the radial temperature and velocity profiles at the torch exit, presented in (Figure 11), we can notice that both temperature and velocity regions derived from the centerline at the torch exit decrease along the axial direction due to turbulent mixing of plasma with cold air.

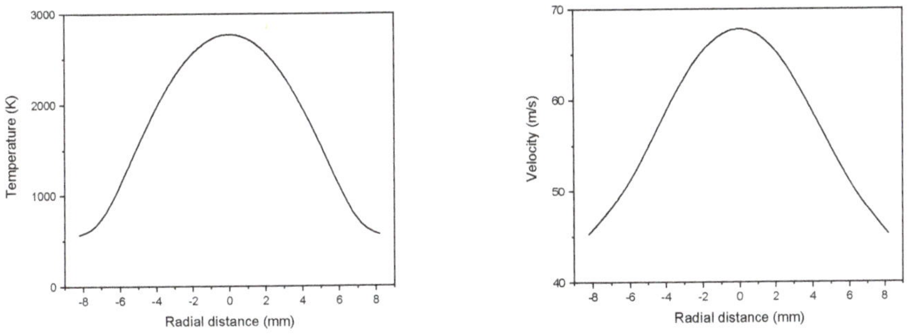

(**a**) (**b**)

Figure 13. The radial profiles of the temperature (**a**) and velocity (**b**) plasma jet at 80 mm from the nozzle torch exit.

The diameter of the plasma jet core increased, and the radial dimension of the core extended gradually. Particles injected into the plasma jet may gain different temperatures and velocities from the plasma. Therefore, an increase in the plasma jet core region implies that additional in-flight particles will be more heated and accelerated, which ultimately increases the efficiency of the deposition and the quality of the coating. Those phenomena were coherent with the actual manufacturing process [13].

4.3. Structure of Nanosilica Particles

X-ray diffraction is an interesting technique to identify the purity, size, and crystalline nature of the materials. Figure 14 depicts the X-ray diffraction patterns of the silica sample. This figure contains, around the angle 2 theta 22–23, a strong broad, which is the characteristic of silica. This result confirms that the state of the synthesized nanosilica was amorphous. The Scherrer formula and the full width at half maximum (FWHM) were used to determine the average particle size of the silica samples. The average size of nanoparticles was calculated using the following formula:

$$G = \frac{K\lambda}{Bcos\Theta_B} \tag{24}$$

where K is a dimensionless shape factor with a typical value of about 0.9, λ is the X-ray wavelength (λ = 1.78901 Å for Co Ka), θ_B is the maximum of Bragg diffraction peak (in rad), and B is the line width at half maximum. Using this formula, the calculated average grain size of nanoparticles was 24 nm.

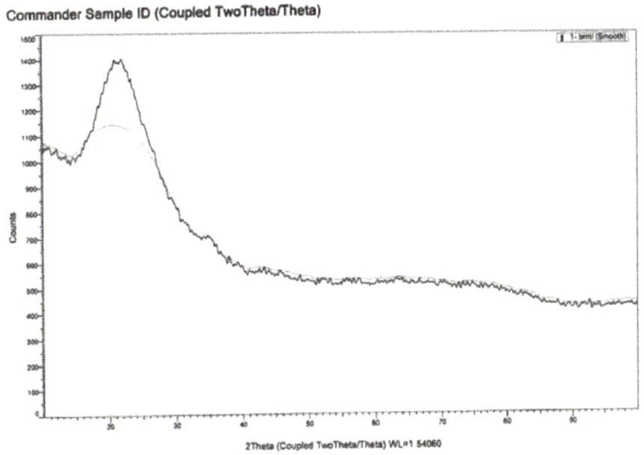

Figure 14. XRD of nanosilica.

The Debye–Scherrer formula was obtained from a model in which the size distribution of the crystallites was ignored; hence, the average grain size obtained from this formula was not precise compared to the size of the nanoparticles measured by TEM. Different images at variable magnifications (50,000–60,000) were recorded for the sample to investigate its average grain size. The recorded TEM images of nanosilica are shown in Figure 15. These images show that the morphology of the nanoparticles had a nearly spherical shape with a diameter ranging from 10 to 20 nm. These results confirm that the average particle dimension of the obtained silica was in nanoscale size and that they are in accordance with the XRD results.

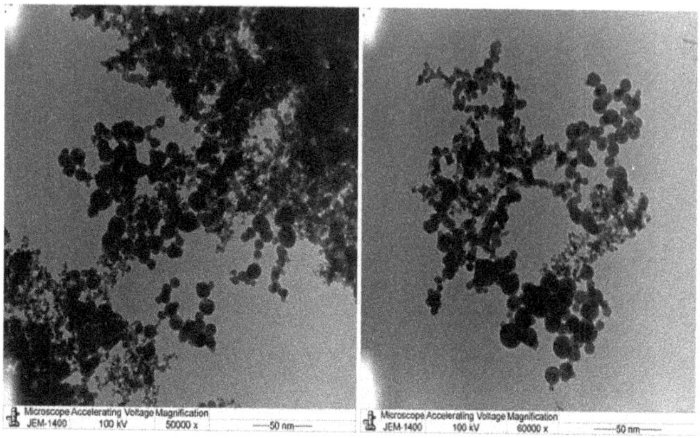

Figure 15. TEM images of nanosilica.

5. Conclusions

In this work, a pilot plasma system, which contained a non-transferred arc system with a power of 30 KW, was used to synthesis nano-sized silica. The plasma operated on nitrogen, and the nitrogen tail flame could be heated to the range of 4273.15 K to 6773.15 K. A 2D numerical model was established to predict the plasma flow and heat transfer inside and outside of the torch. Simulation results showed that the plasma temperature and velocity became higher with increasing current, while the electrothermal efficiency was reduced. Additionally, the thermal efficiency decreased with increasing enthalpy because more energy was removed by cooling water. With increasing current, the plasma jet core with high velocity and temperature was expanded in axial and radial directions. Numerical simulation results were in good accordance with the experimental measurements. In addition, the initial nanosilica particles elaborated in the experimental device were characterized by X-ray diffraction (XRD) and transmission electron microscopy (TEM) to identify the purity, size, and crystalline nature of the materials and to study their mean size. The arc plasma method enabled one to produce spherical silicon ultra-fine powder of about 20 nm in diameter.

Author Contributions: Conceptualization, S.E., I.G. and I.A.A.; methodology, S.E., I.A.A. and I.G.; formal analysis, I.A.A., S.E., S.S.A. and I.G.; investigation, I.A.A., S.E., S.S.A., A.A.A. and I.G.; resources, I.A.A., S.S.A. and A.A.A.; writing—original draft, S.E., I.A.A. and I.G.; writing—review and editing, S.E., I.A.A. and I.G. All authors have read and agreed to the published version of the manuscript.

Funding: This research received no external funding.

Institutional Review Board Statement: Not applicable.

Informed Consent Statement: Not applicable.

Data Availability Statement: Data are contained within the article.

Conflicts of Interest: The authors declare no conflict of interest.

References

1. Hussain, C.-M. *Handbook of Nanomaterials for Industrial Applications*; Elsevier: Amsterdam, The Netherlands, 2018.
2. Jun, B.-M.; Kim, S.; Heo, J.; Park, C.-M.; Her, N.; Jang, M.; Huang, Y.; Han, J.; Yoon, Y. Review of MXenes as new nanomaterials for energy storage/delivery and selected environmental applications. *Nano Res.* **2019**, *12*, 471–487. [CrossRef]
3. Yia, H.; Qina, L.; Huanga, D.; Zenga, G.; Laia, C.; Liua, X.; Lia, B.; Wanga, H.; Zhoua, C.; Huanga, F.; et al. Nano-structured bismuth tungstate with controlled morphology: Fabrication, modification, environmental application and mechanism insight. *Chem. Eng. J.* **2019**, *358*, 480–496. [CrossRef]
4. Kaliannan, D.; Palaninaicker, S.; Palanivel, V.; Mahadeo, M.-A.; Ravindra, B.-N.; Jae-Jin, S. A novel approach to preparation of nano-adsorbent from agricultural wastes (Saccharum officinarum leaves) and its environmental application. *Environ. Sci. Pollut. Res.* **2019**, *26*, 5305–5314. [CrossRef]
5. Bisla, A.; Rautela, R.; Yadav, V.; Singh, P.; Kumar, A.; Ghosh, S.; Kumar, A.; Bag, S.; Kumar, B.; Srivastava, N. Nano-purification of raw semen minimises oxidative stress with improvement in post-thaw quality of buffalo spermatozoa. *Andrologia* **2020**, *52*, e13709. [CrossRef]
6. Aversa, R.; Petrescu, R.V.; Apicella, A.; Petrescu, F.-I. Nano-Diamond Hybrid Materials for Structural Biomedical Application. *Am. J. Biochem. Biotechnol.* **2016**, *13*, 34–41. [CrossRef]
7. Nasrin, S.; Chowdhury, F.-U.-Z.; Hoque, S.-M. Study of hyperthermia temperature of manganese-substituted cobalt nano ferrites prepared by chemical co-precipitation method for biomedical application. *J. Magn. Magn. Mater.* **2019**, *479*, 126–134. [CrossRef]
8. Ananth, A.; Mok, Y.S. Dielectric Barrier Discharge (DBD) Plasma Assisted Synthesis of Ag_2O Nanomaterials and Ag_2O/RuO_2 Nanocomposites. *Nanomaterials* **2016**, *6*, 42. [CrossRef]
9. Post, P.; Jidenko, N.; Weber, A.P.; Borra, J.-P. Post-Plasma SiOx Coatings of Metal and Metal Oxide Nanoparticles for Enhanced Thermal Stability and Tunable Photoactivity Applications. *Nanomaterials* **2016**, *6*, 91. [CrossRef]
10. Dao, V.-D.; Choi, H.-S. Highly Efficient Plasmon-Enhanced Dye-Sensitized Solar Cells Created by Means of Dry Plasma Reduction. *Nanomaterials* **2016**, *6*, 70. [CrossRef]
11. Samokhin, A.; Alekseev, N.; Sinayskiy, M.; Astashov, A.; Kirpichev, D.; Fadeev, A.; Tsvetkov, Y.; Kolesnikov, A. Nanopowders Production and Micron-Sized Powders Spheroidization in DC Plasma Reactors. In *Powder Technology*; IntechOpen: London, UK, 2018.
12. Stein, M.; Kruis, F.-E. Optimization of a transferred arc reactor for metal nanoparticle synthesis. *J. Nanopart. Res.* **2016**, *18*, 258. [CrossRef]
13. Choi, S.; Lee, H.; Park, D.-W. Synthesis of Silicon Nanoparticles and Nanowires by a Non-transferred Arc Plasma System. *J. Nanomater.* **2016**, *2016*, 5849041. [CrossRef]
14. Ghedini, E.; Colombo, V. Time Dependent 3D Large Eddy Simulation of a DC Non-Transferred Arc Plasma Spraying Torch with Particle Injection. In Proceedings of the 34th International Conference on Plasma Science (ICOPS), Santa Fe, NM, USA, 17–22 June 2007; p. 899.
15. Ishigaki, T. Synthesis of Functional Oxide Nanoparticles through RF Thermal Plasma Processing. *Plasma Chem Plasma Process* **2017**, *37*, 783–804. [CrossRef]
16. Santosh, V.S.; Kondeti, K.; Gangal, U.; Yatom, S.; Bruggeman, P.-J. Ag+ reduction and silver nanoparticle synthesis at the plasma-liquid interface by an RF driven atmospheric pressure plasma jet: Mechanisms and the effect of surfactant. *J. Vac. Sci. Technol. A* **2017**, *35*, 061302.
17. Sama, S. Thermal plasma technology: The prospective future in material processing. *J. Clean. Prod.* **2017**, *142*, 3131–3150. [CrossRef]
18. Aboughaly, M.; Gabbar, H.-A.; Damideh, V.; Hassen, I. RF-ICP Thermal Plasma for Thermoplastic Waste Pyrolysis Process with High Conversion Yield and Tar Elimination. *Processes* **2020**, *8*, 281. [CrossRef]
19. Vardelle, A.; Moreau, C.; Themelis, N.-J.; Chazelas, C. A perspective on plasma spray technology. *Plasma Chem. Plasma Process* **2015**, *35*, 491–509. [CrossRef]
20. Li, H.-P.; Chen, X. Three-dimensional modelling of a dc non-transferred arc plasma torch. *J. Phys. D Appl. Phys.* **2001**, *34*, L99–L102. [CrossRef]
21. Trelles, J.-P.; Chazelas, C.; Vardelle, A.; Heberlein, J.-V.-R. Arc Plasma Torch Modeling. *J. Therm. Spray Technol.* **2009**, *18*, 728–752. [CrossRef]
22. Selvan, B.; Ramachandran, K.; Sreekumar, K.-P.; Thiyagrajan, T.-K.; Ananthapadmanabhan, P.-V. Three-Dimensional Numerical Modeling of an Ar-N_2 Plasma Arc inside a Non-Transferred Torch. *Plasma Sci. Technol.* **2009**, *11*, 679. [CrossRef]
23. Guo, Z.; Yin, S.; Qian, Z.; Liao, H.; Gu, S. Effect of Asymmetrical Distribution of Current Density on the Three-Dimensional Non-Transferred Arc Plasma Torch. *Comput. Fluids* **2015**, *114*, 163–171. [CrossRef]
24. Modirkhazeni, S.-M.; Trelles, J.-P. Non-transferred Arc Torch Simulation by a Non-equilibrium Plasma Laminar-to-Turbulent Flow Model. *J. Therm. Spray Technol.* **2018**, *27*, 1447–1464. [CrossRef]
25. Frolov, V.; Ivanov, D. Development of mathematical models of thermal plasma processes. *Mater. Science. Non-Equilib. Phase Transform.* **2017**, *3*, 56–59.

26. Kim, T.-H.; Lee, Y.-H.; Kim, M.; Oh, J.-H.; Choi, S. Thermal Flow Characteristics of the Triple Plasma Torch System for Nanoparticle Synthesis. *IEEE Trans. Plasma Sci.* **2019**, *47*, 3366–3373. [CrossRef]
27. Boulos, M.I.; Fauchais, P.; Pfender, E. *Thermal Plasmas: Fundamentals and Applications*; Plenum Press: New York, NY, USA, 1994.
28. Launder, B.-E.; Spalding, D.-B. *Lectures in Mathematical Models of Turbulence*; Academic Press: London, UK, 1972.
29. COMSOL Multiphysics® v. 5.1. *CFD Module User's Guide*; COMSOL AB: Stockholm, Sweden, 2015.
30. COMSOL Multiphysics® v. 5.1. *Heat Transfer Module User's Guide*; COMSOL AB: Stockholm, Sweden, 2015.
31. COMSOL Multiphysics® v. 5.1. *AC/DC Module User's Guide*; COMSOL AB: Stockholm, Sweden, 2015.
32. COMSOL Multiphysics® v. 5.1. *Plasma Module, User's Guide*; COMSOL AB: Stockholm, Sweden, 2015.
33. Chau, S.W.; Lu, S.Y.; Wang, P.J. Study on arc and flow characteristics of a non-transferred DC steam torch. *J. Chin. Inst. Eng.* **2021**, *44*, 646–658. [CrossRef]
34. Selvan, B.; Ramachandran, K.; Sreekumar, K.P.; Thiyagarajan, T.K.; Ananthapadmanabhan, P.V. Numerical and experimental studies on DC plasma spray torch. *Vacuum* **2010**, *84*, 444–452. [CrossRef]
35. Wen, K.; Liu, X.; Liu, M.; Zhou, K.; Long, H.; Deng, C.; Mao, J.; Yan, X.; Liao, H. Numerical simulation and experimental study of Ar-H_2 DC atmospheric plasma spraying. *Surf. Coat.* **2019**, *371*, 312–321. [CrossRef]
36. Bora, B.; Aomoa, N.; Kakati, M. Characteristics and temperature measurement of a non- transferred cascaded DC plasma torch. *Plasma Sci. Technol.* **2010**, *12*, 181. [CrossRef]

applied sciences

MDPI

Article

Surface Properties of Silica–MWCNTs/PDMS Composite Coatings Deposited on Plasma Activated Glass Supports

Michał Chodkowski [1,*], Iryna Ya. Sulym [2], Konrad Terpiłowski [1] and Dariusz Sternik [3]

1 Department of Interfacial Phenomena, Faculty of Chemistry, Institute of Chemical Sciences, Maria Curie-Skłodowska University in Lublin (UMCS), pl. Marii Curie-Skłodowskiej 3, 20-031 Lublin, Poland; terpil@umcs.pl
2 Laboratory of Oxide Nanocomposites, Chuiko Institute of Surface Chemistry, NASU, General Naumov Str. 17, 03164 Kyiv, Ukraine; irynasulym@ukr.net
3 Department of Physical Chemistry, Faculty of Chemistry, Institute of Chemical Sciences, Maria Curie-Skłodowska University in Lublin (UMCS), pl. Marii Curie-Skłodowskiej 3, 20-031 Lublin, Poland; dsternik@poczta.umcs.lublin.pl
* Correspondence: michal.chodkowski@poczta.umcs.lublin.pl

Abstract: In this paper, we focus on fabrication and physicochemical properties investigations of silica–multiwalled carbon nanotubes/poly(dimethylsiloxane) composite coatings deposited on the glass supports activated by cold plasma. Air or argon was used as the carrier gas in the plasma process. Multiwalled carbon nanotubes were modified with poly(dimethylsiloxane) in order to impart their hydrophobicity. The silica–multiwalled carbon nanotubes/poly(dimethylsiloxane) nanocomposite was synthesized using the sol–gel technique with acid-assisted tetraethyl orthosilicate hydrolysis. The stability and the zeta potential of the obtained suspension were evaluated. Then, the product was dried and used as a filler in another sol–gel process, which led to the coating application via the dip-coating method. The substrates were exposed to the hexamethyldisilazane vapors in order to improve their hydrophobicity. The obtained surfaces were characterized by the wettability measurements and surface free energy determination as well as optical profilometry, scanning electron microscopy, and transmittance measurements. In addition, the thermal analyses of the carbon nanotubes as well as coatings were made. It was found that rough and hydrophobic coatings were obtained with a high transmittance in the visible range. They are characterized by the water contact angle larger than 90 degrees and the transmission at the level of 95%. The X-ray diffraction studies as well as scanning electron microscopy images confirmed the chemical and structural compositions of the coatings. They are thermally stable at the temperature up to 250 °C. Moreover, the thermal analysis showed that the obtained composite material has greater thermal resistance than the pure nanotubes.

Keywords: multiwalled carbon nanotubes; poly(dimethylsiloxane); silica; coating; hexamethyldisilazane; contact angle; wettability; hydrophobicity; surface free energy; areal roughness; low pressure cold plasma

Citation: Chodkowski, M.; Sulym, I.Y.; Terpiłowski, K.; Sternik, D. Surface Properties of Silica–MWCNTs/PDMS Composite Coatings Deposited on Plasma Activated Glass Supports. *Appl. Sci.* **2021**, *11*, 9256. https://doi.org/10.3390/app11199256

Academic Editor: Bogdan-George Rusu

Received: 28 July 2021
Accepted: 28 September 2021
Published: 5 October 2021

1. Introduction

Silica materials are a large group of functional materials with a wide range of applications [1]. They can be obtained in a polycondensation reaction from silicon alkoxides or other similar precursors using the sol–gel process. The final properties of the product depend on the process parameters such as type of precursor and solvent, catalyst, or temperature. This makes it an effective, simple, and cheap technology characterized by many advantages [2]. Silica-based coatings are one of such materials; they are largely developing and future-oriented because they can impart a wide variety of predetermined properties to a surface [3]. Silica coatings can be doped with various fillers or modifiers in order to improve or change their properties. This makes them a composite material. The composite is produced from two or more constituent materials with different physical and chemical properties [4]. Their combination results in a material with properties dissimilar to those of individual elements. When the two constituents are at the nanometer or molecular level, this is a hybrid material [5]. This combination, consisting of organic and inorganic constituents, makes an interesting material with specific physical, thermal, optical, electrical, and mechanical properties that are promising for various applications [6,7].

Recently, the use of carbon nanotubes (CNTs) [8] has become more common, and they are now one of the most widely used organic additives due to their unique properties such as small density, excellent mechanical properties, and good thermal and electrical conductivity, which make them an ideal component for the organic phase in composites or hybrids [9–12]. CNTs are cylindrical structures consisting of rolled-up sheets of single-layer carbon network with the structure (sp^2) of graphene [13]. In the case of the single-walled carbon nanotubes (SWCNTs), this is a single sheet close to 1 nanometer in diameter [14], whereas for the multiwalled carbon nanotubes (MWCNTs), there are several concentrically interlinked single tubes, and the end diameter of the structure can reach up to 100nm [15]. The length of nanotube ranges from nanometers, through millimeters, up to several centimeters [16]. The popularity of carbon nanotubes applications can be demonstrated by their usage not only for nanocomposites [17,18] but also in many fields—for example, drug delivery systems [19], functional fabrics production [20], medicine [21], electronics [22], solar energy systems [23], road constructions [24], and even spacecrafts [25]. There is a quick and simple method to synthesize doped silica composites—mix an organic additive with one of the precursors (for example tetraethyl orthosilicate) followed by the sol–gel reaction assisted with acid or base catalysis [26]. The hydrogen bonds formed between the two constituents prevent phase separation and result in obtaining a transparent and stable composition or a film [27]. However, so far, there are no reports in the literature on the use of carbon nanotubes as a silica coating modifier, but they have been successfully used, for example, to produce composite polymer materials [28] or different types of hybrid materials [29].

Another possibility to modify the properties of the coatings is to modify the support with plasma. Plasma is commonly defined as a fourth state of matter, distinct from a solid, liquid, or gas, that is composed of high-energy ions, electrons, neutral or excited molecules, and UV light [30]. It was first described by the American chemist Irving Langmuir in the 1920s [31,32]. It is crucial to distinguish between thermal and nonthermal (cold) plasmas, and the classification is based on the relative temperatures of their constituents. In the case of the cold plasma, there will not be a local thermodynamic equilibrium between the highly energetic electrons generating plasma and other particles ($T_{electrons} >> T_{plasma}$) because the density of the electrons in the plasma is small compared to that of other constituents. Thus, the term "cold" refers to the plasma with the temperature between 40 °C and 70 °C [33]. This plays a key role if plasma is used to modify heat-sensitive materials because plasma modification of a solid surface is one of its common applications. It can be used for food decontamination [34] and in medicine [35], nanotechnology [36], and surface engineering [37]. The high-energy constituents of the plasma interact with a surface and can change a wide range of its properties such as surface free energy, wettability, roughness, surface charge, and biocompatibility. The ability of plasma modification to induce any changes in the bulk of a solid is still an open question.

The aim of this study was to obtain a new silica–multiwalled carbon nanotubes/poly (dimethylsiloxane) (silica–MWCNTs/PDMS) composite coating. The hydrophobic properties of the product were to be ensured by the modification of carbon nanotubes with poly(dimetylsiloxane) (PDMS) as well as hydrophobization of the surfaces with hexamethyldisilazane. The influence of cold plasma modification of the support on the surface properties of the coating was investigated. The physicochemical properties of the obtained coatings were comprehensively studied using scanning electron microscopy, X-ray diffraction, optical profilometry, thermal analysis, contact angle measurements, and surface free energy evaluation.

2. Materials and Methods

2.1. Materials and Reagents

During the investigation, the following reagents and materials were used:

- demineralized water (SPRING 20 from Hydrolab, Straszyn, Poland)
- ultrapure water (Milli-Q™ system from Merck, Darmstadt, Germany; 18.2 MΩ·cm^{-1} at 298 K)
- multiwalled carbon nanotubes, MWCNTs
- tetraethyl orthosilicate, TEOS (98%, Aldrich, St. Louis, USA)
- hydrochloric acid, HCl (35–38%, POCH S.A., Lublin, Poland)
- ethanol, EtOH (96%, POCH S.A., Lublin, Poland)
- hexamethyldisilazane, HMDS (98%, Aldrich, St. Louis, USA)
- potassium chloride, KCl (reagent grade, POCH S.A., Lublin, Poland)
- glass microscope slides with the dimensions of 76 × 26 × 1 mm (ChemLand, Stargard, Poland)

2.2. Samples Preparation

2.2.1. Synthesis of the Filler

The multiwalled carbon nanotubes were obtained in another experiment using the catalytic chemical vapor deposition (CCVD) method as described by Kartel et al. [38], using pyrolysis of propylene on the complex metal oxide catalysts [39]. The product was hydrophobized by physical adsorption of poly(dimethylsiloxane) as follows. Before the process, the samples were dried at 110 °C for 2 h; then, the hexane solution of PDMS (1 wt% PDMS) was prepared and 5 wt% of the solution was added to the determined amount of dried MWCNTs. After that, the suspension was mechanically stirred and finally dried at room temperature for 48 h and then at 80 °C for 3 h, obtaining the powder form (similar to that of unmodified MWCNTs). The detailed description of the synthesis and study on physicochemical properties of these MWCNTs is available in another paper [40].

The silica–MWCNTs/PDMS hybrid filler was synthesized via the acid-assisted tetraethoxysilane hydrolysis at the molar ratio 1.0:4.6 × 10^{-2}:3.45 (TEOS:HCl:H_2O). The composition was stirred using a magnetic stirrer at 300 rpm at 50 °C for 2 h. Then, the MWCNTs suspension in ethanol (3‰ m/v) was instilled, which corresponds to the volume dilution of 1:3, and the composition was stirred for 30 min. After that, a portion of the sample was submitted to stability testing while the rest was dried at room temperature for 24 h (gelation and solvent evaporation). Sequentially, the powder was suspended in 5 mL of ultrapure water and centrifuged at 5000 rpm for 10 min at room temperature; the procedure was repeated three times. Then, the product was dried at room temperature for 48 h, ground gently in the agate mortar for 2 min into a powder form and heated at 150 °C for 24 h.

2.2.2. Plasma Activation of the Supports

The glass microscope slides, which are factory cleaned, degreased, and ready to use, were taken as the supports for the coatings. They were activated by air or argon cold plasma by means of PICO Low Pressure Plasma System (Diener Electronic GmbH, Germany) using the parameters in Table 1.

Table 1. Plasma process parameters for the activation of the glass supports.

Parameter	Value
plasma type	low pressure cold plasma (LPCP)
process duration	5 min
carrier gas	air or argon
gas flow	50 sccm
pressure	0.2 mbar (controlled via gases)
generator model	LFG40
generator frequency	40 kHz (RF)
generator power [1]	100%/1000 W
flushing/venting gas	air

[1] Efficiency > 90% at the nominal power and accuracy better than ±5% of final value.

2.2.3. Synthesis and Coating Application

The coating was synthesized by the sol–gel method as it was described in our previous paper [41] with the difference that the synthesis proceeded at 50 °C. TEOS was used as the precursor and HCl as a catalyst of the hydrolysis at the molar ratio of 1.0:4.6 $\times$ 10^{-2}:3.45 for TEOS:HCl:H_2O, respectively. The filler (silica–MWCNTs/PDMS composite) suspension in EtOH was prepared at the concentration 3% (m/v). After the synthesis completion, a sample of the product was taken for stability testing (parallel with the coating process).

The KSV NIMA KN4001 Dip Coater (Biolin Scientific, Sweden) was used for the glass supports covering. The withdrawal speeds of the samples as well as the methods of the support activation are presented in Table 2. Between the successive coatings of the samples the sol was still being stirred at 300 rpm and its temperature was maintained at 50 °C. The sample #7 was coated by manual immersion while #8 by spreading of 5 mL of the sol on the support.

Table 2. Parameters of individual samples.

Sample Number	Support Activation	Withdrawal Speed [mm/min]
#1	nonmodified	50
#2	air plasma	50
#3	argon plasma	50
#4	nonmodified	20
#5	air plasma	20
#6	argon plasma	20
#7	nonmodified	n/a (manually)
#8	nonmodified	n/a (spread)

2.2.4. Hydrophobization of the Coatings

To impart the surface hydrophobicity, the substrates were modified with hexamethyldisilazane. They were kept in a desiccator under the HMDS saturated vapor at ambient temperature and pressure for 24 h. Then, the residual modifier (unbound hexamethyldisilazane) and the byproduct (ammonia) were dismissed by heating the substrates at 100 °C for 1 h.

2.3. Samples Study

2.3.1. Stability

The stability measurements were made by the Turbiscan^{LAB} (Formulaction, Toulouse, France) apparatus equipped with the cooler unit, which is a cooling/heating module. The silica–MWCNTs/PDMS hybrid material suspension as well as the sol used for the surface coating with the dip-coating technique were tested. The products were put into the Turbiscan vessel immediately when the synthesis was over, and the measurements were made at 50 °C (the synthesis temperature). The transmission profiles were collected for 3 h every minute and then for 9 h every 30 min. Based on these data, the Turbiscan Stability

Index (TSI) was calculated by the TurbiSoft 2.3 software as it was described in our previous paper [42].

The zeta potential was determined using the Zetasizer Nano ZS90 (Malvern Instruments Ltd., Malvern, United Kingdom) with the automatic measurement procedure that uses the modified PALS (phase analysis light scattering) signal processing technique called M3-PALS based on the electrophoretic mobility. The sample in its native pH was prepared as follows: about 0.02 g of the silica–MWCNTs/PDMS composite was dissolved in 6 mL of the 32.5% aqueous ethanol solution and 10 mL of 1 mM KCl was added in order to improve conductivity in the continuous phase. Finally, the alcohol concentration in the water solution (masses of CNTs and KCl are negligible) was about 12%. The measurements were made at 20 °C using the universal dip cell (Pd electrodes with 2 mm spacing, 40 µL disposable microcuvette) and the Smoluchowski approximation [43,44] was applied in order to transform the measured electrophoretic mobilities into the zeta potential. The appropriate parameters for the dispersant were established in the software: the viscosity equal to 2.16 cP [45], the refractive index equal to 1.3410 at a wavelength (589.29 nm) close to the laser wavelength (632.8 nm) [46], and the dielectric constant equal to 75.67 [47].

2.3.2. Thermal Analysis

The thermogravimetric (TG) study of the carbon nanotubes was carried out using a Derivatograph MOM Q-1500 D (Paulik–Paulik–Erdey, Budapest, Hungary) with registration of the differential TG (DTG) and differential thermal analysis (DTA) data. The measurements were made under atmospheric pressure, at 30–1000 °C, in the static air atmosphere, at a heating rate of 10 °C/min.

The TG/MS/FTIR studies of coating were carried out using STA 449 F1 Jupiter (Netzsch, Selb, Germany) in the range of 30–1000 °C with the heating rate of 10 °C/min, in the synthetic air atmosphere with the gas flow 50 cm^3/min and the mass of the sample was about 4 mg. The apparatus was coupled simultaneously with Tensor 27 (Bruker, Karlsruhe, Germany) FTIR spectrometer as well as QMS 403 D Aëolos Quadro (Netzsch, Selb, Germany) quadrupole mass spectrometer in order to detect volatile products evolved during the analysis.

2.3.3. Wettability and Surface Free Energy

The contact angle measurements were made using the DigiDrop Contact Angle Meter (GBX, Romans-sur-Isère, France) equipped with a closed and thermostated chamber. The Milli-Q ultrapure water ($\gamma_l \cong 72.8$ mN/m at 20 °C) was used as the probe liquid. The sessile droplet technique was used as follows: a 6 µL droplet was settled on the examined surface and the advancing contact angle was measured, then 3 µL of liquid was sucked and the receding contact angle was measured. The contact angle values were calculated by the WinDrop++ software using the polynomial algorithm based on the droplet shape using the contour mode. Ten water droplets were measured and averaged along each surface in order to increase the measurement accuracy.

The surface free energy (SFE) of each sample was estimated using the contact angle hysteresis (CAH) approach proposed by Chibowski [48]:

$$\gamma_s = \gamma_l \frac{(1+\cos\theta_a)^2}{(1+\cos\theta_r)^2 - (1+\cos\theta_a)^2} \tag{1}$$

where: γ_s—the surface free energy, γ_l—the surface tension of the probe liquid, θ_a—the advancing contact angle, θ_r—the receding contact angle. This allows us to determine the SFE as the function of three directly measurable parameters: liquid surface tension and both advancing and receding contact angles.

2.3.4. Surface Topography and Thickness of the Coatings

The surfaces height maps were made using the ContourGT-K1 3D Optical Profiler (Bruker, Germany) in order to evaluate the surface roughness and to obtain information about its topography. The measurements were made with 5× objective at 1× magnification using the white light and VXI technique. The sampling area was 1261 μm × 946 μm. The roughness parameters were calculated using the Vision64 (ver. 5.41) software. The same equipment and procedure were used to estimate the thicknesses of the obtained coatings.

2.3.5. Scanning Electron Microscopy

The morphology of the carbon nanotubes as well as the obtained surfaces were studied using scanning electron microscopy. The images were taken using the Quanta 3D FEG (FEI, Hillsboro, USA) apparatus equipped with the secondary electron detector (SED)—an Everhart-Thornley detector (ETD). The beam operated at 20 kV in the case of CNTs samples or 30 kV in the case of coated surfaces (accelerating voltage for the electrons). The other specific parameters are shown in the SEM images. In the case of the carbon nanotubes samples, the quantitative SEM/EDS (energy dispersive X-ray spectroscopy) analysis was also performed.

2.3.6. X-Ray Diffraction Analysis (XRD)

The surface obtained by the dip-coating with the largest contact angle was examined by the Empyrean multipurpose diffractometer (Malvern Panalytical, Almelo, The Netherlands) with CuKα radiation. The small angle X-ray diffraction patterns were scanned at room temperature in the angular range 2θ from 6° to 95° with a step size of 0.02°.

2.3.7. Optical Properties

The Helios Gamma UV-Vis Spectrophotometer (Thermo Electron Corporation, Beverly, USA) was used in order to make the transmission measurements of the samples. The apparatus was equipped with the quartz-coated single-beam optical system with the 2 nm spectral bandwidth. The tungsten lamp and the deuterium lamp were used as light sources. The measurements were made at room temperature in the wavelength range from 190 nm to 800 nm with the 0.5 nm step, which corresponds to the ultraviolet C (UV-C) and visible (VIS) light. The obtained data were recorded by the VISION software and the baseline subtraction was made automatically.

3. Results and Discussion

The Turbiscan transmission profiles of the silica–MWCNTs/PDMS hybrid filler suspension are shown in Figure 1. Just after the synthesis, the transmission along the entire length of the flask was equal to zero because of the formation of an opaque, black product (the color comes from the carbon nanotubes). The increase in transmission at the top of the vessel over the time is due to the start of the gelling process and the phase separation—formation of a transparent solvent (alcohol) layer. To estimate the stability of the sample, the Turbiscan Stability Index (TSI) was calculated. This is a dimensionless indicator that allows one to compare the samples with each other and can vary in the range of 0–100. The value of the TSI is inversely proportional to the system stability [49]. The Turbiscan brochure states that up to the Turbiscan Stability Index equal to 1, the system is stable (referred to as Visually Excellent for TSI < 0.5 or Visually Good for TSI < 1.0). In this case, the TSI exceeded the value of 0.5 after 8 h 20 min. This means detecting the beginning of destabilization, but in a very early stage, this can be particles migration or size variation. The global TSI after 12 h is equal to 0.9, which allows to confirm the stability of the system during this time. It exceeded the value of 1.0 after 13 h 15 min, but the destabilization remains still invisible for the eye. The red curve shows the transmission profile for the system with complete gelling. The lowering of the upper meniscus of the sample is noteworthy. This confirms the formation of particle agglomerates and the reduction of their mobility, and thus the contraction of the system volume.

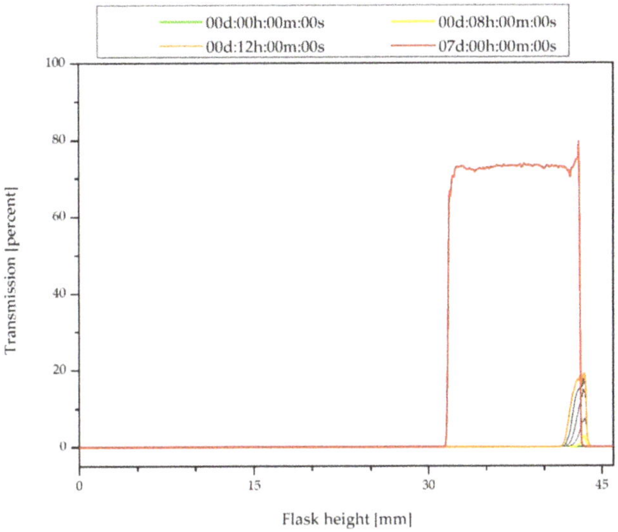

Figure 1. Transmission profiles of the silica–MWCNTs/PDMS hybrid filler suspension just after the synthesis.

As it can be observed in Figure 2, in the case of a composition for the dip-coating, the destabilization occurs faster. The TSI exceeded the value of 0.5 just after 6 min 28 s and 1.0 after 12 min 54 s. The value of 3.0 was reached after 38 min 32 s, which means that important stability destabilization occurs due to large sedimentation. In this stage, the destabilization may not be visible yet, but based on the transmission profiles in Figure 2, it can be concluded that the filler particles fall (sedimentation) to the bottom of the flask. If the composition is used for the spray coating, its stabilization should be considered.

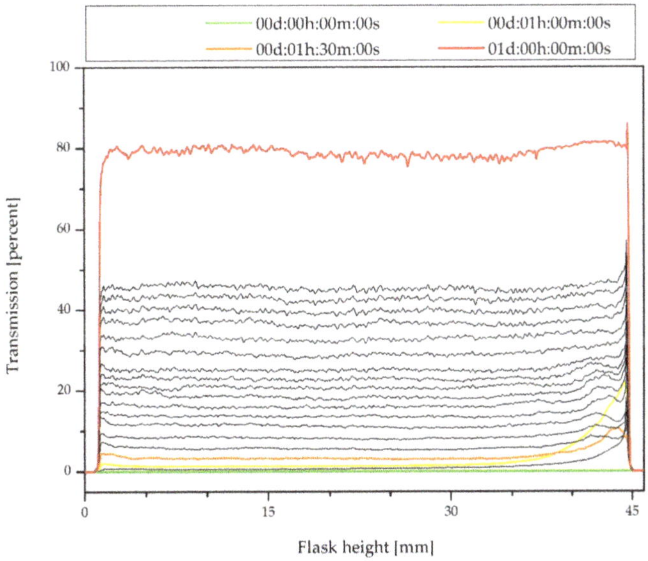

Figure 2. Transmission profiles of the coating composition just after the synthesis.

The zeta potential (ZP) of the obtained filler (dried gel) suspension in the 32.5% ethanol solution was equal to −11.1 mV. The negative value indicates the presence of negative charges on the nanoparticles surface. Therefore, it can be concluded that the surface silanol groups (Si-OH) take the form of the ionized Si-O⁻ species. They can initiate a cross-linking reaction of the silanol groups, which will result in the formation of the oxygen bridging between the nanoparticles and could induce its agglomeration [50]. The ability to create bonds with nanoparticles of the filler is desirable in the synthesis of a coating composition. The information about the surface charge and its structure also allows for the stabilization of the filler nanoparticles suspension.

The results of the thermal analysis of nonmodified multiwalled carbon nanotubes, PDMS, and the MWCNTs/PDMS composite are shown in Figure 3.

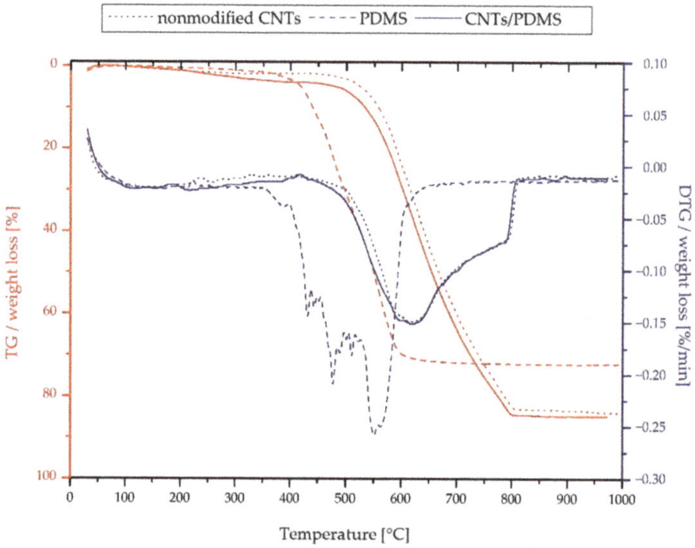

Figure 3. Thermal analysis of the MWCNTs, PDMS, and silica–MWCNTs/PDMS composite.

The first step of weight loss of the PDMS starts from about 290 °C and corresponds to the depolymerization reaction resulting in the volatile cyclic oligomers.

A significant weight loss in the second step from approximately 500 °C is caused by oxidation, which leads to the polymer residue decrease to even about 10% of its previous mass [51,52]. The pristine MWCNTs are thermally stable up to about 400 °C, but above 500 °C, the decomposition process proceeds relatively fast. It corresponds to the sample combustion and can be confirmed by the DTG curve due to the appearance of a high peak [53]. Figure 3 shows that the MWCNTs/PDMS composite decomposes at a much higher temperature than pure PDMS but not much lower than that of the unmodified carbon nanotubes. However, there is a slight initial weight loss at lower temperatures up to 500 °C, which can correspond to the depolymerization of PDMS.

The thermal analysis results of the coating material can be observed in Figure 4. In the first step, from about 60 °C to 200 °C, the adsorbed water is removed. This is confirmed by the DTG peak at 99.1 °C and the DSC peak corresponding to the heat necessary to evaporate the water (endothermic process). Moreover, in the mass spectrum in Figure 5, a strong signal at m/z equal to 17 and 18 can be observed as well as wide peaks in the range of 3000–3400 cm^{-1} in the FT-IR spectrum. The process in the range of 200–500 °C can be associated with decomposition of the surface methyl group due to hydrophobization by HMDS, which is confirmed by the peak in the FT-IR spectrum (Figure 5) in the range of 2800–3000 cm^{-1}. The combustion process of the material begins at a temperature above

600 °C, which confirms the release of carbon dioxide in both spectra in Figure 5. This can be confirmed by the DSC curve, which shows the exothermic peak in the range of 600–700 °C. In the case of the coating, the effects of earlier PDMS depolymerization cannot be clearly observed because the filler is predominantly built in the bulk phase of the material. This will be confirmed also by the SEM images of the surface as well as the XRD analysis further in this paper.

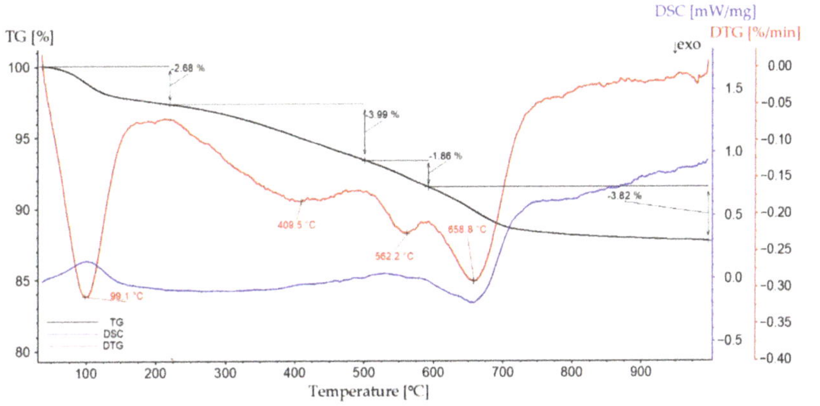

Figure 4. TG, DTG, and DSC curves of the coating.

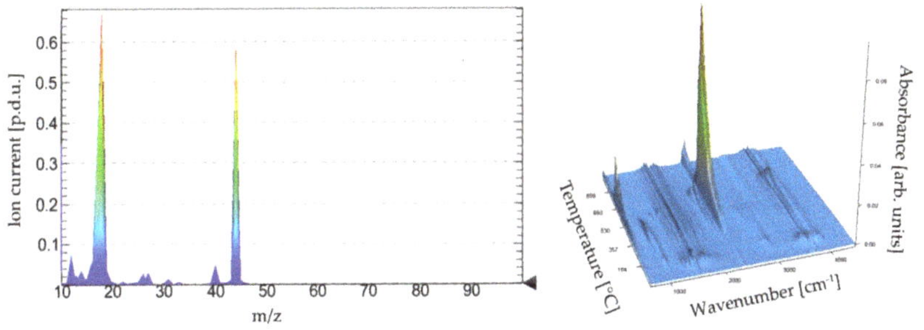

Figure 5. Mass and FT-IR spectra of volatile products of the thermal analysis of the coating.

The total weight loss is equal to 12.35%, of which 2.68% is adsorbed water. This is a significant difference compared to the decomposition of the main filler component, carbon nanotubes with adsorbed PDMS. Thus, it can be concluded that the obtained composite coating is characterized by better stability and thermal resistance.

The water contact angles (WCAs) on each sample are presented in Figure 6. On each real surface, the advancing contact angle is the highest one and the receding contact angle is the smallest contact angle possible to measure. Young's contact angle is somewhere between them, and its experimental measurements are practically impossible [54,55]. For this reason, in order to describe the wettability of the surfaces better, the equilibrium contact angles were calculated using Tadmor's approach [56].

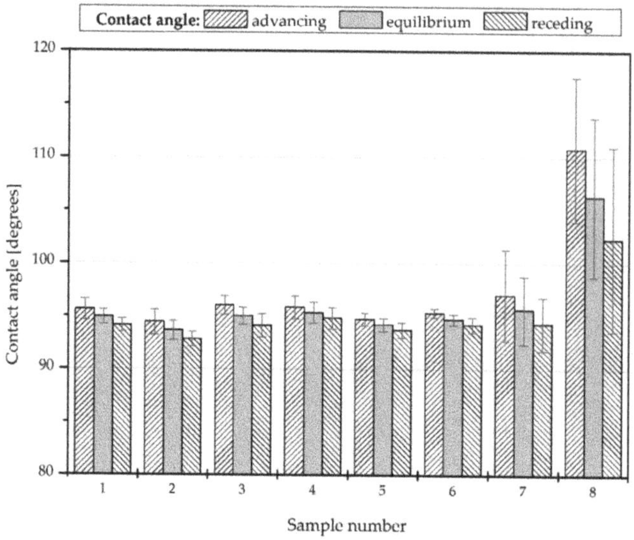

Figure 6. Water wettability of the obtained coatings.

The highest WCA, equal to 106.3 ± 7.5 degrees, can be observed in the case of sample #8. As shown in Figure 7, this surface is also characterized by the largest contact angle hysteresis (8.5 ± 4.1 degrees) and the smallest surface free energy (21.2 ± 3.8 mJ/m^2). This results from the method of applying the coating; the layer with the largest thickness and heterogeneity was obtained, which confirms its roughness parameters and the surface height map. The high standard deviations of the contact angles, contact angles hysteresis, and surface free energies indicate a wide physical and chemical heterogeneity of surfaces #7 and #8.

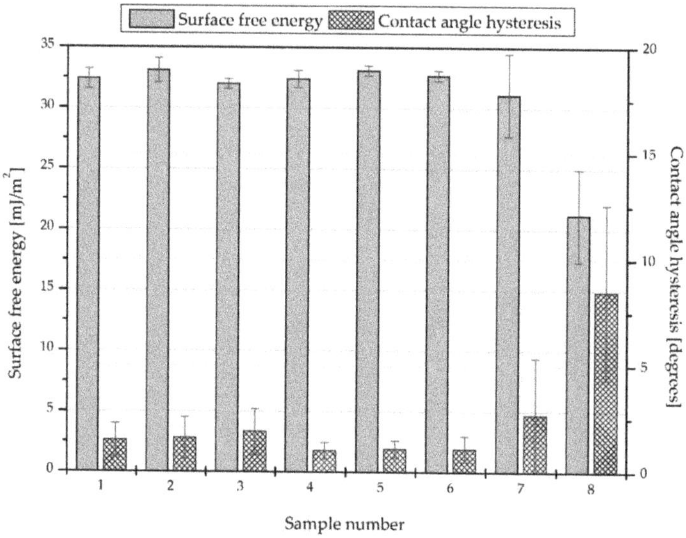

Figure 7. Surface free energies of the obtained surfaces.

Sample #4 has the largest contact angle (95.3 ± 1 degrees) among the samples obtained with the dip coating. However, the difference in the withdrawal speed in the critical range does not affect the surface properties of the produced coatings significantly; the equilibrium contact angles of the corresponding samples only differ by about one degree.

In the case of the air plasma modification of the support, a slight decrease in the water contact angle on the coating can be observed (sample #1 compared to #2 and sample #4 compared to #5), while argon plasma modification causes a slight increase of the contact angle (sample #1 compared to #3) or does not affect surface wettability (sample #4 compared to #6). Moreover, plasma activation will improve the coatings adhesion [57,58]. However, it is necessary to carry specialized durability tests out in order to investigate this phenomenon.

The linear (R) as well as the areal (S) roughness parameters of the obtained surfaces are presented in Table 3. The arithmetic mean deviation of the roughness profile (R_a) and the root mean square deviation of the roughness profile (R_q) are commonly used to describe surface roughness [59,60]. However, they are linear roughness parameters and do not take the entire sampling area into account, only the roughness profile along one of the arbitrary selected axes. As can be seen in Table 3, the linear parameters (R_a and R_q) differ significantly from the corresponding areal parameters (arithmetical mean height—S_a, and root mean square height—S_q). It is postulated that the areal parameters provide more information about the complexity of surfaces and allow for better understanding of surface morphology than the profile (linear) parameters [61]. Thus, the areal parameters were calculated, and they will be analyzed for better surface description.

Table 3. Linear and areal roughness parameters of the obtained surfaces.

	#1	#2	#3	#4	#5	#6	#7	#8
R_a [nm]	3.61	8.51	6.48	2.68	5.40	7.36	703.45	2.670×10^3
R_q [nm]	4.81	11.41	14.23	4.78	9.88	12.09	795.61	4.280×10^3
S_a [nm]	1.69	4.289	5.48	2.06	4.11	5.13	703.00	2.674×10^3
S_q [nm]	3.05	6.473	13.83	4.36	9.11	10.37	796.00	4.277×10^3
S_{sk}	6.77	1.426	−8.57	6.72	7.91	7.07	0.24	2.89
S_{ku}	104.25	25.253	730.91	81.48	142.70	118.27	5.23	18.70
S_{dq} [deg]	0.04	0.06	0.27	0.06	0.14	0.16	9.82	48.19
S_{dr} [%]	0	0	0.001	0	0	0	1.14	46.04
S_{ds} [1/mm^2]	339.01	546.797	162.36	467.72	350.79	418.09	1417.47	1195.38
S_{tr}	0.68	0.819	0.74	0.73	0.74	0.77	0.78	0.73

S_a and S_q are significantly higher in the case of samples #7 and #8—they differ by several orders of magnitude. This explains the different methods of applying the coatings, and thus obtaining a layer with a greater thickness and heterogeneity, compared to the other samples. This is reflected in the surface height maps in Figure 8, where there are more peaks and high flat areas compared to samples #1–#6. This is also the reason for the larger contact angles and contact angles hysteresis values on surfaces #7 and #8 as it was mentioned above. It should be kept in mind that the S_a and the S_q parameters can be specious for the surfaces with different spatial and height symmetries. They can have the same S_a or S_q while the texture will be completely different. Thus, other height, spatial or hybrid parameters for the obtained surfaces were calculated. The skewness (S_{sk}) for all surfaces, except #3, is a positive value. This indicates the predominance of peaks structures, while the negative value for sample #3 points out to predominance of the surface comprising valleys. The kurtosis (S_{ku}) evaluates sharpness in the height distribution; its value above 3.0 for all the samples means that there are excessively high peaks and/or deep valleys on these surfaces. The root mean square gradient (S_{dq}) represents the mean magnitude of the local slopes forming the surface—the greater the value of S_{dq}, the more steeply the surface is inclined. This is useful for differentiating surfaces with similar S_a values. Samples #2 and #5 are such an example. They are both deposited on the support activated by air plasma and characterized by similar S_a values (4.289 nm and 4.11 nm, respectively). However, coating #5 is described by a larger S_{dq} value (0.14°) than #2 (0.06°), which corresponds to the height maps in Figure 8; visually, there are more peaks on surface #5.

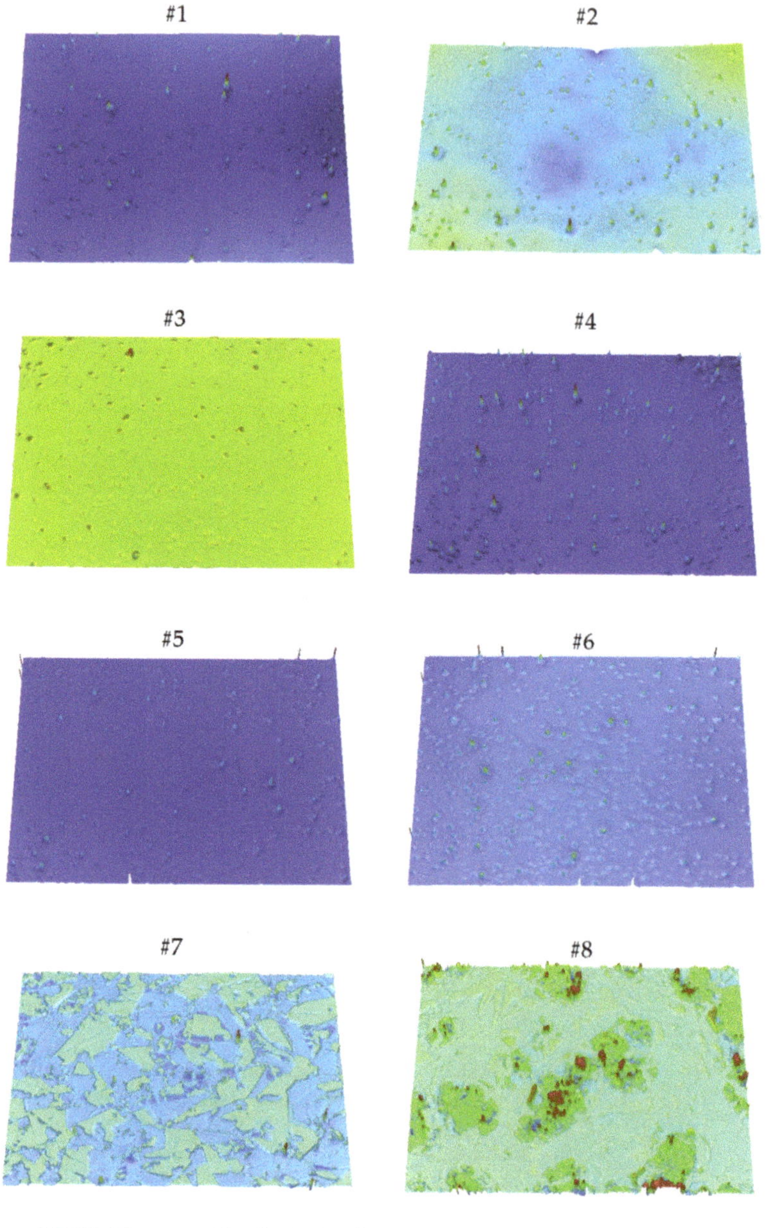

Figure 8. 3-D height maps of the obtained surfaces (sample number above the image).

S_{dq} can be also associated to the wetting degree of surface by various fluids. The developed interfacial area ratio (S_{dr}) describes in percentage the increasing surface area after applying coating compared to the flat surface of the support. It can be concluded that in the case of the samples produced by dip-coating, there are only microroughness due to small S_{dr} values, while on surfaces #7 and #8, there is macroroughness resulting from an increase in the surface area of up to about 10% and 50%, respectively. This confirms the summit density (S_{ds}) parameter, which corresponds to the number of summits per unit area making up the surface. Samples #1–#6 are described by smaller values of the S_{ds} due to single and sharp peaks, while samples #7 and #8 have wider summits. The texture aspect ratio (S_{tr}) evaluates directionality of the surface texture. For all samples, the S_{tr} values are greater than 0.5 with an average of 0.75, which indicates that the surfaces textures do not have periodicity in the specific direction. Regardless of the type of plasma, the modification of the substrate causes an increase in the surface roughness (characterized by the R_q or S_q parameter), and the effect is the most noticeable in the case of argon plasma.

Coatings #1–#3 and #4–#6 were applied with the dip-coating technique with the withdrawal speed equal to 50 mm/min and 20 mm/min, respectively. The differences in the withdrawal speed result in various thicknesses of the obtained layers [62]. In the case of the silica coatings prepared by the acid-assisted TEOS hydrolysis, the withdrawal speed in the range of 20–80 mm/min is referred to as the critical withdrawal speed. The value of 50 mm/min allows to get homogeneous, transparent, and crack-free silica coatings of a minimum film thickness [63]. The approximate thickness of the coatings in the case of its deposition by the dip-coating technique is about 0.46 μm, while for the manual immersion or spreading, it is about 0.79 μm.

The scanning electron microscopy images of the multiwalled carbon nanotubes are shown in Figure 9. In Figure 9a, the pristine nanotubes with a diameter of about 20 nm are presented. In Figure 9b, the MWCNTs/PDMS composite is presented. An increase in the diameter of the nanotubes and characteristic shading can be observed as a result of the PDMS adsorption.

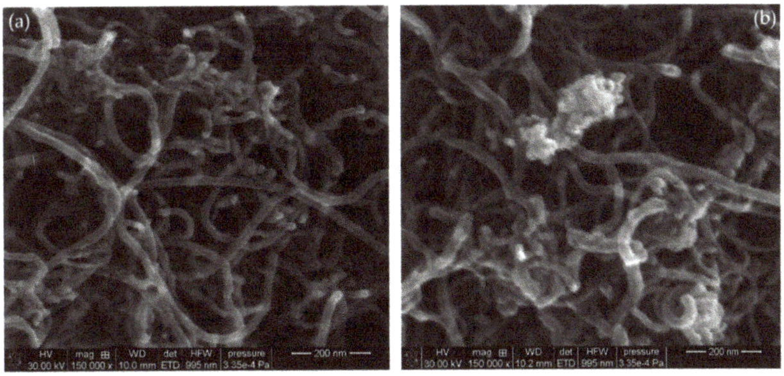

Figure 9. SEM images of MWCNTs: nonmodified (**a**) and modified with PDMS (**b**).

The SEM-EDS elementary analysis results of the carbon nanotubes are shown in Table 4. The effectiveness of PDMS adsorption is evidenced by the decrease in the carbon content from 92.96% to 88.37% with the simultaneous increase in the contents of oxygen and silicon, which are the polymer constituents. The remaining elements such as Mo or Fe are probably impurities left over from the nanotube synthesis process or introduced during the analysis.

The SEM images of samples #4 and #7 are shown in Figure 10. Both images show amorphous silica nanoparticles formed on the surface. More regular arrangement and larger sizes were obtained on surface #4 produced by the dip-coating method (Figure 10a). In the case of surface #7, which was coated manually, the nanoparticles are smaller, and the coverage of the support is heterogeneous. In both cases, the carbon nanotubes (filler particles) cannot be seen on the surface; this means that they are built into the bulk structure of the coating, which will be also confirmed by the XRD analysis (Figure 11).

Table 4. SEM-EDS elementary analysis of carbon nanotubes (MWCNTs): nonmodified and modified with PDMS.

Element [1]	MWCNTs	MWCNTs + PDMS
C	92.96	88.37
O	5.14	7.01
Si	0.46	3.13
Mo	0.39	0.45
Fe	1.06	0.89

[1] Element content in the carbon nanotubes in weight percent (wt%).

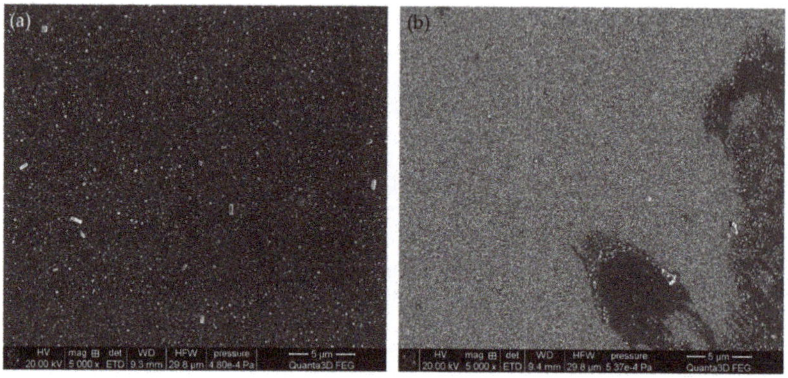

Figure 10. SEM images of the sample #4 (**a**) and #7 (**b**).

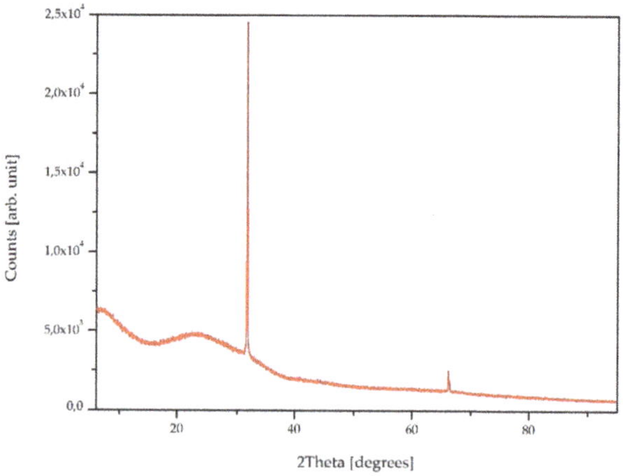

Figure 11. XRD pattern of the sample #4.

The XRD pattern of sample #4 is presented in Figure 11. There can be observed as a much broadened peak over the 2θ range of 20–30°, which corresponds to the amorphous silica structures on the surface [64]. However, the peaks at 32° (100 plane) and 66° also indicate the presence of trigonal silica [65]. This means that during the coating fabrication by the TEOS hydrolysis under the applied conditions, two forms of silica are created. As it was mentioned above, the XRD analysis showed no nanotubes in the top layer of the coating. The XRD patterns for the MWCNTs should appear at around 26° (indexed as 002 reflection of the hexagonal graphite structure) and 43° (100 graphitic planes) [66,67], but there is a lack of them.

As it is presented in Figure 12, the optical properties of the samples investigations show the formation of largely transparent composite films in the case of the samples produced by the dip-coating technique. The transmittance values of samples #1–#6 remain at about 95%. This value is a few percent smaller than for silica (pure polysiloxane coatings) without any filler [42]. However, it should be emphasized that the coatings include carbon nanotubes, the suspension of which during the stability tests revealed no transmission. Moreover, the differences are not significant, and furthermore, the transmission values are greater than for the uncoated glass substrate [42]. For manually applied coatings, the transmission is equal to 70% and only 30% for samples #7 and #8, respectively. This is due to the greater thickness and structure of the coatings, which was confirmed by the above optical profilometry, and therefore more nanotubes concentration in the optical path. The effects observed in the wavelength range of 190–350 nm and at 580 nm [68] were described in detail in our previous paper [42].

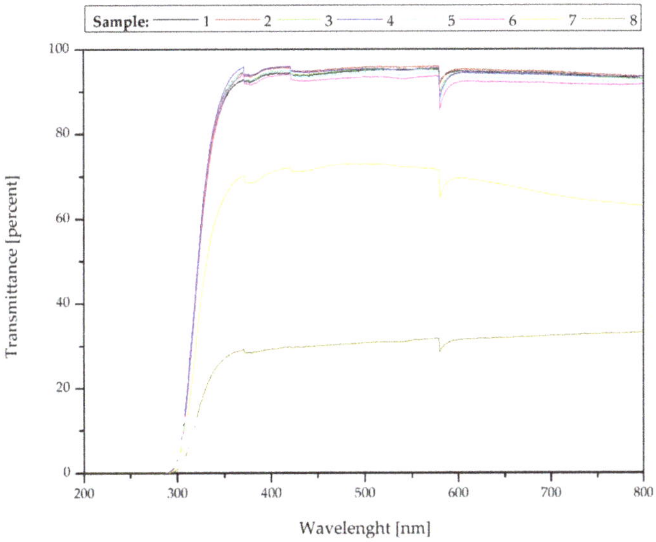

Figure 12. Optical properties—transmittance of the samples.

4. Conclusions

The silica–MWCNTs/PDMS composite coatings on the glass supports modified with cold plasma were fabricated using the quick and simple sol–gel method. The surfaces with water contact angles larger than 90 degrees were obtained; therefore, they can be described as hydrophobic ones. The influence of the type of plasma on the surface properties of the deposited coating was found. The thin films are largely transparent and rough, and the composite is thermally stable up to 250 °C. The SEM images, thermal analysis, and XRD analysis showed that the silica–MWCNTs/PDMS filler is in the bulk phase of the material, not on the surface. Additional investigations are required in order to study the effect of withdrawal speed on the coating thickness and composition. The results will be reported in a due course.

Author Contributions: Conceptualization and methodology, M.C. and K.T.; nanotubes design and synthesis, I.Y.S.; coating synthesis and application, M.C.; investigation, M.C., I.Y.S., K.T., and D.S.; writing—original draft preparation, M.C.; writing—review and editing, M.C. and K.T.; supervision, K.T. All authors have read and agreed to the published version of the manuscript.

Funding: This research received no external funding.

Institutional Review Board Statement: Not applicable.

Informed Consent Statement: Not applicable.

Data Availability Statement: Data are available within the sources mentioned in the references as well as collected by the authors during the experiments and included in this paper (raw data can be available on request from the corresponding author).

Acknowledgments: Not applicable.

Conflicts of Interest: The authors declare no conflict of interest.

References

1. Ciriminna, R.; Fidalgo, A.; Pandarus, V.; Béland, F.; Ilharco, L.; Pagliaro, M. The Sol-Gel Route to Advanced Silica-Based Materials and Recent Applications. *Chem. Rev.* **2013**, *113*, 6592–6620. [CrossRef] [PubMed]
2. Almeida, R.M.; Gonçalves, M.C. Chapter 8.8: Sol-Gel Process and Products. In *Encyclopedia of Glass Science, Technology, History, and Culture*; Richet, P., Conradt, R., Takada, A., Dyon, J., Eds.; John Wiley & Sons: Hoboken, NJ, USA, 2021.
3. Carrera-Figueiras, C.; Pérez-Padilla, Y.; Estrella-Gutiérrez, M.A.; Uc-Cayetano, E.G.; Juárez-Moreno, J.A.; Avila-Ortega, A. Surface Science Engineering through Sol-Gel Process. In *Applied Surface Science*; Injeti, G., Ed.; IntechOpen: London, UK, 2019.
4. Soyaslan, İ.İ. Thermal and sound insulation properties of pumice/polyurethane composite material. *Emerg. Mater. Res.* **2020**, *9*, 859–867. [CrossRef]
5. Salmi, L.D. Atomic Layer Deposition of Inorganic—Organic Hybrid Material Thin Films. Ph.D. Thesis, University of Helsinki, Helsinki, Finland, 2020.
6. Ozkazanc, E.; Ozkazanc, H. Multifunctional polyaniline/chloroplatinic acid composite material: Characterization and potential applications. *Polym. Eng. Sci.* **2019**, *59*, 66–73. [CrossRef]
7. Belardja, M.S.; Djelad, H.; Lafjah, M.; Lafjach, M.; Chouli, F.; Benyoucef, A. The influence of the addition of tungsten trioxide nanoparticle size on structure, thermal, and electroactivity properties of hybrid material–reinforced PANI. *Colloid Polym. Sci.* **2020**, *298*, 1455–1463. [CrossRef]
8. Iijima, S. Helical microtubules of graphitic carbon. *Nature* **1991**, *354*, 56–58. [CrossRef]
9. Salehi, S.; Maghmoomi, F.; Sahebian, S.; Zebarjad, S.; Lazzeri, A. A study on the effect of carbon nanotube surface modification on mechanical and thermal properties of CNT/HDPE nanocomposite. *J. Thermoplast. Compos. Mater.* **2021**, *34*, 203–220. [CrossRef]
10. Shi, X.; Hassanzadeh-Aghdam, M.K.; Ansari, R. A comprehensive micromechanical analysis of the thermoelastic properties of polymer nanocomposites containing carbon nanotubes with fully random microstructures. *Mech. Adv. Mater. Struct.* **2021**, *28*, 331–342. [CrossRef]
11. Gawęda, M.; Długoń, E.; Sowa, M.; Jeleń, P.; Marchewka, J.; Bik, M.; Mroczka, K.; Bezkosty, P.; Kusz, K.; Simka, W.; et al. Polysiloxane-Multiwalled Carbon Nanotube Layers on Steel Substrate: Microstructural, Structural and Electrochemical Studies. *J. Electrochem. Soc.* **2019**, *166*, D707–D717. [CrossRef]
12. Guo, C.; Itoh, K.; Sun, D.; Kondo, Y.; Fuji, M. Carbon Nanotube/Polysiloxane Foams with Tunable Absorption Bands for Electromagnetic Wave Shielding. *ACS Appl. Nano Mater.* **2020**, *3*, 5944–5954. [CrossRef]
13. Li, Y.; Li, Z.; Lei, L.; Lan, T.; Li, Y.; Li, P.; Lin, X.; Liu, R.; Huang, Z.; Fen, X.; et al. Chemical vapor deposition-grown carbon nanotubes/graphene hybrids for electrochemical energy storage and conversion. *FlatChem* **2019**, *15*, 100091. [CrossRef]
14. Raval, J.P.; Joshi, P.; Chejara, D.R. Carbon nanotube for targeted drug delivery. In *Applications of Nanocomposite Materials in Drug Delivery*; Woodhead Publishing: Sawston, UK, 2018; pp. 203–216.
15. Korri-Youssoufi, H.; Zribi, B.; Miodek, A.; Haghiri-Gosnet, A.M. Carbon-Based Nanomaterials for Electrochemical DNA Sensing. In *Nanotechnology and Biosensors*; Elsevier: Amsterdam, The Netherlands, 2018; pp. 113–150.
16. Husen, A.; Siddiqi, K.S. Carbon and fullerene nanomaterials in plant system. *J. Nanobiotechnol.* **2014**, *12*, 16. [CrossRef] [PubMed]
17. Basheer, B.V.; George, J.J.; Siengchin, S.; Parameswaranpillai, J. Polymer grafted carbon nanotubes—Synthesis, properties, and applications: A review. *Nano-Struct. Nano-Objects* **2020**, *22*, 100429.
18. Sulym, I.; Zdarta, J.; Ciesielczyk, F.; Sternik, D.; Derylo-Marczewska, A.; Jesionowski, T. Pristine and Poly(Dimethylsiloxane) Modified Multi-Walled Carbon Nanotubes as Supports for Lipase Immobilization. *Materials* **2021**, *14*, 2874. [CrossRef] [PubMed]
19. Afzal, M.; Ameeduzzafar; Alharbi, K.S.; Alruwaili, N.K.; Al-Abassi, F.A.; Al-Malki, A.A.L.; Kazmi, I.; Kumar, V.; Kamal, M.A.; Nadeem, M.S.; et al. Nanomedicine in treatment of breast cancer—A challenge to conventional therapy. *Semin. Cancer Biol.* **2021**, *69*, 279–292. [CrossRef]
20. Xue, C.H.; Wu, Y.; Guo, X.J.; Liu, B.Y.; Wang, H.D.; Jia, S.T. Superhydrophobic, flame-retardant and conductive cotton fabrics via layer-by-layer assembly of carbon nanotubes for flexible sensing electronics. *Cellulose* **2020**, *27*, 3455–3468. [CrossRef]
21. Ungvári, K.; Mészáros, S.; Szabó, A.; Hernádi, K.; Tóth, Z. In Vitro Biocompatibility Test of Multiwall Carbon Nanotubes with Human Osteoblast Cells: Potential Application for Bone Implant Interface Reinforcement. *J. Nanosci. Nanotechnol.* **2021**, *21*, 2394–2403. [CrossRef]
22. Gaviria, W.A.; Hersam, M.C. Chirality-Enriched Carbon Nanotubes for Next-Generation Computing. *Adv. Mater.* **2020**, *32*, 1905654. [CrossRef]
23. Ghalandari, M.; Maleki, A.; Haghighi, A.; Safdari Shadloo, M.; Alhuyi Nazari, M.; Tlili, I. Applications of nanofluids containing carbon nanotubes in solar energy systems: A review. *J. Mol. Liq.* **2020**, *313*, 113476. [CrossRef]

24. Wu, S.; Tahri, O. State-of-art carbon and graphene family nanomaterials for asphalt modification. *Road Mater. Pavement Des.* **2021**, *22*, 735–756. [CrossRef]
25. Shifa, M.; Tariq, F.; Chandio, A.D. Mechanical and electrical properties of hybrid honeycomb sandwich structure for spacecraft structural applications. *J. Sandw. Struct. Mater.* **2021**, *23*, 222–240. [CrossRef]
26. Rangelova, N.; Radev, L.; Nenkova, S.; Miranda Salvado, I.M.; Vas Fernandes, M.; Herzog, M. Methylcellulose/SiO_2 hybrids: Sol-gel preparation and characterization by XRD, FTIR and AFM. *Open Chem.* **2011**, *9*, 112–118. [CrossRef]
27. Li, S.; Liu, M. Synthesis and conductivity of proton-electrolyte membranes based on hybrid inorganic–organic copolymers. *Electrochim. Acta* **2003**, *48*, 4271–4276. [CrossRef]
28. Dul, S.; Ecco, L.G.; Pegoretti, A.; Fambri, L. Graphene/Carbon Nanotube Hybrid Nanocomposites: Effect of Compression Molding and Fused Filament Fabrication on Properties. *Polymers* **2020**, *12*, 101. [CrossRef] [PubMed]
29. Pachekoski, W.M.; Amico, S.C.; Pezzin, S.H.; Moraes d'Almeida, J.R. Carbon nanotube hybrid polymer composites: Recent advances in mechanical characterization. In *Hybrid Polymer Composite Materials: Properties and Characterisation*; Thakur, V.K., Thakur, M.K., Pappu, A., Eds.; Woodhead Publishing: Sawston, UK, 2017; pp. 133–150.
30. What Is Plasma Technology and What Are Its Applications? Available online: https://www.azonano.com/article.aspx?ArticleID=5280 (accessed on 30 August 2021).
31. Goldston, R.; Rutherford, P. *Introduction to Plasma Physics*; Institute of Physics Publishing: Bristol, UK, 1995.
32. Morozow, A.I. *Introduction to Plasma Dynamics*; CRC Press: Boca Raton, FL, USA, 2013.
33. Cocktail Party Physics. Chilling Out with Cold Plasmas. Available online: https://blogs.scientificamerican.com/cocktail-party-physics/chilling-out-with-cold-plasmas/ (accessed on 30 August 2021).
34. Misra, N.N.; Kaur, S.; Tiwari, B.K.; Kaur, A.; Singh, N.; Cullen, P.J. Atmospheric pressure cold plasma (ACP) treatment of wheat flour. *Food Hydrocoll.* **2015**, *44*, 115–121. [CrossRef]
35. Park, G.Y.; Park, S.J.; Choi, M.Y.; Koo, I.G.; Byun, J.H.; Hong, J.W.; Sim, J.Y.; Lee, J.K.; Collins, G.J. Atmospheric-pressure plasma sources for biomedical applications. *Plasma Sources Sci. Technol.* **2012**, *21*, 043001. [CrossRef]
36. Ananth, A.; Gandhi, M.S.; Mok, Y.S. A dielectric barrier discharge (DBD) plasma reactor: An efficient tool to prepare novel RuO_2 nanorods. *J. Phys. D Appl. Phys.* **2013**, *46*, 155202. [CrossRef]
37. Baklanov, M.R.; de Marneffe, J.F.; Shamiryan, D.; Urbanowicz, A.M.; Shi, H.; Rakhimova, T.V.; Huang, H.; Ho, P.S. Plasma processing of low-k dielectrics. *J. Appl. Phys.* **2013**, *113*, 041101. [CrossRef]
38. Kartel, M.; Sementsov, Y.I.; Mahno, S.; Trachevskiy, V.; Bo, W. Polymer composites filled with multiwall carbon nanotubes. *Univ. J. Mater. Sci.* **2016**, *4*, 23–31. [CrossRef]
39. Melezhyk, A.V.; Sementsov, Y.I.; Yanchenko, V.V. Synthesis of Fine Carbon Nanotubes on Coprecipitated Metal Oxide Catalysts. *Russ. J. Appl. Chem.* **2005**, *78*, 917–923. [CrossRef]
40. Sulym, I.; Kubiak, A.; Jankowska, K.; Sternik, D.; Terpiłowski, K.; Sementsov, Y.; Borysenko, M.; Deryło-Marczewska, A.; Jesionowski, T. Superhydrophobic MWCNTs/PDMS-nanocomposite materials: Preparation and characterization. *Physicochem. Probl. Miner. Process.* **2019**, *55*, 1394–1400.
41. Chodkowski, M.; Terpiłowski, K.; Goncharuk, O. Surface properties of the doped silica hydrophobic coatings deposited on plasma activated glass supports. *Physicochem. Probl. Miner. Process.* **2019**, *55*, 1450–1459.
42. Chodkowski, M.; Terpiłowski, K.; Pasieczna-Patkowska, S. Fabrication of transparent polysiloxane coatings on a glass support via the sol-gel dip coating technique and the effect of their hydrophobization with hexamethyldisilazane. *Physicochem. Probl. Miner. Process.* **2020**, *56*, 76–88. [CrossRef]
43. Smoluchowski, M. *Handbuch der Electrizität und des Magnetismus, Band II*; Barth-Verlag: Leipzig, Germany, 1921; pp. 366–427.
44. Delgado, A.V.; González-Caballero, F.; Hunter, R.J.; Koopal, L.K.; Lyklema, J. Measurement and interpretation of electrokinetic phenomena. *Pure Appl. Chem.* **2005**, *77*, 1753–1805. [CrossRef]
45. González, B.; Calvar, N.; Gómez, E.; Domínguez, Á. Density, dynamic viscosity, and derived properties of binary mixtures of methanol or ethanol with water, ethyl acetate, and methyl acetate at T = (293.15, 298.15, and 303.15) K. *J. Chem. Thermodyn.* **2007**, *39*, 1578–1588. [CrossRef]
46. Refractive Index of Ethanol Solutions. Available online: http://www.refractometer.pl/refraction-datasheet-ethanol (accessed on 28 June 2021).
47. Wyman, J. The dielectric constant of mixtures of ethyl alcohol and water from −5 to 40°. *J. Am. Chem. Soc.* **1931**, *53*, 3292–3301. [CrossRef]
48. Terpiłowski, K.; Hołysz, L.; Chodkowski, M.; Clemente Guinarte, D. What Can You Learn about Apparent Surface Free Energy from the Hysteresis Approach? *Colloids Interfaces* **2021**, *5*, 4. [CrossRef]
49. Matusiak, J.; Grządka, E. Stability of colloidal systems—A review of the stability measurements methods. *Annales Universitatis Mariae Curie-Sklodowska Sectio AA-Chemia* **2017**, *72*, 33–45. [CrossRef]
50. Xu, P.; Wang, H.; Tong, R.; Du, Q.; Zhong, W. Preparation and morphology of SiO_2/PMMA nanohybrids by microemulsion polymerization. *Colloid Polym. Sci.* **2006**, *284*, 755–762. [CrossRef]
51. Camino, G.; Lomakin, S.M.; Lazzari, M. Polydimethylsiloxane thermal degradation Part 1. Kinetic aspects. *Polymer* **2001**, *42*, 2395–2402. [CrossRef]
52. Sulym, I.; Klonos, P.; Borysenko, M.; Pissis, P.; Gun'ko, V.M. Dielectric and Thermal Studies of Segmental Dynamics in Silica/PDMS and Silica/Titania/PDMS Nanocomposites. *J. Appl. Polym. Sci.* **2014**, *131*, 1236–1246. [CrossRef]

53. Bužarovska, A.; Stefov, V.; Najdoski, M.; Bogoeva-Gaceva, G. Thermal analysis of multi-walled carbon nanotubes material obtained by catalytic pyrolysis of polyethylene. *Maced. J. Chem. Chem. Eng.* **2015**, *34*, 373–379. [CrossRef]
54. Chodkowski, M.; Terpiłowski, K. Significance of the receding contact angle in the determination of surface free energy. *Annales Universitatis Mariae Curie-Sklodowska Sectio AA-Chemia* **2018**, *73*, 61–80. [CrossRef]
55. Bormashenko, E. Wetting of real solid surfaces: New glance on well-known problems. *Colloid Polym. Sci.* **2013**, *291*, 339–342. [CrossRef]
56. Tadmor, R. Line energy and the relation between advancing, receding, and young contact angles. *Langmuir* **2004**, *20*, 7659–7664. [CrossRef]
57. Cui, L.; Ranade, A.N.; Matos, M.A.; Dubois, G.; Dauskardt, R.H. Improved Adhesion of Dense Silica Coatings on Polymers by Atmospheric Plasma Pretreatment. *ACS Appl. Mater. Interfaces* **2013**, *5*, 8495–8504. [CrossRef]
58. Soma Raju, K.R.C.; Sowntharya, L.; Lavanya, S.; Subasri, R. Effect of plasma pretreatment on adhesion and mechanical properties of sol-gel nanocomposite coatings on polycarbonate. *Compos. Interfaces* **2012**, *19*, 259–270. [CrossRef]
59. Webb, H.K.; Truong, V.K.; Hasan, J.; Fluke, C.; Crawford, R.J.; Ivanova, E.P. Roughness Parameters for Standard Description of Surface Nanoarchitecture. *Scanning* **2012**, *34*, 257–263. [CrossRef]
60. Raghavendra, C.R.; Basavarajappa, S.; Sogalad, I.; Saunshi, V.K.K. Study on surface roughness parameters of nano composite coatings prepared by electrodeposition process. *Mater. Today Proc.* **2021**, *38*, 3110–3115. [CrossRef]
61. He, B.; Ding, S.; Shi, Z. A comparison between profile and areal surface roughness parameters. *Metrol. Meas. Syst.* **2021**, *28*, 413–438.
62. Faustini, M.; Louis, B.; Albouy, P.A.; Kuemmel, M.; Grosso, D. Preparation of Sol−Gel Films by Dip-Coating in Extreme Conditions. *J. Phys. Chem. C* **2010**, *114*, 7637–7645. [CrossRef]
63. Figus, C.; Patrini, M.; Floris, F.; Fornasari, L.; Pellacani, P.; Marchesini, G.; Valsesia, A.; Artizzu, F.; Marongiu, D.; Saba, M.; et al. Synergic combination of the sol–gel method with dip coating for plasmonic devices. *Beilstein J. Nanotechnol.* **2015**, *6*, 500–507. [CrossRef]
64. Zhou, Z.H.; Xue, J.M.; Wang, J.; Chan, H.S.O.; Yu, T.; Shen, Z.X. $NiFe_2O_4$ nanoparticles formed in situ in silica matrix by mechanical activation. *J. Appl. Phys.* **2002**, *91*, 6015–6020. [CrossRef]
65. Martínez, J.R.; Palomares-Sánchez, S.; Ortega-Zarzosa, G.; Ruiz, F.; Chumakov, Y. Rietveld refinement of amorphous SiO_2 prepared via sol–gel method. *Mater. Lett.* **2006**, *60*, 3526–3529. [CrossRef]
66. He, X.; Xu, X.; Bo, G.; Yan, Y. Studies on the effects of different multiwalled carbon nanotube functionalization techniques on the properties of bio-based hybrid non-isocyanate polyurethane. *RSC Adv.* **2020**, *10*, 2180–2190. [CrossRef]
67. Nie, P.; Min, C.; Song, H.J.; Chen, X.; Zhang, Z.; Zhao, K. Preparation and Tribological Properties of Polyimide/Carboxyl-Functionalized Multi-walled Carbon Nanotube Nanocomposite Films Under Seawater Lubrication. *Tribol. Lett.* **2015**, *58*, 7. [CrossRef]
68. Carter, S.F.; France, P.W. Drawing induced absorption loss in multicomponent glass fibres. *J. Non-Cryst. Solids* **1983**, *58*, 47–55. [CrossRef]

applied sciences

MDPI

Article

The Effect of Oxygen Admixture with Argon Discharges on the Impact Parameters of Atmospheric Pressure Plasma Jet Characteristics

Atif H. Asghar [1] and Ahmed Rida Galaly [2,3,*]

1 Department of Environmental and Health Research, The Custodian of the Two Holy Mosques Institute for Hajj and Umrah Research, Umm Al-Qura University, Makkah 24381, Saudi Arabia; ahasghar@uqu.edu.sa
2 Department of Engineering Science, Faculty of Community, Umm Al-Qura University, Makkah 24381, Saudi Arabia
3 Department of Physics, Faculty of Science, Beni-Suef University, Beni-Suef 62521, Egypt
* Correspondence: argalaly@uqu.edu.sa

Abstract: Dry argon (Ar) discharge and wet oxygen/argon (O_2/Ar) admixture discharge for alternating current atmospheric pressure plasma jets (APPJs) were studied for Ar discharges with flow rates ranging from 0.2 to 4 slm and for O_2/Ar discharges with different O_2 ratios and flow rates ranging from 2.5 to 15 mslm. The voltage–current waveform signals of APPJ discharge, gas flow rate, photo-imaging of the plasma jet length and width, discharge plasma power, axial temperature distribution, optical emission spectra, and irradiance were investigated. Different behavior for varying oxygen content in the admixture discharge was observed. The temperature recognizably decreased, axially, far away from the nozzle of the jet as the flow rate of dry argon decreased. Similar behavior was observed for wet argon but with a lower temperature than for dry argon. The optical emission spectra and the dose rate of irradiance of a plasma jet discharge were investigated as a function of plasma jet length, for dry and wet Ar discharges, to determine the data compatible with the International Commission on Non-Ionizing Radiation Protection (ICNIRP) data for irradiance exposure limits of the skin, which are suitable for the disinfection of microbes on the skin without harmful effects, equivalent to 30 μJ/mm^2.

Keywords: atmospheric pressure plasma jet; oxygen/argon admixture; electrical and optical properties; emission intensity; dose of irradiance

Citation: Asghar, A.H.; Galaly, A.R. The Effect of Oxygen Admixture with Argon Discharges on the Impact Parameters of Atmospheric Pressure Plasma Jet Characteristics. *Appl. Sci.* **2021**, *11*, 6870. https://doi.org/10.3390/app11156870

Academic Editor: Bogdan-George Rusu

Received: 10 May 2021
Accepted: 12 July 2021
Published: 26 July 2021

1. Introduction

Plasma, in physical science, is the fourth state of matter. In technological applications, plasma can exist in different forms and can be created as thermal and non-thermal plasma. Plasma technology is improving in many applications such as medical, industrial, and environmental applications [1].

The deposition of thin films, the treatment of organic and inorganic surfaces, the surface modification of polymer films, and the processing of materials are commonly conducted using plasma. Using plasma in such applications is considered to provide the most uniform and controlled treatment [2].

Plasma technology is very rich in its applications, especially in the killing of microorganisms on rigid or smooth surfaces [3]. Many researchers have studied glow discharge plasma at atmospheric pressure because of its technological simplicity; no vacuum system is needed, a greater choice of supply gases is available, and the technology is inexpensive [4].

Cold plasma applications are acceptable from an ecological and economical point of view. The physical application of cold plasma as a modern disinfection method is of great importance because of increasingly strict environmental demands [5].

Low-temperature gas plasma applications dealing with the protocols of killing microorganisms have opened new fields in biotechnology applications. Recently, glow discharge plasma at atmospheric pressure has attracted significant attention, leading to many evaluations of the disinfection of bacteria by air plasmas at atmospheric pressure such as medical, environmental, and industrial evaluations [6].

The configurations, characteristics, and applications of a cold plasma jet emerging by APPJ have attracted much attention: (i) configurations [7,8], such as electrode design, gas type, emerging plasma frequency, and flow rate; (ii) characteristics of the jet [9,10], such as length, width, temperature, emission spectra, irradiance, direct and indirect exposure, consumed energy, and consumed power; (iii) applications [11,12], such as the inactivation of microbes (water purification, sterilization, and wound healing), coating and etching (polymeric surface modification and synthesis of nanostructures), and medical applications (teeth bleaching, skin treatments, and cancer treatment).

Moreover, there are important factors that affect the APPJ performance, such as tube dimensions and powering characteristics: (i) tube dimensions include material, shape, length, and the outer and inner diameter of the tube [13]; (ii) powering characteristics include power source, applied voltage, and frequency [14].

Many publications have discussed the various applications of APPJs, such as the effect of the antimicrobial agent ratio on *Escherichia coli* and its application in fresh-cut cucumbers by studying the survival curve shapes of different microbes, using the effects of different impact parameters on the characteristics of the plume emerging from the APPJ [15–17].

The present work represents the characteristics of the cold plasma plume emerging from the APPJ under an alternating current (AC); these characteristics were studied by measuring the optical and electrical properties of the APPJ. These properties included the discharge voltage and current, output plasma power, axial distribution of temperature, flow rate, jet length, jet width, emission intensity of the plume, emission spectra, and the amount of energy emitted at each wavelength per unit area from the plasma jet using different gases, such as pure argon and an admixture of oxygen and argon at different ratios.

2. Experimental Set-Up and Procedures

Figure 1a shows a systematic diagram of a non-thermal APPJ using Ar and O_2/Ar admixture discharges. The ceramic tube is the main part in the APPJ, with 2 mm and 1.5 mm for the outer and inner diameters, respectively. The APPJ dimensions and powering characteristics are given in Table 1. The APPJ consists of three electrodes: two isolated hollow cylindrical copper electrodes around the ceramic tube, with 20 mm separation from each other, one electrode powered by an AC high-voltage power source with a voltage ranging from 2.5 to 25 kV and a variable frequency of up to 60 kHz, and another electrode grounded at 40 mm away from the nozzle and 20 mm from the high voltage electrode. Moreover, the aluminum inner capillary with a 1.5 mm diameter represents the third electrode of the discharge, with the whole ceramic tube length ended with the nozzle and described in Figure 1a with the dotted line inside the tube, also described briefly in our previous work [18]. Gas flows into the ceramic tube from two gas inlets, one for argon gas and the other for oxygen to admix inside the aluminum capillary tube, which is maintained in a floating potential.

The flow rates were measured using a volumetric flow meter connected to a needle valve to control the flow rates. The APPJ system creates discharges using: (i) flow rates ranging from 0.2 to 4 slm for Ar discharges (dry argon); (ii) O_2/Ar admixture discharges (wet argon) with different O_2 ratio admixtures, as shown in Table 2.

(a)

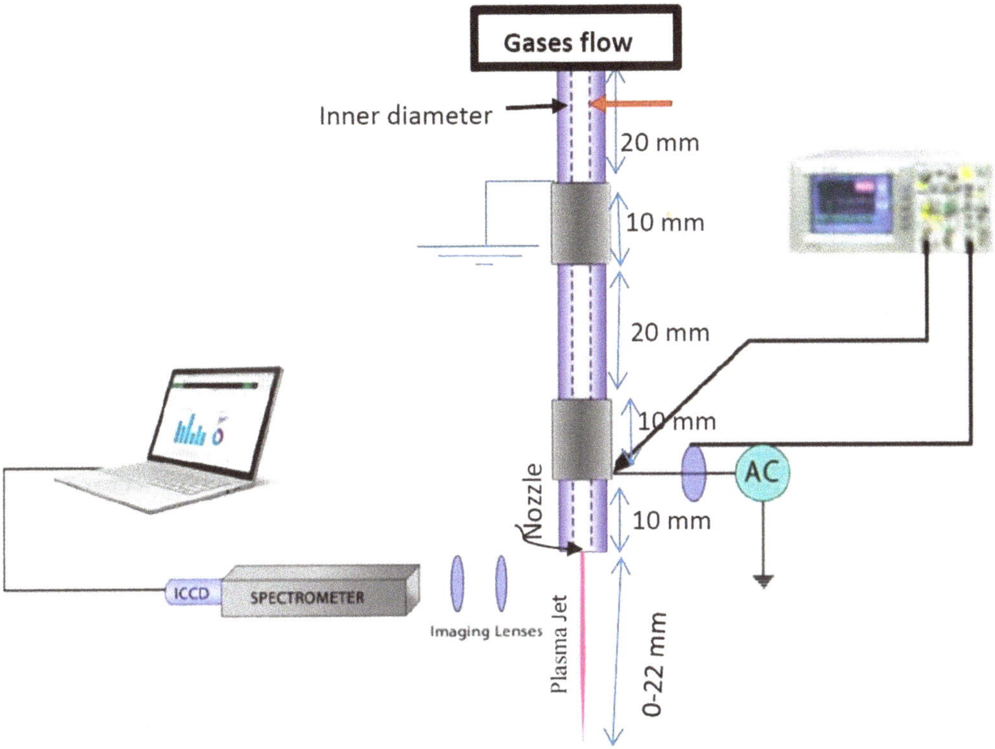

(b)

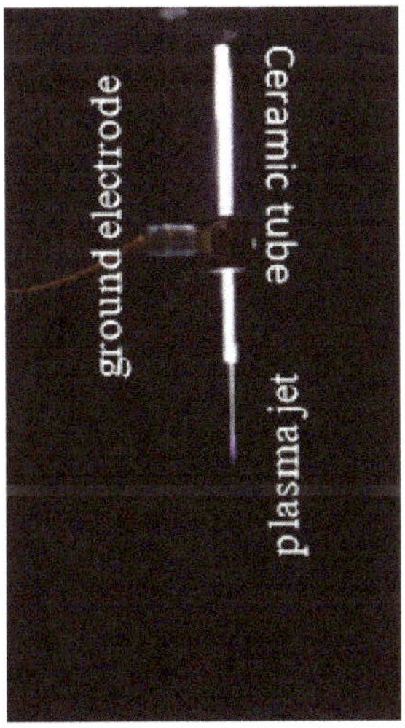

Figure 1. *Cont.*

(c)

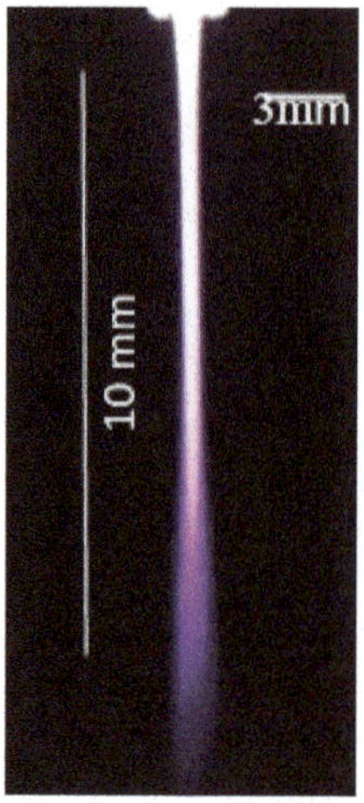

Figure 1. (**a**) Schematic diagram of APPJ experimental set-up; (**b**) Typical example of a ground electrode; (**c**) Plasma jet width and length as calibration scale.

Table 1. Tube dimensions and powering characteristics.

Tube dimensions	Ceramic	Material
	Cylindrical	Shape
	70 mm	Length
	2 mm	Outer diameter
	1.5 mm	Inner diameter (Nozzle)
Powering characteristics	AC high voltage	Power source
	2.5 to 25 kV	Applied voltage
	60 kHz	Frequency

Table 2. Equivalent O_2 flow rate ratio.

O_2 Flow Rate	Equivalent O_2 Ratio
2.5 mslm	0.25%
5 mslm	0.50%
10 mslm	1%
15 mslm	1.5%

The thermal, electrical, spectroscopical, and photographical characteristics of plasmas generated by the APPJ were measured: (i) measurements used a digital Canon camera (Ota City, Tokyo, Japan) with an exposure time of 40 ms for fast-imaging the emerging jet afterglow discharge in a darkened laboratory. The length and width of the jet measurements can be accurately measured relative to the ground electrode as a reference (the ground electrode with length and width 10 and 3 mm, respectively), as shown in Figure 1b. (ii) Jet dimensions can be calculated from APPJ images according to the dimensions of the ground electrode, as a calibration scale, using Microsoft Paint, as shown in Figure 1c. The calibrations and measurements are discussed briefly in our previous work, ref. [18]. (iii) An avaspec-2048 spectrometer (Louisville, CO, USA) with a charge coupled device (CCD) detector was used to measure the axial distribution emission spectra of the APPJ, from the nozzle to far away. The spectral range of the spectrometer was 200 to 1100 nm with a spectral resolution of 1.4 nm. A Fiber Optics Cable (FOC) was connected to the spectrometer and collected emitted light from the APPJ via a lens at the end of the FOC. (iv) A Fluoroptic thermometer (Model No.604, Luxtron Corporation, Santa Clara, CA, USA) was used to measure the average plasma temperature for Ar and O_2/Ar discharges. (v) A Tektronix P6015A probe (Beaverton, OR, USA) equipped with a high voltage probe and a current probe was used to measure the applied voltage U (kV) and discharge current I (mA) of the jet. (v) The dose rate of the APPJ plume irradiance per unit area was measured using an 818-RAD irradiance and dosage sensor (MKS/Newport, Model No.: 818-RAD, Newport Beach, CA, USA), compatible with a 1919-R optical power meter with the following characteristics: 8 mm aperture, 200–850 nm spectral wavelength range, 100–250 mW/cm^2 irradiance range, and 30 W/cm^2 maximum power density.

Different gas admixtures were used: a mixture of oxygen with argon at different ratios, where the mass flow rate of each gas was controlled and the gases flowed into a ceramic tube. Waveform signals of APPJ discharge were recorded using a 350 MHz digital oscilloscope, for which the applied voltage was measured using a Tektronix P6015A high-voltage probe; the discharge current was observed by measuring the voltage over a resistance equivalent to 33 kΩ. The average discharge power can be calculated using the voltage–current waveforms of the discharges and integrating the product of the discharge voltage U (kV) and discharge current I (mA) over one cycle as in Equation (1):

$$P = f \int_{t_0}^{t_0+T} U(t)\, I(t)\, dt. \qquad (1)$$

P is the average power of the discharge, and $f = \frac{1}{T}$; f and T are the frequency and period of the discharge, respectively. In the case of a sinusoidal waveform, Equation (1) can be written [19]:

$$P = I_{\text{rms}}\, U_{\text{rms}}\, \cos(\varphi), \qquad (2)$$

where $I_{\text{rms}} = \frac{I_0}{\sqrt{2}}$ and $U_{\text{rms}} = \frac{U_0}{\sqrt{2}}$ are the root mean square (rms) current and rms voltage, respectively. I_0 and U_0 are the peak values of current and voltage, respectively, and φ is the phase angle between the discharge voltage and current.

The recent study in this article represents the control parameters of the plume generated by the APPJ using cold plasma. The measured jet parameters included length and width, power, applied voltage, pure argon concentration, and different admixtures of oxygen and argon plasma discharge.

The 3rd electrode with the narrow diameter, the powering characteristics, and gas flow rate contribute to:

a. Control in the jet dimensions such as width, length, and covered area;
b. Control in the lifetime of the discharge process mode, whether laminar flow mode or turbulent flow mode;
c. Control in the heat impact emerging from the nozzle;
d. Control in the antibacterial effect factors of culture media down the nozzle such as exposure time, optical emission spectra, and irradiance.

3. Results and Discussion

3.1. Voltage–Current Waveform Signals of APPJ Discharge

The electrical properties of APPJ discharge for dry argon (pure Ar) and different oxygen/argon admixtures (wet argon) were investigated. Figure 2a–d show the current–voltage waveform of the APPJ discharge where: (i) Figure 2a shows the voltage waveform, plus the current waveforms of the APPJ discharge as follows: (ii) Figure 2b shows an Ar flow rate of 1 slm and discharge plasma power of 2.5 W; (iii) Figure 2c shows an admixture of 1 slm Ar flow rate with 0.25% (O_2) and a discharge plasma power of 1.77 W; and (iv)

Figure 2d shows an admixture of 1 slm Ar flow rate with 1.5% (O_2) and a discharge plasma power of 1.65 W.

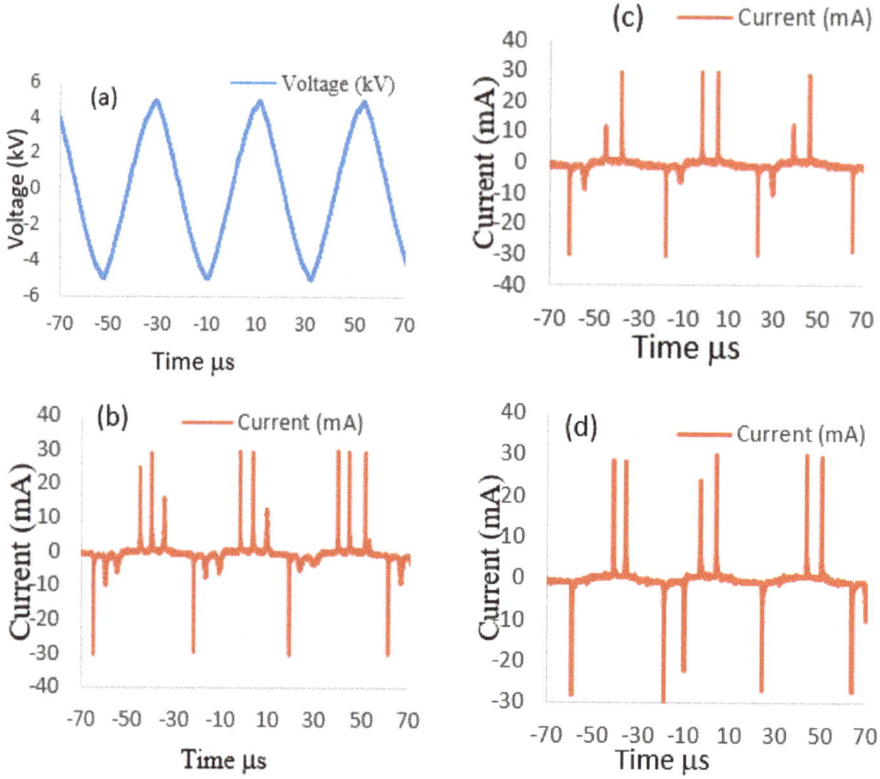

Figure 2. (**a**) Voltage waveform and current waveforms for (**b**) 1 slm argon gas, (**c**) admixture of argon 1 slm/0.25% oxygen, and (**d**) admixture of argon 1 slm/1.5% oxygen.

Figure 2a shows that the applied voltage is sinusoidal with 11.2 kV as the peak-to-peak voltage. The discharge current (I mA) consists of a displacement current (Figure 2b–d) [20,21], three short peaks for pure argon (Figure 2b), and one or two peaks for the O_2/Ar admixture (Figure 2c,d), appearing at every half cycle. Generally, these peaks appear because of the glow-like discharge when the plasma is formed [22,23]. The number of the current peaks decreased when the admixture of oxygen increased, as shown from Figure 2b to Figure 2d, due to the reduction in the sheath creation around the jet. The decreasing average discharge plasma power for increasing oxygen/argon ratios is attributed to increasing numbers of collisions among particles with an increasing flow rate; moreover, additional particles will contribute to energy exchange [24,25].

3.2. Gas Flow Rate

The discharge plasma power does not depend only on the applied peak-to-peak voltage, but also on the gas flow rate. The applied peak-to-peak voltage is limited to 11.2 kV for our experiment. Figure 3a shows the influence of the flow rate on the discharge plasma power for the emerging jet of pure argon discharge: the flow rate increases from 0.2 to 3 slm, and the argon discharge plasma power increases from 1.95 to 2.4 W. By increasing the argon flow rate further to 4 slm, the discharge plasma power begins to decrease, from 2.31 to

1.7 W [26]. Figure 3b shows that for oxygen/argon admixtures (see Table 2), the discharge plasma power of the emerging jet decreases from 1.75 to 1.65 W, for oxygen admixture ratios increasing from 0.25% to 1.5% [27]. As the oxygen percentages increases, ions, atoms, and free radicals are produced due to inelastic collisions, leading to losses in the discharge process and lower power than in the case of argon discharges. This is useful in sterilization and inactivation because of the longer interaction between the jet and the sample.

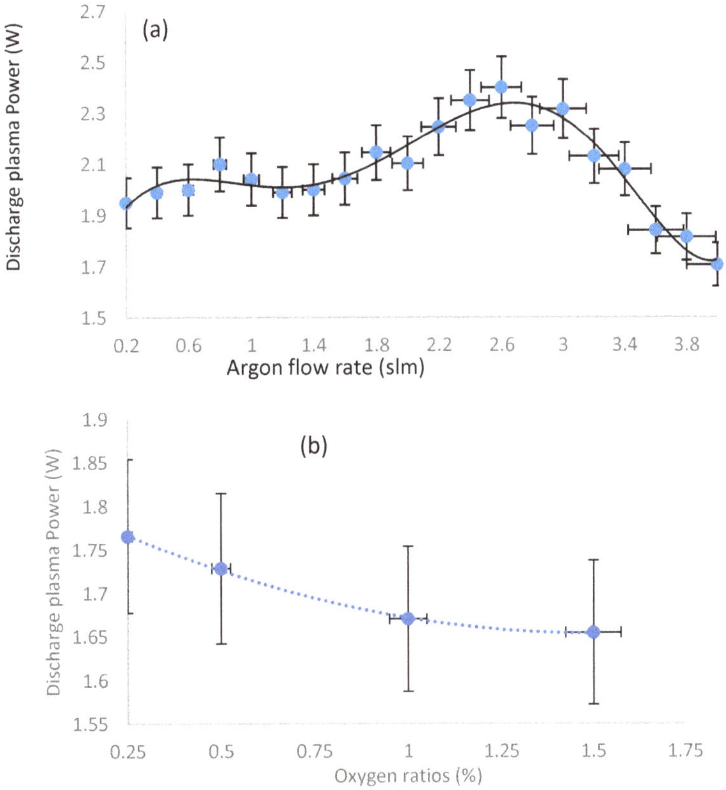

Figure 3. Influence of different flow rates on discharge plasma power (**a**) for pure argon, (**b**) for different oxygen ratios.

3.3. Length and Width of the Jet

Measurement of the length and width of the jet of argon and oxygen/argon admixture discharges, for different flow rates and different discharge plasma powers of the emerging jet, can be performed by photo-imaging the plasma jet. Figure 4a represents eight photo images of an argon discharge as a function of flow rate (from 0.2 to 4 slm). Figure 4b represents four photo images of an oxygen/argon discharge as a function of oxygen ratio (from 0.25% to 1.5%). The images were taken in a darkened laboratory. All the photo images, depending on the calibrated length and width of the ground electrode (10 and 3 mm, respectively), as shown in Figure 1c, were taken as a reference for measuring the length and the width of the emerging jet. As shown in Figure 4, the jet is tilted and not vertical, which may be due to the sheath around the jet besides the edge effect of the jet.

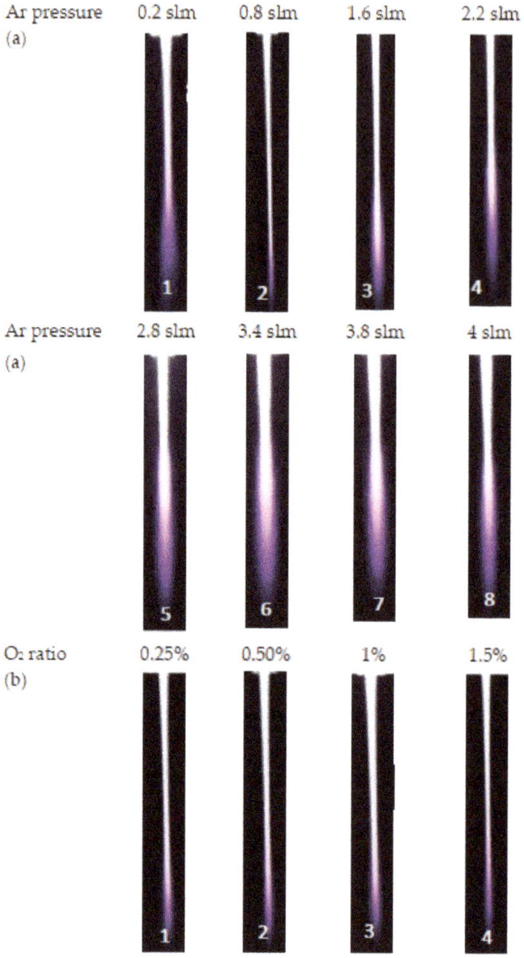

Figure 4. (**a**) Photo-imaging of the plasma jet lengths for argon discharge as a function of flow rate from 0.2 slm to 4 slm, and (**b**) Photo-imaging of the plasma jet lengths for oxygen ratio from 0.25% to 1.5%.

Figure 5a shows the plasma jet length for an argon discharge as a function of flow rate from 0.2 to 4 slm. The plasma jet length decreases from 20.6 to 10.7 mm with increasing flow rate from 0.2 to 2 slm and begins to stabilize at an average jet length of 9.8 mm when the flow rate increases from 2.2 to 4 slm. Figure 5b shows the plasma jet length of an oxygen/argon discharge as a function of the oxygen ratio admixture with 1 slm of Ar; with increasing oxygen concentration using oxygen ratios from 0.25% to 1.5%, the plasma length decreases from 17.9 to 15.6 mm. This may be because of an electronegative property of oxygen, to attract electrons, meaning that the effects on the discharge intensity diminish, as does the plasma jet length [28].

The width of the jet is an active and interesting parameter that depends on plasma jet length and the applied flow rates of argon and oxygen. The width is a guideline for the maximum area of irradiance emerging from the jet and reaching the exposed sample.

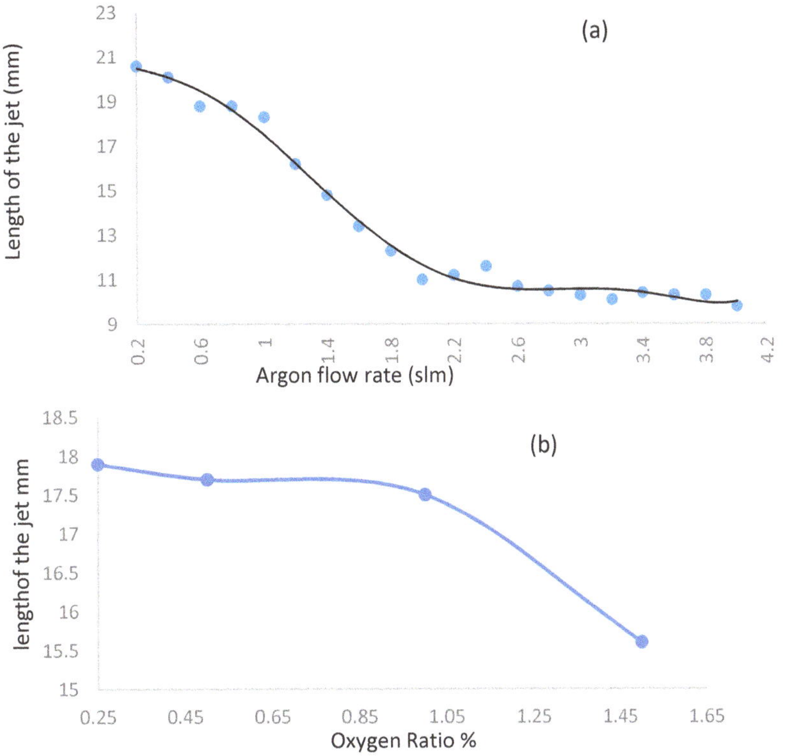

Figure 5. Influence of different flow rates on the length of the emerging plasma jet (**a**) for pure argon, (**b**) for oxygen ratios with argon flow rate 1 slm.

For the argon discharge, Figure 6a shows that in group I_{Ar}, as the flow rate increases from 1.2 to 2 slm, the jet width increases axially to a maximum of 1.39 to 2.07 mm, for a plasma jet length of 13.2 mm; the jet length then begins to decrease recognizably to between 0.56 and 1.5 mm, for a plasma jet length of 15.4 mm. Figure 6b shows that in group II_{Ar}, as the flow rate increases from 2.8 slm to 4 slm, the jet width increases axially to a maximum of 1.88 to 1.1 mm, for a plasma jet length of 8.8 mm; the jet width begins to decrease recognizably to between 1.4 and 0.6 mm, for a plasma jet length of 11 mm.

Figure 6a,b show that the best flow rates of dry argon, which obtain maximal irradiance that emerges from the jet and reaches the exposed samples, are moderate flow rates (2–2.8 slm). These moderate flow rates represent the maximum transition region from the laminar flow mode to the turbulent flow mode to obtain the largest widths, help to cover the largest exposure area of sample and accelerate the antibacterial process by dry argon, as discussed and applied in our previous work [29].

Figure 7a,b show the influence of the flow rate ratio of oxygen on the width and the length of the jet, from 0.25%, 0.5%, and 1% to 1.5% admixture with 1 slm of Ar, where two phases will be observed as follows:

(a) Figure 7a shows the jet width for wet argon as a function of plasma jet length less than 10 mm, at different applied flow rate ratios of oxygen, ranging from 0.25% to 1.5%. As the flow rate ratio of oxygen increases, the jet width recognizably decreases axially to a minimum of 0.609 to 0.366 mm, for a plasma jet length of 8.8 mm.
(b) Figure 7a shows the jet width for wet argon as a function of plasma jet length, ranging from 11 to 18 mm, at different applied flow rate ratios of oxygen, ranging from 0.25% to 1.5%. As the flow rate ratio of oxygen increases, the jet width begins to

increase, reaching a wider scale from 0.561 to 1.196 mm, for a plasma jet length of 17.6 mm. This means that, as in Figure 7b, as the admixture values of oxygen flow rates increase, elongating the axial length dimension of the jet, and increase the width dimensions of the plasma jet. Tables 3 and 4 give the largest width dimension values at the equivalent length dimensions of jet for an argon and oxygen/argon admixture discharge, respectively. The optical emission spectra and irradiances of the atmospheric pressure plasma jets can be obtained using these dimensions, as briefly presented below in Sections 3.5 and 3.6.

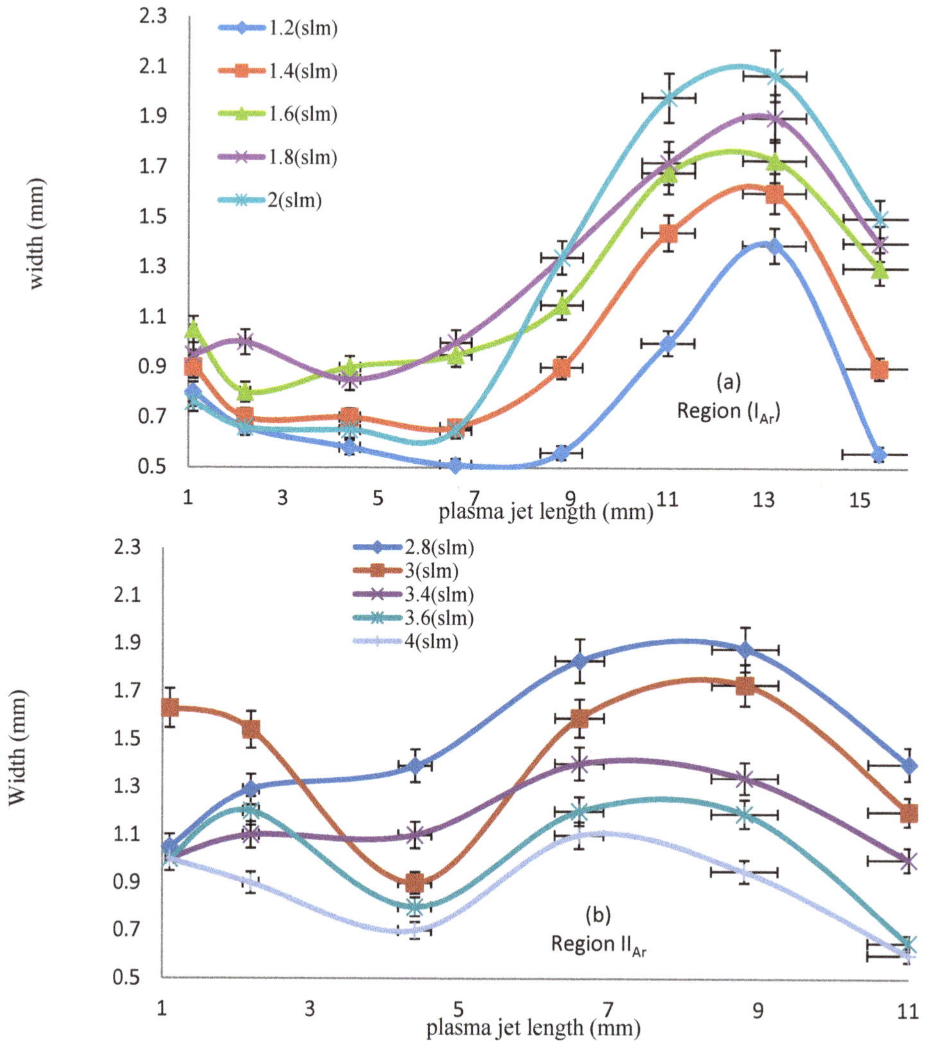

Figure 6. Relation between the plasma jet length and the width of the jet of dry argon for a flow rate (**a**) from 1.2 to 2 slm, (**b**) from 2.8 to 4 slm.

(**a**)

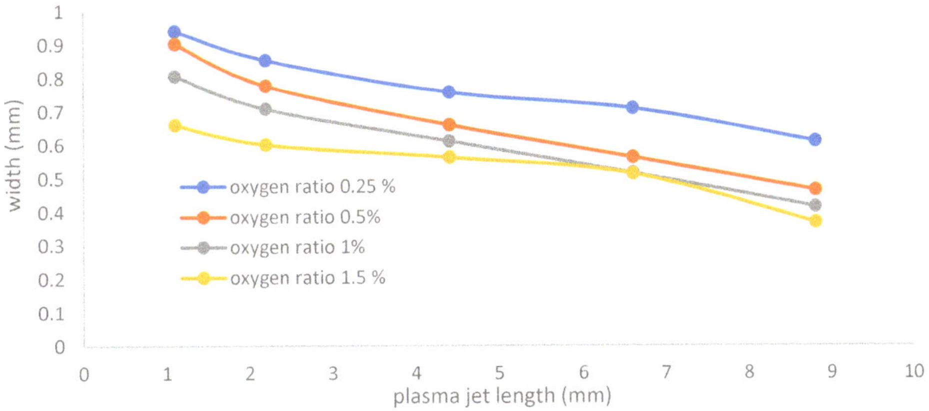

(**b**)

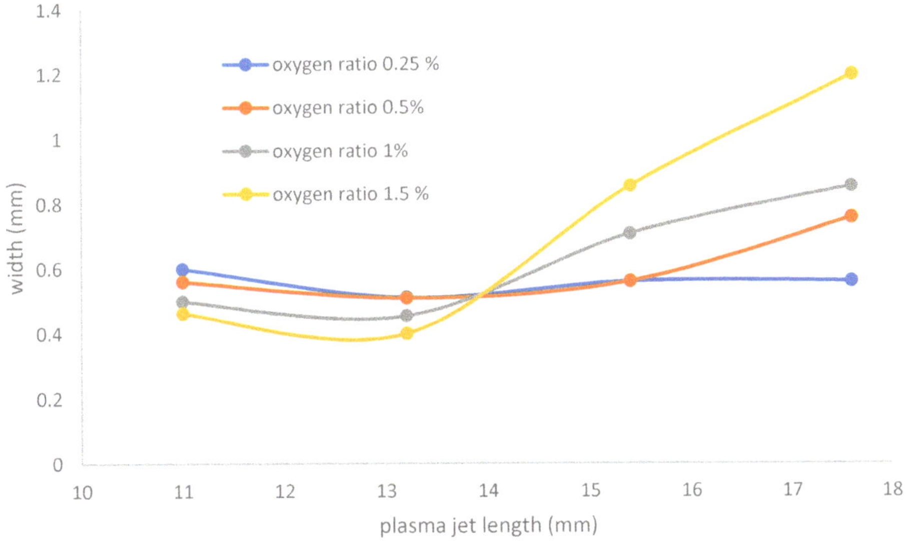

Figure 7. (**a**) Jet width for wet argon as a function of plasma jet length less than 10 mm and at different applied flow rate ratios of oxygen. (**b**) Jet width for wet argon as a function of plasma jet length ranging from 11 to 18 mm and at different applied flow rate ratios of oxygen.

Table 3. Largest width of the jet for dry argon discharge and the equivalent length.

Flow Rate slm	Width mm	Length mm
1.8	1.9	13.2
2	2.07	13.2
2.8	1.8	8.8
3	1.73	8.8

Table 4. Largest width of the jet for oxygen/argon admixture discharge and the equivalent length.

Axial Length of the Jet (mm)		Oxygen Ratio 0.25%	Oxygen Ratio 0.50%	Oxygen Ratio 1%	Oxygen Ratio 1.5%
13.2	Width (mm)	0.455	0.51	0.455	0.4
15.4		0.561	0.561	0.707	0.854
17.6		0.561	0.756	0.853	1.196

3.4. Axial Temperature Distribution

Since this paper deals with non-thermal plasma (cold plasma), the temperature of the emerging jet from the APPJ is a critical factor in inactivation processes [30,31]. Figure 8 shows the axial distribution of temperature from the nozzle of the APPJ to a far away axial distance, at different powers of argon discharge using 1 slm of argon flow rate. The temperature depends on the input power, which ranges from 1 to 2.5 W. The temperature recognizably decreases far away—321 and 332 K at the nozzle (0 mm) to values from 310 to 319 K at 22 mm from the nozzle. The variation in the axial temperature distribution for argon discharge at different applied flow rates is shown in Figure 9. As the flow rate increases from 0.2 to 4 slm, the axial temperature decreases from 487 to 364 K at the nozzle, and from 396 to 364 K at 14 mm from the nozzle.

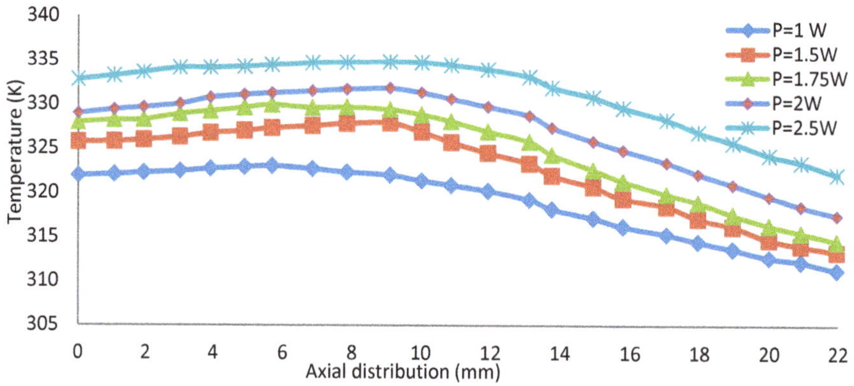

Figure 8. Axial distribution of temperatures from the nozzle of the plasma source at different powers for argon discharge.

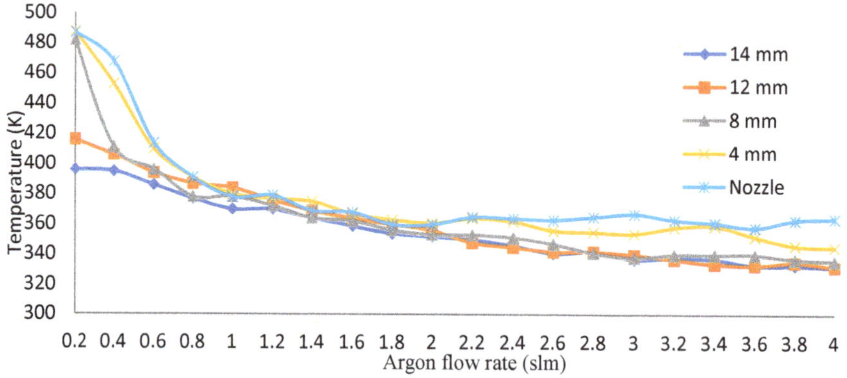

Figure 9. Axial temperature distributions for argon at different applied flow rates.

Figure 10 shows the relation between the oxygen ratio (with 1 slm of argon flow rate) and the axial temperature of the emerging jet at different axial locations. When the flow rate of oxygen increases, the temperature increases to reach a stable value. At the nozzle, the temperature ranges from 395 K to a stable value of 409 K, and at 12 mm from the nozzle the temperature ranges from 376 to 380 K.

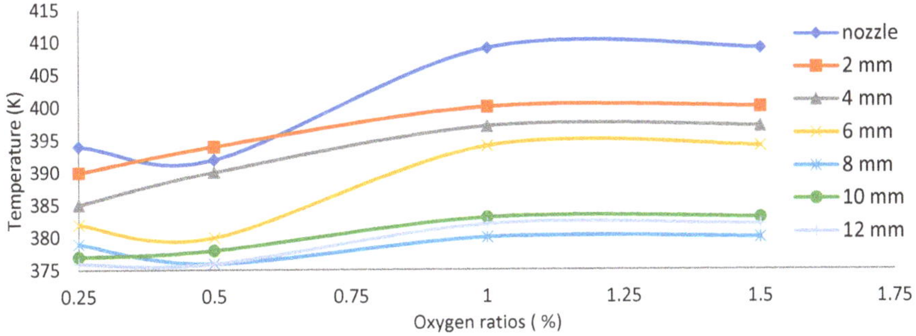

Figure 10. Oxygen ratio (with 1 slm of argon flow rate) vs. temperature of the emerging jet for different axial distributions.

As shown in Figures 9 and 10, the gas temperatures of the plume in O_2/Ar admixtures (with 1 slm of argon flow rate) are slightly lower than those in pure argon discharges. However, as the oxygen ratio increases, the temperature begins to increase and then becomes stable. The reason for this difference between the temperatures of Ar/O_2 and Ar plasmas might be because, as the oxygen ratio increases, the numbers of collisions among particles increase with the flow rate, and more particles participate in energy exchange and dissipating power processes [32]. Therefore, the rotational temperature and vibrational temperature decrease as a result of processes that occur due to adding oxygen to the argon during discharge. Furthermore, adding oxygen accelerates the disinfection process, since a large quantity of thermal energy is transferred from the jet to the alive culture compared with the case for pure argon—the thermal conductivity of oxygen (0.0238 W m^{-1} K^{-1}) is higher than that of argon (0.0162 W·m^{-1} K^{-1}) [33].

3.5. Optical Emission Spectra of APPJ

Optical emission spectroscopy (OES) of the APPJ was performed at the core of the jet's vertical axis using fiber optics with the following parameters: (i) the intensity of the emission spectra (IES) of the emitted jet versus the wavelength; (ii) the peak-to-peak voltage was 11.2 kV, with a 25 kHz frequency; (iii) the wavelength ranged from 250 to 850 nm; (iv) detection was carried out at two different axial locations—the nozzle and 10 mm apart from the nozzle; (v) the investigated flow rates for dry argon discharges were 1.8 and 3.2 slm and for wet argon discharges were 1 slm of argon with different ratios of oxygen admixture: 0.25% and 1.5%.

Figure 11 shows the OES of dry argon discharge with an applied flow rate of 1.8 slm taken from the two axial locations: nozzle and 10 mm apart from the nozzle. The dry argon APPJ emission spectrum at the nozzle is presented in Figure 11a. A high emission intensity with a strong line is found for the hydroxide band (OH) at 309.6 nm (($A^2\Sigma^+$-$X^2\Pi$) transition), for argon lines as follows: ArI: {696.7, 727.3, 738.46, 751.47, 763.76, 772.53, 795.53, 801.47, 811.53, 826.45, and 842.46 nm} ($3s^23p^5(^2P^\circ_{3/2})4p$ transition), and for the nitrogen band (N_2): {337.26, 357.77, 380.36 nm} (($C^3\Pi_u$-$B^3\Pi_g$) transition).

Figure 11b shows the emission spectrum detected at 10 mm from the jet nozzle for dry argon, a moderate emission intensity lower than that of the nozzle measurements. The OH band appears lower with 80% than IES at the nozzle, and the nitrogen band (N_2) with higher IES than at the nozzle by 90%, and with lines, as follows: {337.26, 357.77,

380.36, 405.22, and 433.62 nm} (($C^3\Pi_u$-$B^3\Pi_g$) transition); besides argon lines appeared at the jet nozzle.

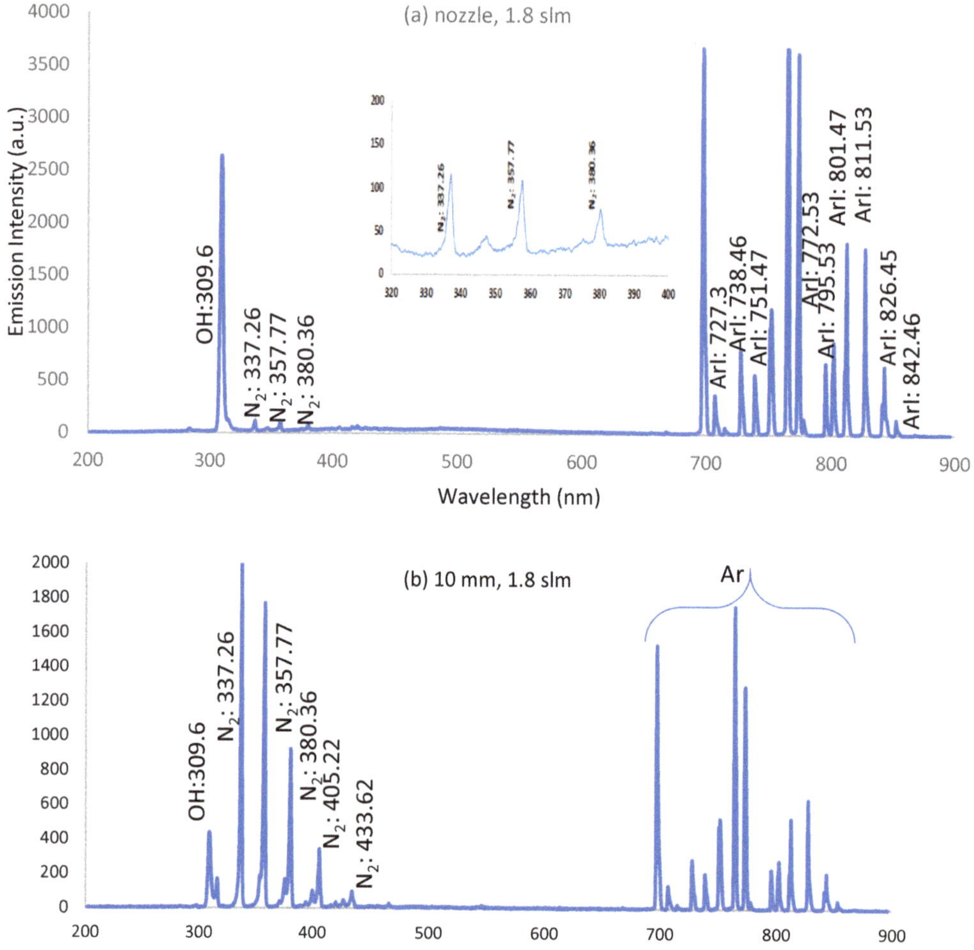

Figure 11. Optical emission spectra of APPJ using argon discharge at an applied flow rate of 1.8 slm for (**a**) nozzle and (**b**) 10 mm.

The intensity of APPJ emission spectra decreased when the argon flow rate increased to 3.2 slm for all spectra measured at the two different axial locations (nozzle and 10 mm), as shown in Figure 12a,b. A reduction in the APPJ emission spectra was measured when the dry argon flow rate increased to more than 2.4 slm for all spectra measured due to a transition from the laminar flow mode to the turbulent flow mode.

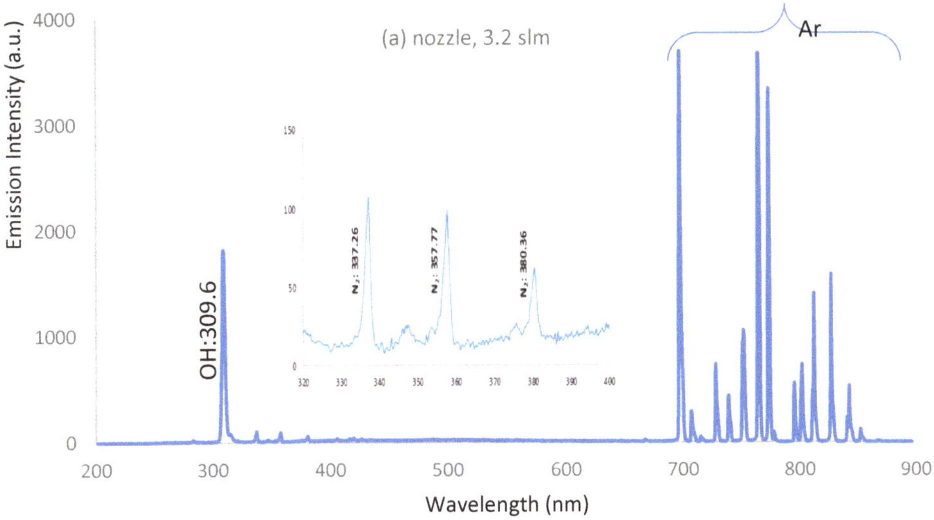

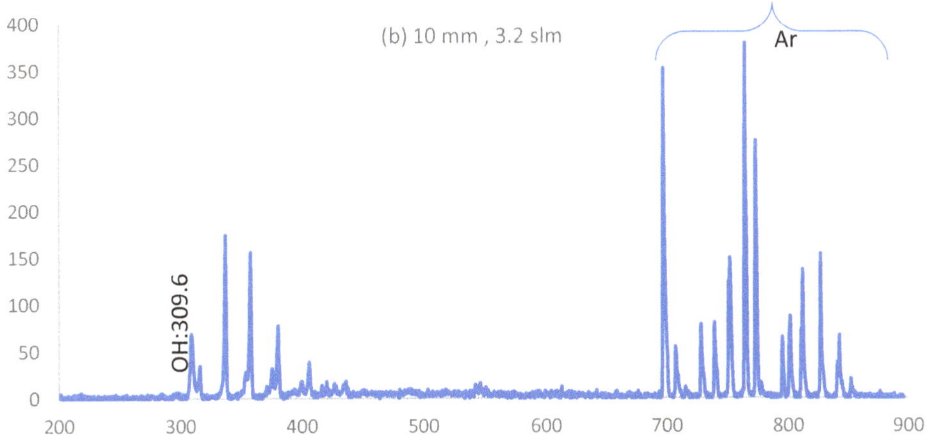

Figure 12. Optical emission spectra of APPJ using argon discharge at an applied flow rate of 3.2 slm for (**a**) nozzle and (**b**) 10 mm.

Figure 13a displays the optical emission spectra of wet argon discharges with ratios of 0.25% of oxygen admixture with 1 slm of argon at the two different axial locations (nozzle and 10 mm). A high IES with a strong OH band at 309.6 nm was measured at the nozzle location; a low IES for weak N_2 bands was measured: {337.26, 357.77, 380.36, 380.36, 405.22, 415.85, 420.19, 427.3, and 433.62 nm} (($C^3\Pi_u$-$B^3\Pi_g$) transition); Ar lines appeared as presented in Figure 11a for the case of a dry argon discharge; and oxygen (O) radical lines were observed: {777.84 and 843.8 nm} ($3s^23p^5(^2P°_{3/2})4s$ transition).

For a wettability with 0.25% of oxygen and at 10 mm from the nozzle, as shown in Figure 13b, the same lines and bands appeared in the emission spectra recorded at the nozzle, but IES decreased by 60% for the OH band and increased by 80% for the N_2 bands: {337.26, 357.77, 380.36, 380.36, 405.22, and 433.62 nm} (($C^3\Pi_u$-$B^3\Pi_g$) transition), where the wavelengths of the Ar lines were as follows: ArI: {696.7, 727.3, 738.46, 751.47,

763.76, 795.53, 801.47, 811.53, and 826.45 nm} ($3s^2 3p^5 (^2P^\circ_{3/2}) 4p$ transition), with a 27% lower emission spectrum intensity; oxygen lines at 777.84 and 843.8 nm ($3s^2 3p^5 (^2P^\circ_{3/2})$ $4s$ transition) were recorded.

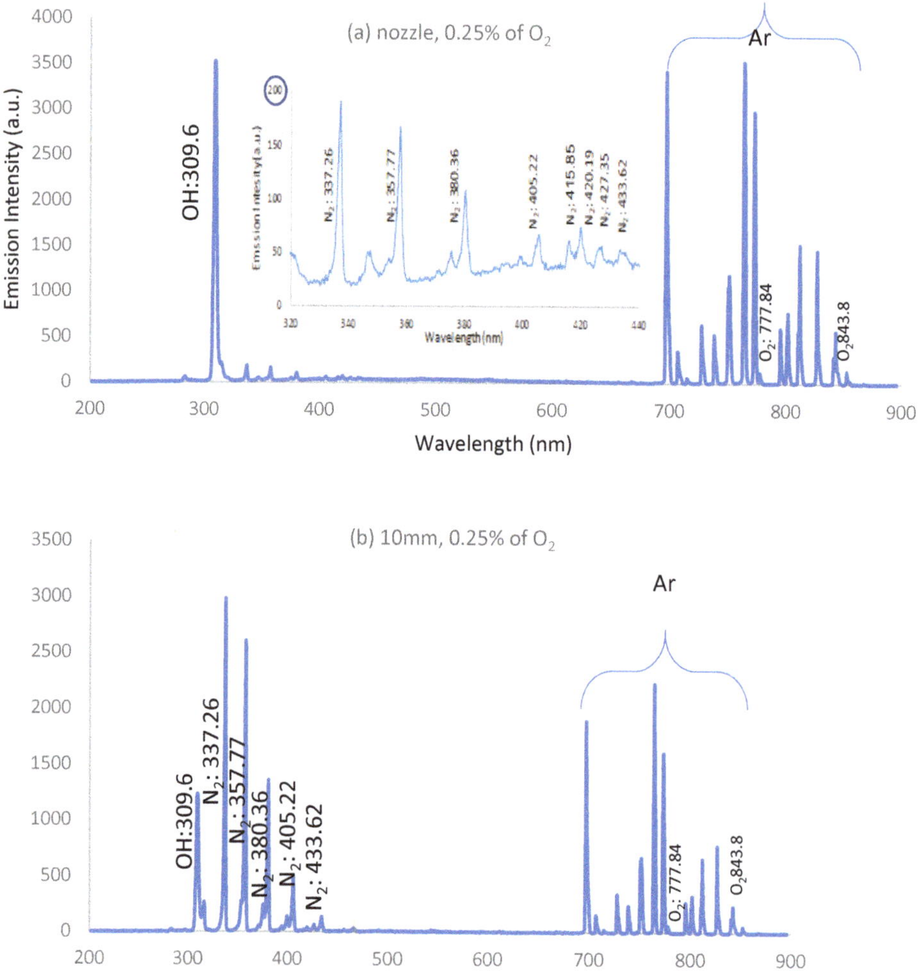

Figure 13. Optical emission spectra of APPJ using oxygen/argon admixture discharge at an applied flow rate of 0.25% of O_2 for (**a**) nozzle and (**b**) 10 mm.

For wet argon discharges when the O_2 percentage increased to 1.5%, as depicted in Figure 14a,b, at the two observed locations (nozzle and 10 mm), IES was measured for a wettability of 1.5% for O_2 at 10 mm from the nozzle (Figure 14b), giving the same lines and bands as those observed at the nozzle, but IES increased by 37% for (OH) band and decreased by 33% for (N_2) bands.

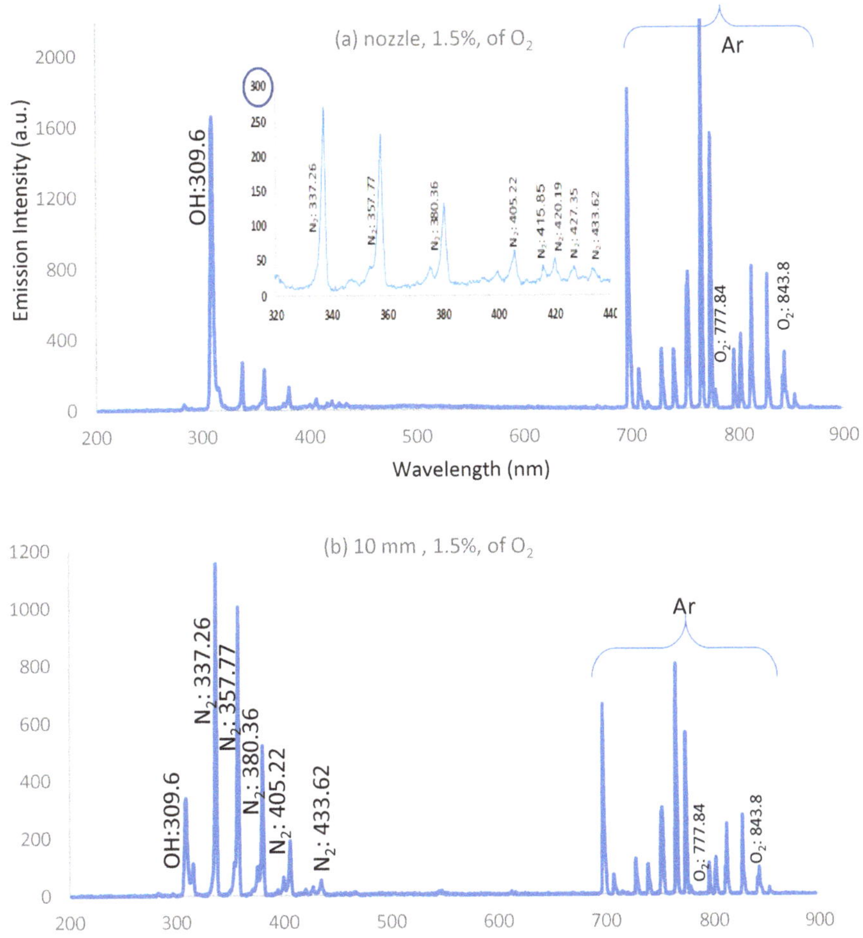

Figure 14. Optical emission spectra of APPJ using oxygen/argon admixture discharge at an applied flow rate of 1.5% of O_2 for (**a**) nozzle and (**b**) 10 mm.

Generally:

a- IES decreases along the jet length and decreases apart from the nozzle due to the presence of the strong electric field near the nozzle and because of the high rate of charge carrier generation by electron impacts near the nozzle.

b- As the admixture of oxygen increases, IES decreases due to the decrease in electron density and temperature resulting from significant dissociation of the oxygen molecules in the discharge processes [34].

c- As the admixture of oxygen increases, IES for the concentration of O, OH, and NO radicals increases far away from the nozzle, compared with the dry argon case.

d- There are many reactions for dry argon discharge, as follows [35]:

i- Argon reacts with an energetic electron (e^*) to produce metastable argon (Ar^m):

$$Ar + e^* \rightarrow Ar^m + \bar{e} \quad (3)$$

ii- Ar^m reacts with e* to produce excited argon (Ar*):

$$e^* + Ar^m \rightarrow Ar^* + \bar{e} \quad (4)$$

iii- Ar* reacts with water to generate $OH^\bullet$:

$$H_2O + Ar^* \rightarrow H^\bullet + OH^\bullet + Ar \quad (5)$$

iv- For the oxygen admixture in wet argon, there are many dissociation reactions in addition to the reactions for dry argon [36,37]:

$$O_2 + e^- \rightarrow 2O + e^- \quad (6)$$

$$N_2 + e^- \rightarrow 2\,N + e^- \quad (7)$$

$$N + O_2 \rightarrow NO + O \quad (8)$$

$$N_2{}^* + O \rightarrow NO + N^* \quad (9)$$

$$O_2 + O \rightarrow O_3 \quad (10)$$

From the dissociation reactions (6) to (10), it is concluded that: (i) The dissociation reactions, the degree of gas ionization, and the production of ozone, O_3, play an important role in the inactivation process. (ii) Due to the oxygen admixture in wet argon, there are dissociation reactions that produce radicals and charged particles under high-energy electron bombardment [38]. (iii) The bonding energy $B.E_{N\equiv N}$ (9.79 eV) > $B.E_{O=O}$ (5.15 eV) and the dissociation and concentration of active species of $O_2 > N_2$ lead to an inactivation process by O_2 higher than for N_2 [39]. (iv) $OH^\bullet$ and $O^\bullet$ radical emission results due to impurities in the gas or due to the entry of air into the discharge zone [40]. (v) The presence of OH, O, and N_2 bands and lines is attributed to the interaction of ambient air with excited argon species, as well as high-energy electrons in the plasma.

Reactive species, such as O, OH, and NO, are the most effective agents in biomedical applications; the plume interacts with ambient gases and molecules. The spectral lines of other elements will be investigated in our future experimental study on APPJ impact parameters that affect the microbial inactivation process of bacteria [41].

3.6. *Irradiance*

The amount of energy (radiant power) emitted per unit area from the plasma jet is the irradiance (W/m^2). The optical emission spectra, the measured dimensions (length and width) of the emerging APPJ (for argon and oxygen/argon admixture discharges) at different flow rates, and the constant applied voltage are important parameters in determining the exposed irradiance, suitable for disinfection processes in medical applications.

The dose rate of irradiance of the APPJ plume per unit area [42] can be calculated by the plume power (W) measured with a power meter detector divided by the cross-sectional area of the effective window of the detector (70×10^{-6} m^2).

Figure 15a,b show that the dose rate of irradiance per unit area ($\mu J/mm^2$) decreases as the jet length increases:

a- Figure 15a shows the influence of the flow rate on the discharge plasma power of the emerging jet for pure argon discharge; by increasing the flow rate from 1.8 to 3 slm, the irradiance per unit area of the plasma jet discharge decreases from 55 to 13 $\mu J/mm^2$ for a plasma jet distance with 8 mm. With increasing plasma jet length to 18.4 mm, the irradiance decreases to between 15 and 6.09 $\mu J/mm^2$.

b- Figure 15b shows the influence of different oxygen ratios; whereas the oxygen ratios increase from 0.25% to 1.5%, the irradiance per unit area of plasma jet discharge decreases from 28.57 to 5.68 $\mu J/mm^2$ for a plasma jet length of 8 mm. By increasing the plasma jet length to 18.4 mm, the irradiance decreases to between 6.9 and 4.02 $\mu J/mm^2$. The dose rate of irradiance per unit area is lower for the oxygen/argon admixture discharges than for the argon discharges. The oxygen percentages increase; inelastic collisions lead to losses in the discharge process and lower irradiance compared with the case for argon discharges.

c- According to the measured data and the Guidelines of the International Commission on Non-Ionizing Radiation Protection (ICNIRP), the limits of irradiance exposure of the skin must not exceed 30 μJ/mm^2 [43,44]. From the results, it is concluded that the measured irradiances under the drawn dashed line in Figure 15a for argon discharges and the irradiances for all oxygen/argon admixture discharges in Figure 15b are compatible with ICNIRP irradiance limits.

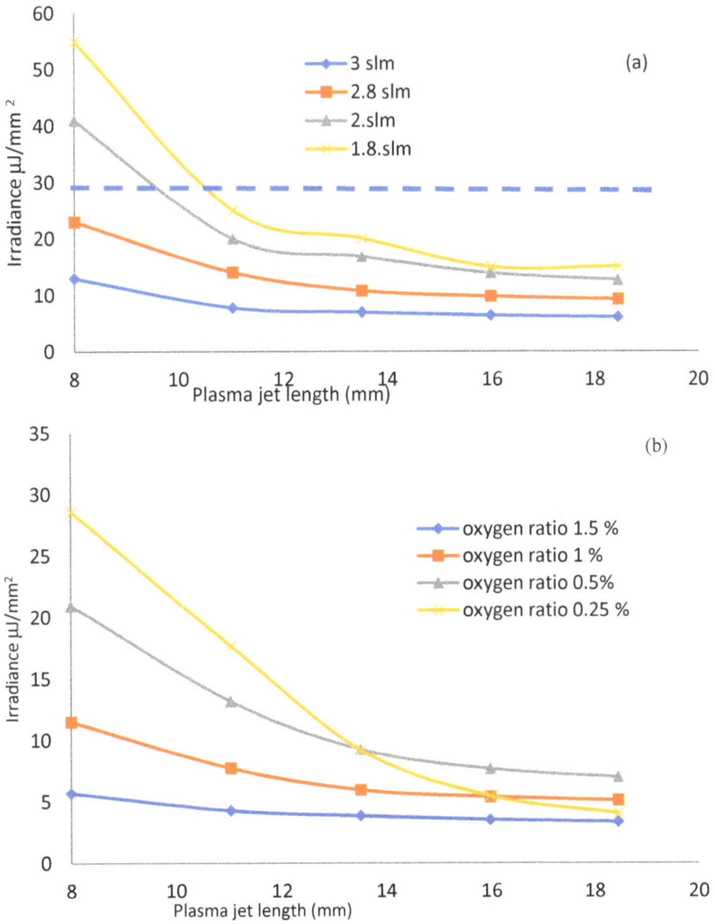

Figure 15. Dose rate of irradiance per unit area (μJ/mm^2) of plasma jet discharge as a function of plasma jet length (**a**) for argon discharge with different flow rates and (**b**) for oxygen/argon admixture discharge for different oxygen ratios.

4. Conclusions

The impact of a non-thermal atmospheric pressure plasma jet (APPJ) using different working gases, powered by an AC high-voltage source with a variable frequency reaching 60 kHz, and with a voltage ranging from 2.5 to 25 kV, has been determined. The optical and electrical characteristics of APPJ discharges for Ar and Ar/O_2 working gases have been determined, such as: voltage–current waveform signals, gas flow rates, discharge plasma powers, lengths, widths, the axial temperature distribution, optical emission spectra, and irradiance.

The discharge plasma power values of oxygen admixture discharges decrease, from 1.75 to 1.65 W, for oxygen admixture ratios increasing from 0.25% to 1.5%, and are lower than those of argon discharges, and the plasma power values increase from 1.95 to 2.4 W when the argon flow rate increases from 0.2 to 3 slm. This is useful in sterilization and inactivation processes, since it prolongs the interaction processes between the plasma jet and the sample.

The width of the jet is an interesting parameter that depends on the plasma jet length and the applied flow rate of argon and oxygen. The width is a guideline for the maximum irradiance area emerging from the jet and reaching the sample. As the oxygen flow rates increase, the width of the plasma jet increases and elongates the axial length of the jet. In general, the temperature of the jet reaching the sample must not exceed the threshold of room temperature. As the oxygen ratio increases, the numbers of collisions among particles increase, and the jet temperatures decrease as a result of processes during discharge.

For discharges with oxygen admixture ratios between 0.25% and 1.5% with argon, the emission spectra of APPJ give a behavior similar to that of pure argon discharges, but with low values of intensity due to the decrease in electron density and temperature and higher dissociation and ionization of the oxygen molecules in the discharges processes in the case of oxygen admixture.

The optical emission spectra and the dose rate of irradiance of plasma jet discharge were investigated as a function of plasma jet length for dry argon discharge and for wet argon discharge. This investigation delivered data compatible with the International Commission on Non-Ionizing Radiation Protection (ICNIRP) for irradiance exposure limits of the skin, 30 $\mu J/mm^2$. This limit is suitable for the disinfection of microbes on the skin without harmful effects.

Our future work will involve an experimental study on the impact parameters affecting the microbial disinfection process of bacteria on skin in a wound area. The study will use different distances between the jet of the APPJ and the treated samples and the required knowledge to avoid toxic gas formation, damage, and heat radiation production in the sample. Moreover, the Reynolds numbers of argon and oxygen/argon admixture discharges for various gas flow rates will be considered.

Author Contributions: Conceptualization, methodology, validation, formal analysis, investigation, resources, data curation, writing (original draft preparation, review, and editing), visualization, supervision, project administration, and funding acquisition, all tasks done by the two authors. Both authors have read and agreed to the published version of the manuscript.

Funding: The research work was funded by the Deanship of Scientific Research—Umm Al-Qura University, Makkah, Saudi Arabia, where the project was setup with funding No. 18-sci-1-01-0022.

Institutional Review Board Statement: Not applicable.

Informed Consent Statement: Not applicable.

Data Availability Statement: Data are contained within the article.

Acknowledgments: The authors acknowledge the support of the Deanship of Scientific Research-Umm El-Qura University-Makkah-Saudi Arabia where the project was set up with funding no. 18-sci-1-01-0022, as well as the full support by the Department of Applied Physics of Ghent University (Belgium) and in particular that of Rino Morent and Iuliia Onyshchenko.

Conflicts of Interest: The authors have no conflict of interest to declare.

References

1. Van Oost, G. Plasma for environment. *J. Phys. Conf. Ser.* **2017**, *941*, 012014. [CrossRef]
2. Laroussi, M.; Leipold, F. Evaluation of the roles of reactive species, heat, and UV radiation in the inactivation of bacte-rial cells by air plasmas at atmospheric pressure. *Int. J. Mass Spectrom.* **2004**, *233*, 81–86. [CrossRef]

3. Laroussi, M.; Mendis, D.A.; Rosenberg, M. Plasma interaction and microbes. *New J. Phys.* **2003**, *5*, 41. [CrossRef]
4. Morent, R.; De Geyter, N.; Van Vlierberghe, S.; Dubruel, P.; Leys, C.; Gengembre, L.; Schacht, E.; Payen, E. Deposition of HMDSO-based coatings on PET substrates using an atmospheric pressure dielectric barrier discharge. *Prog. Org. Coat.* **2009**, *64*, 304. [CrossRef]
5. Laroussi, M. Nonthermal decontamination of biological media by atmospheric-pressure plasmas: Review, analysis, and prospects. *IEEE Trans. Plasma Sci.* **2002**, *30*, 1409–1415. [CrossRef]
6. Lee, H.W.; Nam, S.H.; Mohamed, A.-A.; Kim, G.C.; Lee, J.K. Atmospheric Pressure Plasma Jet Composed of Three Electrodes: Application to Tooth Bleaching. *Plasma Process. Polym.* **2010**, *7*, 274–280. [CrossRef]
7. Morent, R.; De Geyter, N.; Verschuren, J.; De Clerck, K.; Kiekens, P.; Leys, C. Non-thermal plasma treatment of textiles. *Surf. Coat. Technol.* **2008**, *202*, 3427–3449. [CrossRef]
8. Machala, Z.; Hensel, K.; Akishev, Y. *Plasma for Bio-Decontamination, Medicine and Food Security*; Springer: Dordrecht, The Netherlands, 2011; pp. 417–430.
9. Lee, M.-H.; Min, B.K.; Son, J.S.; Kwon, T.-Y. Influence of Different Post-Plasma Treatment Storage Conditions on the Shear Bond Strength of Veneering Porcelain to Zirconia. *Materials* **2016**, *9*, 43. [CrossRef] [PubMed]
10. Wu, C.-C.; Wei, C.-K.; Ho, C.-C.; Ding, S.-J. Enhanced Hydrophilicity and Biocompatibility of Dental Zirconia Ceramics by Oxygen Plasma Treatment. *Materials* **2015**, *8*, 684–699. [CrossRef]
11. Nam, S.H.; Lee, H.J.; Hong, J.W.; Kim, G.C. Efficacy of Nonthermal Atmospheric Pressure Plasma for Tooth Bleaching. *Sci. World J.* **2015**, *2015*, 1–5. [CrossRef]
12. Laroussi, M. Low-Temperature Plasma Jet for Biomedical Applications: A Review. *IEEE Trans. Plasma Sci.* **2015**, *43*, 703–712. [CrossRef]
13. Xiong, Q.; Lu, X.P.; Jiang, Z.H.; Tang, Z.Y.; Hu, J.; Xiong, Z.L.; Pan, Y. An Atmospheric Pressure Nonequilibrium Plasma Jet Device. *IEEE Trans. Plasma Sci.* **2008**, *36*, 986–987. [CrossRef]
14. Seo, Y.S.; Mohamed, A.-A.; Woo, K.C.; Lee, H.W.; Lee, J.K.; Kim, K.T. Comparative Studies of Atmospheric Pressure Plasma Characteristics between He and Ar Working Gases for Sterilization. *IEEE Trans. Plasma Sci.* **2010**, *38*, 2954–2962. [CrossRef]
15. Sun, Y.; Zhang, Z.; Wang, S. Study on the Bactericidal Mechanism of Atmospheric-Pressure Low-Temperature Plasma against Escherichia coli and Its Application in Fresh-Cut Cucumbers. *Molecules* **2018**, *23*, 975. [CrossRef] [PubMed]
16. Weltmann, K.-D.; Brandenburg, R.; von Woedtke, T.; Ehlbeck, J.; Foest, R.; Stieber, M.; Kindel, E. Antimicrobial treatment of heat sensitive products by miniaturized atmospheric pressure plasma jets (APPJs). *J. Phys. D Appl. Phys.* **2008**, *41*. [CrossRef]
17. Mohamed, A.-A.H.; Aljuhani, M.M.; Almarashi, J.Q.M.; Alhazime, A. The effect of a second grounded electrode on the atmospheric pressure argon plasma jet. *Plasma Res. Express* **2020**, *2*, 015011. [CrossRef]
18. Galaly, A.R.; Ahmed, O.B.; Asghar, A.H. Antibacterial effects of combined non-thermal plasma and photocatalytic treatment of culture media in the laminar flow mode. *Phys. Fluids* **2021**, *33*, 043604. [CrossRef]
19. Dünnbier, M.; Becker, M.M.; Iséni, S.; Bansemer, R.; Loffhagen, D.; Reuter, S.; Weltmann, K.-D. Stability and excitation dynamics of an argon micro-scaled atmospheric pressure plasma jet. *Plasma Sources Sci. Technol.* **2015**, *24*, 65018. [CrossRef]
20. Sarani, A.; Nikiforov, A.; Leys, C. Atmospheric pressure plasma jet in Ar and Ar/H2O mixtures: Optical emission spectroscopy and temperature measurements. *Phys. Plasmas* **2010**, *17*, 063504. [CrossRef]
21. Morent, R.; De Geyter, N.; Leys, C.; Vansteenkiste, E.; De Bock, J.; Philips, W. Measuring the wicking behavior of textiles by the combination of a horizontal wicking experiment and image processing. *Rev. Sci. Instrum.* **2006**, *77*, 093502. [CrossRef]
22. Morent, R.; De Geyter, N.; Leys, C.; Gengembre, L.; Payen, E. Surface Modification of Non-woven Textiles using a Dielectric Barrier Discharge Operating in Air, Helium and Argon at Medium Pressure. *Text. Res. J.* **2007**, *77*, 471–488. [CrossRef]
23. Vicoveanu, D.; Ohtsu, Y.; Fujita, H. Pulsed Discharge Effects on Bacteria Inactivation in Low-Pressure Radio-Frequency Oxygen Plasma. *Jpn. J. Appl. Phys.* **2008**, *47*, 1130–1135. [CrossRef]
24. Singh, M.K.; Ogino, A.; Nagatsu, M. Inactivation factors of spore-forming bacteria using low-pressure microwave plasmas in an N_2 and O_2 gas mixture. *New J. Phys.* **2009**, *11*. [CrossRef]
25. Laroussi, M. Low Temperature Plasma-Based Sterilization: Overview and State-of-the-Art. *Plasma Proc. Polym.* **2005**, *2*, 391. [CrossRef]
26. Deng, X.; Leys, C.; Vujosevic, D.; Vuksanovic, V.; Cvelbar, U.; De Geyter, N.; Morent, R.; Nikiforov, A. Engineering of Composite Organosilicon Thin Films with Embedded Silver Nanoparticles via Atmospheric Pressure Plasma Process for Antibacterial Activity. *Plasma Process. Polym.* **2014**, *11*, 921. [CrossRef]
27. Ploux, L.; Mateescu, M.; Anselme, K.; Vasilev, K. Antibacterial Properties of Silver-Loaded Plasma Polymer Coatings. *J. Nanomater.* **2012**, *2012*, 1–9. [CrossRef]
28. Deng, X.L.; Nikiforov, A.; Vanraes, P.; Leys, C. Direct current plasma jet at atmospheric pressure operating in nitrogen and air. *J. Appl. Phys.* **2013**, *113*, 023305. [CrossRef]
29. Asghar, A.H.; Ahmed, O.B.; Galaly, A.R. Inactivation of *E. coli* Using Atmospheric Pressure Plasma Jet with Dry and Wet Argon Discharges. *Membranes* **2021**, *11*, 46. [CrossRef] [PubMed]
30. Soloshenko, I.; Tsiolko, V.; Khomich, V. Sterilization of medical products in low- pressure glow discharges. *Plasma Phys. Rep.* **2000**, *26*, 792. [CrossRef]
31. Lu, X.; Ye, T.; Cao, Y.; Sun, Z.; Xiong, Q.; Tang, Z.; Xiong, Z.; Hu, J.; Jiang, Z.; Pan, Y. The roles of the various plasma agents in the inactivation of bacteria. *J. Appl. Phys.* **2008**, *104*, 053309. [CrossRef]

32. Shen, J.; Cheng, C.; Shidong, F.; Hongbing, X.; Yan, L.; Guohua, N.; Yuedong, M.; Jiarong, L.; Xiangke, W. Sterilization of Bacillus subtilis Spores Using an Atmospheric Plasma Jet with Argon and Oxygen Mixture Gas. *Appl. Phys. Express* **2012**, *5*, 3. [CrossRef]
33. Cheng, C. Atmospheric pressure plasma jet utilizing Ar and Ar/H2O mixtures and its applications to bacteria inactivation. *Chin. Phys. B* **2014**, *23*, 7. [CrossRef]
34. Lu, X.; Naidis, G.V.; Laroussi, M.; Reuter, S.; Graves, D.B.; Ostrikov, K. Reactive species in non-equilibrium atmospheric-pressure plasmas: Generation, transport, and biological effects. *Phys. Rep.* **2016**, *630*, 1–84. [CrossRef]
35. Bruggeman, P.; Schram, D.; González, M.A.; Rego, R.; Kong, M.G.; Leys, C. Characterization of a direct dc-excited discharge in water by optical emission spectroscopy. *Plasma Sources Sci. Technol.* **2009**, *18*, 5–17. [CrossRef]
36. Dodet, B.; Odic, E.; Goldman, A.; Goldman, M.; Renard, D. Hydrogen Peroxide Formation by Discharges in Argon/Water Vapor Mixtures at Atmospheric Pressure. *J. Adv. Oxid. Technol.* **2005**, *8*, 91–97. [CrossRef]
37. Kirkpatrick, M.; Dodet, B.; Odic, E. Atmospheric pressure humid argon DBD plasma for the application of sterilization measurement and simulation of hydrogen, oxygen, and hydrogen peroxide formation. *Int. J. Plasma Environ. Sci. Technol.* **2007**, *1*, 96–101.
38. Taghizadeh, L.; Brackman, G.; Nikiforov, A.; van der Mullen, J.; Leys, C.; Coenye, T. Inactivation of biofilms using a low power atmospheric pressure argon plasma jet; the role of en-trained nitrogen. *Plasma Process. Polym.* **2015**, *12*, 75–81. [CrossRef]
39. Galaly, A.R.; Zahran, H.H. Disinfection of Microbes by Magnetized DC Plasma. *J. Mod. Phys.* **2014**, *5*, 781–791. [CrossRef]
40. Galaly, A.R.; Zahran, H.H. Inactivation of Bacteria using Combined Effects of Magnetic Field, Low Pressure and Ultra Low Frequency Plasma Discharges (ULFP). *J. Phys. Conf. Ser. (IOP)* **2013**, *431*, 012014. [CrossRef]
41. Lam, Y.L.; Kan, C.W.; Yuen, C.W. Effect of oxygen plasma pre-treatment and titanium dioxide overlay coating on flame retardant finished cotton fabrics. *Bioresources* **2011**, *6*, 1454–1474.
42. Deng, X.; Nikiforov, A.; Coenye, T.; Cools, P.; Aziz, G.; Morent, R.; De Geyter, N.; Leys, C. Antimicrobial nano-silver non-woven polyethylene terephthalate fabric via an atmospheric pressure plasma deposition process. *Sci. Rep.* **2015**, *5*, 10138. [CrossRef] [PubMed]
43. The International Commission on Non-Ionizing Radiation Protection. Guidelines on limits of exposure to ultraviolet radiation of wavelengths between 180 nm and 400 nm incoherent optical radiation. *Health Phys.* **2004**, *87*, 171–179. [CrossRef] [PubMed]
44. The International Commission on Non-Ionizing Radiation Protection. General approach to protection against non-ionizing radiation. *Health Phys.* **2002**, *82*, 540–545. [CrossRef] [PubMed]

applied sciences

MDPI

Review

Applications of Cold Atmospheric Pressure Plasma Technology in Medicine, Agriculture and Food Industry

Mária Domonkos [1,*], Petra Tichá [1], Jan Trejbal [1] and Pavel Demo [1,2]

1 Department of Physics, Faculty of Civil Engineering, Czech Technical University in Prague, Thákurova 7, 166 29 Praha 6, Czech Republic; petra.ticha@fsv.cvut.cz (P.T.); jan.trejbal@fsv.cvut.cz (J.T.); pavel.demo@fsv.cvut.cz (P.D.)
2 Institute of Physics, Czech Academy of Sciences, Cukrovarnická 10/112, 162 00 Praha 6, Czech Republic
* Correspondence: maria.domonkos@fsv.cvut.cz

Abstract: In recent years, cold atmospheric pressure plasma (CAPP) technology has received substantial attention due to its valuable properties including operational simplicity, low running cost, and environmental friendliness. Several different gases (air, nitrogen, helium, argon) and techniques (corona discharge, dielectric barrier discharge, plasma jet) can be used to generate plasma at atmospheric pressure and low temperature. Plasma treatment is routinely used in materials science to modify the surface properties (e.g., wettability, chemical composition, adhesion) of a wide range of materials (e.g., polymers, textiles, metals, glasses). Moreover, CAPP seems to be a powerful tool for the inactivation of various pathogens (e.g., bacteria, fungi, viruses) in the food industry (e.g., food and packing material decontamination, shelf life extension), agriculture (e.g., disinfection of seeds, fertilizer, water, soil) and medicine (e.g., sterilization of medical equipment, implants). Plasma medicine also holds great promise for direct therapeutic treatments in dentistry (tooth bleaching), dermatology (atopic eczema, wound healing) and oncology (melanoma, glioblastoma). Overall, CAPP technology is an innovative, powerful and effective tool offering a broad application potential. However, its limitations and negative impacts need to be determined in order to receive regulatory approval and consumer acceptance.

Keywords: atmospheric pressure plasma; low temperature plasma; disinfection; pathogen inactivation; plasma medicine; plasma agriculture

Citation: Domonkos, M.; Tichá, P.; Trejbal, J.; Demo, P. Applications of Cold Atmospheric Pressure Plasma Technology in Medicine, Agriculture and Food Industry. *Appl. Sci.* **2021**, *11*, 4809. https://doi.org/10.3390/app11114809

Academic Editor: Bogdan-George Rusu

Received: 28 April 2021
Accepted: 19 May 2021
Published: 24 May 2021

1. Introduction

Applications of plasma technology have a long history in electronics, semiconductor industry and materials science (e.g., etching, chemical vapor deposition, plasma polymerization, surface structuring) [1–5]. In recent decades, cold atmospheric pressure plasma (CAPP) technology has been actively used in several industrial sectors, because it is suitable for surface treatment of many different materials (such as metal, wood, paper, glass, polymer, ceramic, nonwoven textile, etc.), while striving to retain favorable bulk properties of the material [6–9]. CAPP has recently been extended to animal and human medicine, agriculture and food industry [10,11]. In this paper, several emerging applications of CAPP are briefly reviewed, and current trends are highlighted.

2. Plasma

Plasma is considered the fourth state of matter after solid, liquid and gas. It can be defined as a partially or fully ionized quasi-neutral substance, composed of electrons, ions, neutral particles, molecules in the ground or excited state, radical species and quanta of electromagnetic radiation (UV photons and visible light). These particles exhibit collective behavior [9]. Plasma exists in many forms in nature and constitutes more than 99% of the matter in the visible universe (stars, interstellar and interplanetary media, solar wind, tail of a comet, Aurora Borealis and Australis, quark-gluon plasma, etc.). Man-made plasma systems use heat, apply high voltage or inject electromagnetic waves to a gas for plasma generation. Plasmas are classified as equilibrium and nonequilibrium according to the relative temperature of electrons, ions and neutrals [9,12]. Equilibrium forms (e.g., torch, plasma spraying, arc jet) are known as thermal (hot) plasmas, since the temperatures of neutrals, ions and electrons are approximately of the same order maintaining a thermal equilibrium [12,13]. Nonequilibrium plasmas are known as nonthermal plasmas (cold), with the temperature of the particles varying from each other [1,14]. The electron (light particles) temperature (≈10,000 K) is much higher compared to the temperature (≈300–1000 K) of heavy species (ions and neutrals) [15,16]. Cold plasmas are weakly ionized gases, which can be generated at low as well as atmospheric pressures. They are usually excited and sustained electrically by applying radio frequency (RF) power, microwave (MW) power, alternating current (AC) and direct current (DC) [12,17,18].

2.1. Benefits of Cold Atmospheric Pressure Plasma

Nowadays, cold atmospheric pressure plasma is considered more advantageous over low-pressure (<100 Pa) plasma for industrial applications, due to its technological and economic advantages [19]. First of all, CAPP is able to generate stable plasma at atmospheric pressure, i.e., there is no vacuum and the reactor is frequently open [6]. The application thus requires lower investment and operational cost compared to low-pressure plasma systems due to the absence of costly time-, space- and energy-consuming vacuum systems [20]. Moreover, the simplest CAPP reactors use only ambient air as working gas, which is converted into plasma (i.e., gas supply is not required) [6]. Thus, CAPP systems are easy to handle with excellent scalability and industrial applicability (integrable in existing process lines, capable of continuous surface modification, etc.) [11]. Another advantage of cold plasma is the ability to treat thermally labile samples (soft and organic materials, polymers) without any surface damage because the substrate temperature remains close to room temperature (in general < 50 °C) [15,21]. The treatment time is relatively short (from seconds to minutes) [9,15]. The efficiency of CAPP treatment depends on the reactor configuration (electrode arrangement, distance from the substrate surface) and the operating parameters of the device (gas composition, flow rate, power, temperature, process duration, etc.) [22–24].

2.2. Plasma Sources

There are several methods for generating CAPP from various gases such as (i) dielectric barrier discharge, (ii) plasma jet, (iii) corona discharge, (iv) gliding arc discharge, etc. (Figure 1) [10,25]. Commonly used working gas includes air, oxygen, nitrogen, helium, argon and their mixtures [14,18,21,26].

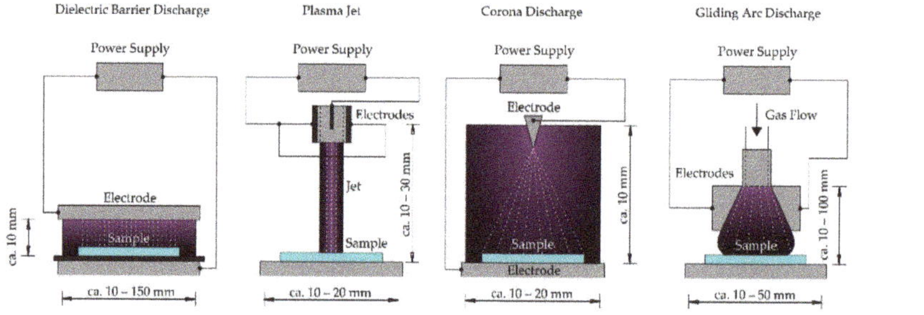

Figure 1. Schematic drawing of diverse cold atmospheric pressure plasma devices.

Dielectric barrier discharge (DBD) is generated by applying a high voltage (~kV) electric DC or AC current at high frequency (~kHz) across an adjustable gap (ranging from tens of microns to several cm) between two electrodes separated by an insulating dielectric barrier. The geometry of DBDs usually consists of two parallel plates in planar or cylindrical arrangements. DBDs use a dielectric material (e.g., quartz, glass, ceramics, enamel, silicon rubber, teflon, mica, plastic) to cover at least one of the electrodes [27]. The nonconducting coating eliminates the transition of the discharge to an electrical arc [10,28–30].

The atmospheric pressure plasma jet (APPJ) is a type of cold plasma discharge that produces a high velocity stream of highly reactive chemical species with weak emitted light [31,32]. APPJs typically consist of two concentric cylindrical electrodes, where the inner electrode is connected to a RF or MW power source at high frequency, causing ionization of the working gas (mainly noble gases such as helium or argon). The gas exits through a nozzle, which gives a "jet-like" appearance [20]. Based on the configuration and used materials, APPJs can be divided into single electrode jets, dielectric-free electrode jets, DBD jets, etc. Miniature plasma jets are known as plasma pens, plasma torches or plasma needles [28,30,33]. The main component of plasma needles is an electrode with a sharpened tip inside of a tube. The feed gas (most frequently helium) is flowing through a tube and is mixed with air at the needle tip where a micro discharge is created [34]. The diameter of the generated plasma glow is a few millimeters [35].

Corona discharge is generated by the application of high voltage between two or more sharp electrodes. The coronizing electrode is usually realized as a needle or a thin wire. The ionization process creates a crown around this active electrode. Coronas are very weak discharges, having very low electron and ion densities [36,37].

Gliding arc discharge plasma reactors are known as hot plasma sources, however, under specific conditions they may also produce cold plasma. The gliding arc plasma can combine the advantages of both thermal and nonthermal plasmas (nonthermal plasma conditions at higher power). The discharge is formed by a high voltage at the spot where the distance between diverging electrodes is the shortest (~ in the range of millimeters). Electrodes are placed in a fast gas flow and the discharge increases its volume and length in the flow direction [38–40].

The plasma sources can be applied directly (the target is in direct contact with the active plasma region) or indirectly (plasma afterglow or storable plasma-activated medium is used which contains various reactive species) to the object [41].

3. Applications of Cold Atmospheric Pressure Plasma

3.1. Medicine

In the past 20 years, cold plasma treatment has been extended to medicine, mainly as a tool for the inactivation of pathogens (bacteria, fungi, viruses, biofilms) on medical or laboratory equipment (e.g., surgical instruments, pharmaceutical devices, implants, dialysis tubes, glassware, plastic tubes, pipette tips, beds, floors, etc.) [42–44]. Conventional methods for disinfection (inactivation of pathogenic organisms) and sterilization (elimination of all viable microorganisms), such as steam and heat treatment, autoclaves, irradiation, wet chemical treatment (ethylene oxide, ozone, chlorine, hydrogen peroxide, sodium hypochlorite, alcohol or any carbohydrate solutions, superoxidized water, various kind of acids, etc.) and UV light exhibit several drawbacks [45]. They are often slow-acting, flammable or unstable at ambient conditions [46]. Moreover, they can cause irreversible damage to the modified material and irritate the skin and eyes of humans [47]. On the contrary, CAPP can be utilized for heat labile or chemically reactive materials (e.g., heat sensitive biomaterials, polymers, living tissues) to prevent secondary infections.

Two basic types of CAPP systems are dominating in plasma medicine: indirect (e.g., plasma jet, pen, needle) and direct (e.g., dielectric barrier discharge device) plasma sources [26,36,48,49]. In the direct exposure mode, the plasma is in contact with the biological target. Floating electrode DBD (FE-DBD) system allows safe usage of plasma in therapeutic applications. It consists of two electrodes, the first is a dielectric-protected powered electrode and the second electrode is a human or animal body (skin or organ) [41,50]. Direct application of CAPP requires high standards of safety (e.g., homogeneous discharge with permitted values has to be created in order to provide nondestructive treatment). Indirect plasma sources do not use the human tissue as a counter electrode, the afterglow of plasma or plasma-activated liquid (it can be stored and shipped) is used [49,51]. Typically, these devices are portable, and allow efficient treatment of large areas even with uneven surfaces. However, their homogeneity and stability need further improvement [47].

Plasma sources produce reactive species (with a lifetime ranging from nanoseconds to hours), which are known from redox biology and play a pivotal role in biological applications [52–57]. Reactive oxygen-based species (ROS) include, e.g., superoxide ($O_2^{\bullet -}$), hydrogen peroxide (H_2O_2), hydroxyl radical ($^\bullet OH$), singlet oxygen ($^1O_2$), ozone (O_3), alkoxyl ($RO^\bullet$) and peroxyl ($RO_2{}^\bullet$). Nitrogen-based species include (RNS), e.g., nitric oxide ($^\bullet NO$), nitrogen dioxide ($^\bullet NO_2$) and peroxynitrite ($ONOO^-$). These reactive species (ROS/RNS=RONS) also play a crucial role in the pathogen inactivation mechanism (Figure 2), because they can modulate the environment of cells and affect their behavior [30,48,49,58,59]. RONS can cause cell wall erosion, cell membrane disruption (protein denaturation, virus leakage), functionality changes (oxidation of amino acids), damage to DNA and RNA and apoptosis [43,57,60]. However, it should be pointed out that the precise mechanism of microbial inactivation using CAPP treatment and the contribution of various components (UV, electrons, ion bombardment and reactive species) has not yet been fully understood [61].

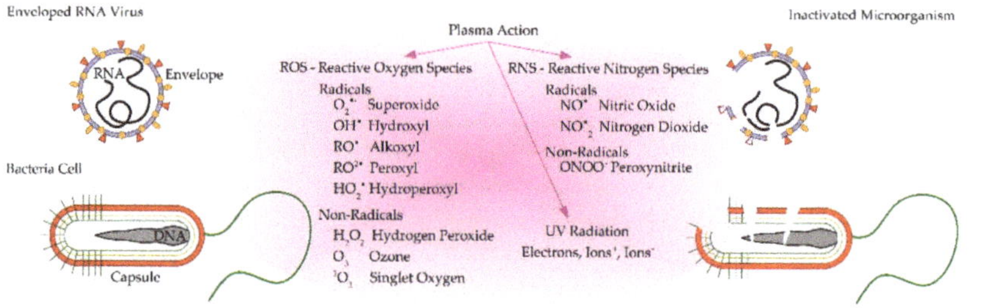

Figure 2. Schematic illustration of plasma inactivation of viruses and bacteria using CAPP treatment.

Drug resistance and incurable bacterial infections are serious public health threats, as the world is heading towards a post-antibiotic era, mainly caused by the misuse and overuse of various medications [62]. It is an urgent need to develop new techniques to treat infectious diseases caused by multidrug-resistant germs. Promising methods include light-based therapies (antimicrobial blue light, antimicrobial photodynamic inactivation, ultraviolet light, pulsed light) and CAPP [63]. CAPP in particular seems to be highly effective against multidrug resistant organisms (e.g., Methicillin-resistant *Staphylococcus aureus*, vancomycin-resistant enterococci), regardless of the kind of germ [42,47,49,64]. Clearly, the efficiency of the elimination process is highly dependent on the plasma device, process parameters and environmental factors (e.g., wound type, extracellular matrix) [65]. CAPP did not show any bacterial adaptation after consecutive treatments [63].

Brun et al. studied two clinically significant ESKAPE (an acronym for six virulent and antibiotic resistant pathogens) bacteria. After the plasma treatment, the decrease in bacterial load (*P. aeruginosa* and methicillin-resistant *S. aureus*) was comparable to the inactivation using biocide (chlorhexidine) and antibiotics (ciprofloxacin, daptomycin). The CAPP device (RF source from two parallel brass grids operating with helium) generated RONS in bacteria, disrupted membrane integrity and reduced the bacterial load. They treated the samples using the plasma afterglow, which inactivated the bacteria independently of their growth mode (planktonic or biofilm) [66].

Safety and bactericidal efficiency of CAPP against *Pseudomonas aeruginosa* was studied by Dijksteel et al. Their DBD plasma treatment (4–6 min) had bactericidal properties, but it did not induce mutations, apoptosis and DNA damage or affected the wound healing process in in vitro and ex vivo rat wound models [65].

The in vitro study of Wang et al. evaluated the bactericidal efficacy of CAPP (plasma jet using air) on a strain of super multidrug-resistant *P. aeruginosa* (aerobic Gram-negative bacillus causing various infections, such as pneumonia, bloodstream, skin and soft tissue infections). Both direct and plasma activated liquid treatments resulted in a decrease in cell growth (based on the colony-forming unit assay). The direct CAPP exposure was more effective, inducing higher intracellular ROS levels. Furthermore, the disruption of membrane integrity was also more effective based on immunofluorescence images [67].

Gas plasma technology has been under research for more than 50 years due to its decontaminating properties and the majority of work has been focused on bacteria. However, contamination with infectious viruses also threatens human and animal health. The antiviral activity of CAPP is a younger but evolving research area. For example, Bunz et al. observed that CAPP has an antiviral effect against herpes simplex virus type 1 (HSV-1). The effect was measurable after reducing the viral load by 100-fold [68]. Guo et al. efficiently inactivated different kinds of bacteriophages (including double-stranded DNA, single-stranded DNA and RNA bacteriophages) using CAPP treatment. Damaging of nucleic acids and proteins was achieved using argon and artificial air. Antiviral ability of plasma-activated water could also be a promising disinfection method to prevent the spread of viral diseases [56]. The paper of Filipić et al. provided a comprehensive overview about the achievements in the plasma-mediated inactivation of viruses. Their review discusses the inactivation of enteric viruses (e.g., norovirus, adenovirus, hepatitis A virus), respiratory viruses (influenza A and B, SARS-CoV-2), sexually transmitted viruses (e.g., HIV) and animal viruses (e.g., avian influenza virus, porcine reproductive and respiratory syndrome virus) [24].

During viral pandemics, like the COVID-19 crisis, respiratory viruses are responsible for over a million deaths [69]. In 2020, there has been an enormous research effort to use CAPP technology as an antiviral treatment [24]. Guo et al. used pseudoviruses with the SARS-CoV-2 S protein as a model (for biosafety limitations), and showed that plasma-activated water effectively inhibited pseudovirus infection through S protein inactivation [70]. Decontamination procedures of pathogenic viruses in different media and on various surfaces could help to limit virus spread [43]. Chen et al. studied SARS-CoV-2 inactivation using APPJ with argon and helium feed gas on various surfaces including plastic, metal and leather (the discharge voltages for argon and helium were 16.8 kV and 16.6 kV at 12.9 kHz and 12.7 kHz frequency, flow rate 6.4 L/min and 16.5 L/min). The roughness, material composition and absorptivity were aspects that influenced surface inactivation of SARS-CoV-2. The argon plasma treatment inactivated all viruses in less than 180 s. Helium plasma did not disinfect all viruses on surfaces even at 300 s because of the much lower RONS concentrations compared to argon plasma for the same operating conditions. The results confirmed the important role played by RONS concentration in virus inactivation. Comprehension of how SARS-CoV-2 interacts with CAPP is essential for future plasma utilization. [71]. The spread of SARS-CoV-2 is mostly via the transmission of respiratory droplets in poorly ventilated closed spaces [72]. It is important to try to improve the indoor air quality, e.g., by reducing the airborne time of SARS-CoV-2 aerosol microdroplets. Bisag et al. used a lab-scale dielectric barrier discharge plasma source to inactivate aerosols containing purified SARS-CoV-2 RNA suspension flowing through the device. Results show that CAP can degrade viral RNA in a short residence time (<0.2 s) [73]. The virus contains nucleic acids encased in a capsid protein coat. Reactive oxygen and nitrogen species have been shown to be responsible for virus inactivation through effects on capsid proteins, which preceded the degradation of nucleic acids. RONS can disrupt virus integrity by etching away the protein protective layer, and then act directly on nucleic acids, damaging the genetic material used for virus genome translation and replication. CAPP treatment can result in loss of viral infectivity [24,74].

Application of cold plasma is expected to decontaminate face masks or shields from SARS-CoV-2 surrogates without affecting their filtration and fitting performance [24,75]. Furthermore, CAPP can be used as an alternative to alcohol-based hand disinfection [76]. Hands are one of the most common transmission routes for many infections because people frequently touch their facial mucous membranes—the eyes, nose and mouth, which are the main portal of entry for germs [24,43]. Sterilization using CAPP is a fast and efficient method, which is essential in healthcare institutions. However, some undesirable effects have to be solved (e.g., ozone is a toxic byproduct) by optimization of the geometry of the hand dispensary system [76]. Based on early and incomplete results, CAPP has potential in inactivating different types of viruses in the near future, but confirmation will be required, because studies are in their infancy at present. Scientists anticipate that CAPP will be an effective and environmentally friendly tool to replace, complement, or upgrade existing sterilization methods, mitigating the economic and public health burdens of the pandemic [43].

Attri et al. analyzed in full theoretical detail the influence of oxidation on the SARS-CoV-2CTD protein structure and the SARS-CoV2-CTD/hACE complex. Via molecular dynamics, the basic statistical characteristics, relative binding free energy of the oxidized complex and the effect of CAPP-induced oxidation on the stability/flexibility have been determined. It was shown that the protein structures are sensitive to radical oxygen and the binding free energy (without entropic term) is lowered as a consequence of the plasma oxidation. However, the inactivation mechanism of SARS-CoV by CAPP is still an open problem, the application of cold plasma seems to be a very prospective method in this field [77].

Besides decontamination, cold plasma technology can also be used for direct therapeutic intervention. With the help of plasma, the medical treatment process could be markedly shortened. Other benefits of CAPP treatment are good tolerability (painless), biocompatibility and biosecurity (it is assumed that CAPP treatment can be applied to living cells and tissues without causing any damage) [47,78].

First of all, CAPP is a promising tool for wound healing because it has antimicrobial effects. Furthermore, it can enhance the proliferation of skin fibroblasts and angiogenesis [49,79]. Wiegand et al. demonstrated that plasma treatment using an open jet plasma device has strong bactericidal and fungicidal properties. Different bacteria strains (*Staphylococcus aureus, Pseudomonas aeruginosa*) and yeasts (*Candida albicans* and *Malassezia pachydermatis*) were treated which are associated with wound and skin infections. After the CAPP treatment, differences were observed due to the diverse structures of the cell wall of the microbes (e.g., Gram-positive bacteria have thicker cell walls then Gram-negative bacteria). The study concentrated on the influence of various process parameters of the plasma treatment. Nitrogen-based plasma was more effective than air. Increased input power and treatment time had higher antimicrobial efficacy against the tested microorganisms. [42].

The CAPP application has been intensively studied in dermatology [47]. Clinical trials have focused on onychomycosis (fungal infection of the nail), oncology (melanoma, actinic keratosis), viral warts (caused by infection with human papillomavirus), wound healing (different kinds of chronic infectious, microbiologically infected/contaminated wounds, herpes zoster-related pain), hair loss (increased hair follicle diameter), biofilm disruption (atopic dermatitis, itch), cosmetic applications (skin rejuvenation, reduction of wrinkles) and other ailments [26,51]. The treatment requires careful dosage (fast treatment and gentle heating) in order to prevent unwanted skin burns or damage deeper tissues. For example, longer exposure of the skin (>43 °C) can cause blisters [47].

CAPP also exhibits a promising future in dentistry for bonding to dentin and ceramics, surface activation of dental implants, tooth bleaching, removing dental plaque/biofilms from teeth, composite restoration and disinfection of root canals [80]. Plasma can reach inaccessible areas of the tooth surface such as fissures and grooves, furthermore the procedure is painless because plasma does not cause thermal damage to the tissue [41,81]. The promising effects of CAPP treatment useful in various areas of dentistry, for instance, cariology (cariogenic microorganisms, e.g., *Streptococcus mutans, Lactobacillus acidophilus*), periodontology (*Porphyromonas gingivalis, Tannerella forsythia* and *Treponema denticola*), endodontics (*Enterococcus faecalis,*) and oral oncology, was reviewed by Borges et al. [82]. Lee et al. investigated the antibacterial effect of CAPP treated dental titanium implants on Gram-positive and Gram-negative bacteria with different cell wall structures. The biofilm formation rate and adhesion of Gram-negative bacteria were significantly lower than Gram-positive bacteria on samples treated with the APPJ. Gram-positive bacteria are more resistant to plasma than Gram-negative bacteria. This is related to the thickness of the peptidoglycan layer in the bacterial cell wall, which may reduce the antibacterial effects [83].

Cold plasma has shown promising results in cancer therapy because it can selectively induce apoptosis in cancer cells, reduce tumor volume and vasculature and halt metastasis [49,58,84]. CAPP has shown substantial anticancer capability over a wide range of cancer cells, for instance, melanoma [47,85], carcinoma [86,87] and osteosarcoma [88]. Cancer cells vary from normal cells, e.g., they produce higher amounts of reactive oxygen species. Thus, cancer cells are more susceptible to plasma-generated ROS than normal cells. ROSs contribute to oxidative stress and can cause cell death [89]. However, it is important to tailor the plasma process parameters to produce a controllable amount of ROS to obtain the desired biological responses. The mechanism of CAPP action in the case of cancer includes the induction of apoptosis, DNA damage, cell cycle arrest at the S-phase and increase of the intracellular ROS concentrations [79]. CAPP can open new horizons in oncology because it seems to be a promising complementary therapy to conventional cancer treatments (chemotherapy, surgery, radiation therapy, immunotherapy and others).

The anti-melanoma activity of a softjet CAPP device was studied by Yadav et al. Three different human melanoma cells (skin cancer) were successfully treated using air and N_2 gases. The results showed preferential killing of melanoma cells, apoptotic pathways by triggering apoptotic genes in all three melanoma cell lines. However, the exact mechanism for the inhibitory effect of CAPP has remained unknown [85].

Mateu-Sanz et al. provided evidence of plasma-activated Ringer's saline (PAR) as a promising therapy option for treating Osteosarcoma (a type of malignant bone cancer). They used two types of plasma jet devices (single-electrode needle device operating in helium and pin-type electrode with a grounded outer electrode operating with argon) to obtain PAR. The cytotoxic effects of PAR in human and mouse osteosarcoma was investigated [88].

Based on the above-mentioned properties, it can be said that plasma medicine holds enormous application and development potential (Figure 3) [47]. CAPP seems to be ready to enter the healthcare area for various medical therapies. However, a lot remains to be done (conduction and evaluation of preclinical and clinical trials with standardized protocols), in order to fully understand the interactions between plasma and biological cells and tissues (both in vitro and in vivo) [26,49].

3.2. Food Industry and Agriculture

Global food demand is significantly increasing due to the rapidly growing world population, changes in diet, limited agricultural land, climate change and increasing water deficiency [22]. Agriculture and the food industry face intense pressure because modern-day consumers desire nutritious, fresh, safe and minimally processed foods and drinks. Nowadays, a plethora of methods is available for food processing, such as pasteurization, high-pressure processing, distillation, ozonation, irradiation (ultraviolet light treatment, pulsed light treatment), ultrasonication and chemical treatments (e.g., chlorine, hydrogen peroxide, peroxyacetic acid, organic acid) [25,61,90]. However, these kinds of treatments could have a negative impact on the food quality, toxicology, sensorial and nutritive characteristics which make them less attractive to customers [25,91]. For these reasons, the food industry is continuously seeking alternative methods to improve food production [11,92].

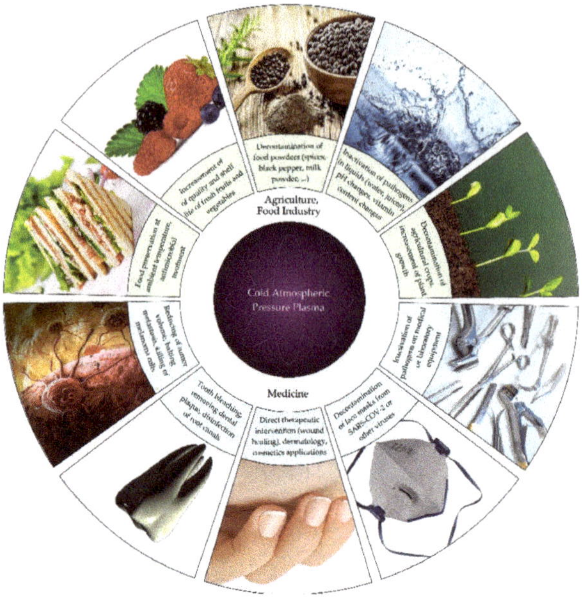
Cold Atmospheric Pressure Plasma
Agriculture, Food Industry
Medicine
Decontamination of food powders (spices, black pepper, milk powder, ...)
Inactivation of pathogens in liquids (water, juices), pH changes, vitamin content changes
Decontamination of agricultural crops, increasement of plant growth
Inactivation of pathogens on medical or laboratory instruments
Decontamination of face masks from SARS-COV-2 or other viruses
Direct therapeutic intervention (wound healing), dermatology, cosmetics applications
Tooth bleaching, removing dental plaque, disinfection of root canals
Reducing of tumor volume, halting metastasis, killing of melanoma cells
Food preservation at ambient temperature, antimicrobial treatment
Increasement of quality and shelf life of fresh fruits and vegetables

Figure 3. Schematic illustration of selected applications of CAPP treatment in medicine, agriculture and food industry.

Inactivation of microorganisms (disinfection of foods, packaging materials and equipment) improves food safety, which is one of the major challenges of this industrial sector (Figure 3) [22]. The major components of food matrices are protein, lipids, carbohydrates, water, minerals and vitamins [10]. The aim of any processing is to impart edibility, palatability and prolong shelf life, while maintaining food quality.

CAPP treatment seems to be an effective technology that achieves food preservation at ambient or sublethal temperatures, which reduces the negative thermal effects on the nutritional and quality properties of food. Cold plasma has great potential to inactivate bacteria, viruses, mycotoxins, yeast, molds, endotoxins, etc., on plant- and animal-based foods (e.g., fresh and dry fruits, vegetables, juices, nuts, egg shells, egg-based products, undercooked meat and fish, dairy products, spices, cereals) [20,23,52,90,91,93–96]. Different types of *Escherichia coli*, *Listeria*, *Salmonella*, *Tulane* virus and hepatitis A virus are the most prevalent foodborne pathogens, which can cause serious health issues [61,94,97–99]. Several pathogens can also survive freezing (*E. coli* for >180 days) [10].

The specific mechanism of microbial inactivation is still under investigation. The inactivation occurs due to various physicochemical processes (emission of UV radiation, generation of ozone and other active species) [25]. The production of reactive species depends on the used working gas. Reactive oxygen and/or nitrogen species have a potent microbicidal effect, they can damage macromolecules by oxidizing nucleic acids, proteins and lipids [24,25,93]. Besides that, the UV radiation can destroy the membranes of microorganisms, structural cell functions and genetic material of pathogens [93]. However, it is worth mentioning that the contribution of UV radiation to the antimicrobial effect is controversial [100]. The resistance to UV light seems to be dependent on the type of microorganism (microbial growth phase, stress conditions, e.g., pH, osmotic concentration and growth temperature) and the plasma device [25]. The most often used reactor configurations are DBD and APPJ. The physicochemical properties (color, texture, pH, acidity, antioxidant activity, amount of proteins, enzymes, carbohydrates, vitamins, lipids, allergens, toxins) could change depending on the plasma treatment process parameters [10,20,22]. Furthermore, the operating cost of plasma processing is an important consideration. It mainly depends on the cost of the working gas (plasma generated from noble gases is much more expensive than air) [23].

The antimicrobial effect of the plasma treatment is also highly dependent on the surface structure and surface to volume ratio of the product [23,25,57]. CAPP treatment on solid/dry foods mainly affects only their surface. The low penetration depth of the plasma components is advantageous because more important nutrients can remain inside the food [10].

Spoilage of ready-to-eat salads (fruits and vegetables) due to microbial growth causes significant food waste. The effect of DBD plasma treatment on the quality (microbial load, hardness, pH value, color) and shelf life of fresh cut, leafy rocket salad was studied by Giannoglou et al. The greatest reduction of the load (*Pseudomonas* spp.) was obtained after 10 min plasma treatment. The pH and color of the leaves were not affected, the shelf life was increased compared to untreated salad [101].

Yadav et al. used DBD plasma treatment for ready-to-eat ham to inactivate *Listeria monocytogenes*, which may occur during slicing and packing. They significantly reduced the cell counts (at least by 2 log) and studied the changes in color and lipid oxidation as a function of ham formulation, plasma treatment time, in-package gas composition and storage conditions [102].

Decontamination of food powders (e.g., onion powder, spices, black pepper, legume flour, milk powder) using plasma is more complex. Usually, it requires high plasma power density, long treatment time compared to flat samples. Pina-Perez et al. published the inactivation efficiency of *Bacillus subtilis* spores using an air surface microdischarge CAPP with low plasma power density (5 mW/cm^2) and relatively short treatment time (7 min). The inhibiting effects on flat glass and corn starch samples were evaluated. Etching of spore hulls using reactive nitrogen species has been reported as a fundamental inactivation principle [103].

In the case of liquids, the penetration depth is less important, because every element comes into contact with the plasma volume, however, not only the pathogens are damaged [10]. Several studies confirmed that CAPP treatment has the ability to inactivate microorganisms (e.g., *Escherichia coli* O157:H7, *Zygosaccharomyces rouxii*, *Salmonella enterica*) in fruit juices (e.g., apple, orange, blueberry) with very good inactivation rate. Although there is some uncertainty in the literature about the operating parameters and their effect on the quality parameters of the juices. Some researchers indicated that increasing treatment time can lead to color changes (ascorbic acid degradation), pH changes and changes in vitamin content (due to oxidation reactions). Moreover, additional research is needed for large scale processing and to prove that plasma does not have any toxic residuals [91].

Many different microorganisms attach to surfaces (e.g., food matrixes, processing equipment) and develop biofilms [57]. These complex microbial ecosystems are more resistant to various environmental stresses, antimicrobials and inactivation treatments (longer treatment time is necessary) than planktonic cells due to their three-dimensional extracellular matrix [25]. Biofilm inactivation process includes various processes, like destruction of extracellular matrix, cells and cell components, etching and reduction of biofilm thickness [57]. Kadri et al. also demonstrated that biofilms are less susceptible to cold plasma treatment. Furthermore, treatment efficiency depends on the biofilm age (mature biofilms are more resistant to CAPP than young biofilms) and the type of bacteria. They presented the inactivation of various single and mixed biofilm systems of *L. innocua* and *E. coli*, which produced an extracellular polymeric substance matrix of different thickness and composition [92].

XU et al. extensively studied yeast cell inactivation at the subcellular level. It was shown that cold plasma may effectively lower the yeast cell physiological activities by the superposition of several mechanisms with different impacts (in particular, cell membrane damage, energy metabolism or DNA fragmentation). Their results showed that $^{\bullet}OH$ (it attacked the cell membrane and increased its permeability) and $^1O_2$ species (it disturbed the cell energy metabolism) contribute most to the yeast inactivation [59].

Attri et al. showed that RONS produced using CAPP is able to inactivate thermophilic bacteria, which can tolerate a wide temperature and pH range (e.g., spores of *Geobacillus* spp. in raw milk can survive pasteurization temperatures, spores of *Bacillus stearothermophilus* can spoil low acid canned foods). Sufficiently high dose (long treatment duration, i.e., 20 min) plasma treatment (using DBD device) caused protein denaturation/modification (model protein: MTH1880 from *Methanobacterium thermoautotrophicum*) [104].

Beyrer et al. studied the effectiveness of a direct contact DBD device against spores (dormant forms of microorganisms, like bacterial endospores), which are very resistant to heat and UV treatments due to their durable coat layers. They compared the inactivation kinetics of spores of *Bacillus* spp. (~3 $\log_{10}$ cycles of inactivation after 10 s exposure time), *Geobacillus* spp. and *Penicillium* spp. on flat glass carriers, native starch granules (non-porous material) and shells of diatoms (highly porous system) [105].

The safety of animal origin foods is an even bigger challenge for the food industry. Microbial inactivation experiments mainly focus on poultry (e.g., *Salmonella* spp. on eggs, chicken meat), meat (e.g., *L. monocytogenes*, *E. coli*, *Salmonella* spp. and *C. jejuni* on beef, pork) and fish (e.g., *Lactobacillus*, *Pseudomonas*) products [25]. CAPP treatment is able to inactivate various pathogens, however, ROS species can cause quality problems, which affects the consumer acceptability and shelf life [93]. For example, changes in color (e.g., loss of color, darkening) are a result of undesirable reactions due to the partial inactivation of enzymes and microorganisms [25,52]. The review of Nasiru et al. summarizes the influence of various DBD plasma device process parameters on microbial inactivation in meat products. They concluded that the use of oxygen or carbon dioxide in the working gas mixture results in enhanced effectiveness of the plasma treatment. Furthermore, increased power/voltage and treatment duration also have a pronounced effect on microbial decontamination [106]. Seafood is considered part of a healthy diet, however these products are responsible for many foodborne disease outbreaks. Seafood is shipped worldwide; the control of pathogenic and spoilage microorganisms is essential to ensure food safety. CAPP has high potential for commercial use in the seafood industry. Ekonomou et al. published a systematic review about the microbiological safety and quality of fish and seafood (squid shreds, mackerel, Asian sea bass). They compared various non thermal methods (high hydrostatic pressure processing, ultrasound, pulsed electric field, electrolyzed water and CAPP treatment) [107].

Plasma treatment is also gaining attention in agriculture since climate change has caused reductions in crop yield (reduction in the quality and quantity of crop products) (Figure 3) [108]. Furthermore, chemical-based methods are becoming less preferred due to the emergence of pathogen resistance (many pests have developed resistance to pesticides, new diseases have emerged) and environmental pollution [98]. CAP has the potential to increase crop plant vitality and production.

Agricultural crops (fruits, vegetables) are often contaminated because they come in contact with dust, insects, animal urine and feces, workers and equipment during harvest and postharvest (transport, storage, cleaning, packaging and food processing) stages [16,108]. Plasma inactivation processes are mostly focusing on bacterial (e.g., *Erwinia carotovora*, *Clavibacter michiganensis*, *Pectobacterium carotovorum*) and fungal pathogens (e.g., *Alternaria*, *Aspergillus*, *Botrytis*, *Colletotrichum*, *Fusarium*, *Penicillium*) in agriculture [109].

The review papers of Attri et al. focused on preharvest applications of CAPP in agriculture. These papers summarize laboratory experiments dealing with the effects of direct (DBD, APPJ) and indirect (plasma-activated water) treatments on the plant (e.g., wheat, corn, chili pepper, lentils, tomato, rice, etc.) growth and development. The CAPP generated RONS can alter the germination rate, plant morphology (shoot and root length, leaf area, etc.), gene expression and biochemical processes (changes in hormones, amino acids, antioxidants, soluble sugar level, chlorophyll content, etc.). For example, higher antioxidant activity, growth hormones and metabolites led to early germination, improved germination percentage, elevated growth (root, shoot, leaves) and increased plant yield [110].

The paper of Takaki et al. described various CAPP treatments to keep the freshness and quality of agricultural products in the postharvest stage. For example, removing ethylene during storage and transportation (fruits and vegetables in storehouses, preservation boxes and transportation containers) is important because ethylene works as a plant hormone and it can induce fruit ripening and undesirable reactions (e.g., bitter flavors, yellowing of green leafy vegetables and increase of vulnerability to disease. Decomposition of ethylene is an oxidation process by atomic oxygen, which can be achieved using CAPP treatment (e.g., corona and DBD discharges) [111].

Plasma and plasma-treated water can also be utilized for controlling plant diseases (e.g., seed-borne, foliage, root and postharvest diseases) by inactivating pathogens (e.g., disinfection of seeds, fertilizer, water, soil) [23,109,112,113]. Review paper of Attri et al. concluded that plasma can also enhance seed germination (e.g., radish sprouts, wheat, sunflower, pea, tomato seeds). They described the possible mechanisms of plasma treatment in agriculture (increased gibberellin level and decreased abscisic acid content, enhanced activity of catalase, superoxide dismutase and peroxidase, improved water absorption, elevated levels of proline, chlorophyll, polyphenols sugar and protein contents) [114]. Seed germination efficiency (speed, percentage) depends on the plasma source, plant species and moisture content. Plasma-induced physicochemical changes in the properties of the seed coat or surface (e.g., elevated hydrophilicity and water permeability) enhance water imbibition, which is essential for seed germination. Adhikari et al. also discussed the beneficial effects of plasma treatment on seed germination, plant growth, and development. RONS can act as signaling molecules, which initiate a germination process and break the dormancy stage [108]. Another critical phase for plant development is the vegetative growth (it determines the overall crop productivity), which can be also regulated using plasma. As indicated by several studies, RONS have a positive effect on plant organs (shoots, roots, leaves and flowers) at different growth stages. Reactive species (H_2O_2 and NO) may disturb redox homeostasis and trigger mild oxidative stress in plants [108].

Another application of CAPP technology is the enhancement of seedling growth, which depends on seed metabolism and external environmental factors. Even 1 min CAPP treatment significantly promoted the seedling growth (fresh weight and length increment) of Arabidopsis thaliana. The results of Wang et al. suggested the plasma treatment accelerates the seedling abscisic acid (ABA) accumulations at the early stages of growth. ABA regulates the concentration of calcium (Ca^{2+}) and RONS (e.g., OH, H_2O_2, NO_3^-, NO_2^-). The reactive species are easily transported through the cell membrane by diffusion and aquaporins. RONS serve as nutrients and also act as signalling molecules involved in the growth process [115].

Kučerová et al. studied the effect of PAW (produced form tap water using self-pulsing transient spark discharge) irrigation on lettuce plants. They concluded that H_2O_2 and NO_3^- are the most important RONS in the PAW. However, proper concentrations must be applied in order to stimulate the growth process and positively affect the physiological parameters (number and quality of leaves, fresh and dry weight of plants, photosynthetic pigment content, photosynthetic rate and activity of antioxidant enzymes) of plants [116].

The study of Hashizume et al. represents the first trial of CAPP treatment in an actual production paddy field. They treated rice plants either directly by direct irradiation, or indirectly by immersing plants in a plasma-activated Ringer's lactate solution (PAL). Their results suggest that the plasma treatment of rice seedlings is effective at improving plant growth, grain yield and grain quality. For example, direct irradiation experiments (plants irradiated during the vegetative growth period) resulted in increased grain yield by as much as 15% [117].

Pesticide (e.g., insecticides, fungicides, rodenticides, herbicides, garden chemicals) residues are toxic to human health and the environment. They have been linked to various illnesses, such as cancer, reproductive disorders and endocrine-system dysfunctions. It is therefore very important to focus attention on this issue and it is widely agreed that the use of pesticides should be regulated worldwide. The Environmental Working Group

(EWG) annually releases the dirty dozen food list, which contains fruits and vegetables with highest traces of pesticides [118]. Results of Ali et al. confirmed that plasma activated water (PAW) and buffer solution were able to reduce ($p < 0.05$) chlorothalonil fungicide and thiram on tomato. Notable negative impact on the quality of the fruit was not observable based on pH value, ascorbic acid, titratable acidity, total soluble solid, lycopene and total phenolic content evaluations. The PAW increased the formation of RONS, which were beneficial to the degradation of various organic and inorganic pesticides [119].

Volkov et al. demonstrated that cold plasma (using plasma jet) can behave as a catalyst for important redox chemical reactions, such as the oxidation of nitrogen, occurring at the plasma/water and plasma/air interfaces, and in the volume of the liquid phase. Due to the reduced activation energy, atmospheric nitrogen can be converted to other forms (e.g., HNO_3) useful in the agriculture industry for nitrogen fixation, production of nitrogen compounds and fertilizers. Plasma treatment of water may provide a promising alternative to current methods (e.g., Birkeland–Eyde, Haber–Bosch and Ostwald processes) which have well-known environmental and ecological issues [120].

Another new approach in plant disease control is the so-called plasma vaccination (RONS enter the plant through wounding or small openings and further penetrate the plant cells), which activate plant immune response [109].

Plant growth in space is under research as a possible technology to be used in future. Plants provide fresh food, oxygen and psychological benefits for astronauts on long -term missions. CAPP as a waterless, chemical-free technology has potential as a disinfection tool in spaceflight, however even stricter regulations are needed [25].

Another branch of agriculture is animal husbandry dealing with animals (e.g., cattle, sheep, goats, pigs, chickens, rabbits and insects) raised for meat, milk, eggs and fiber. Good animal husbandry practices are essential for animal welfare and productivity. CAPP can be helpful in maintaining better health conditions of animals via i) microbial decontamination of air (deactivation of indoor and outdoor bioaerosols), water (E.coli), food, instruments (surface pathogens, such as methicillin-resistant staphylococcus aureus, Klebsiella pneumoniae); ii) wound healing in animals (e.g., wound myiasis caused by blowfly, inactivation of Chlamydia trachomatis); iii) packaging of animal products (sterilization of packages, disinfection the inside of sealed bags) [121].

Newcastle disease and avian influenza are the two most common devastating diseases among poultry (chicken, turkey and duck). It has been already reported that CAPP can be used as an effective and safe agent for inactivated vaccine preparation against viruses [121]. The study of Su et al. indicates that virulent Newcastle disease can be inactivated using plasma-activated solutions (H_2O, NaCl, H_2O_2). The efficiency of the inactivation was confirmed using embryo lethality assay and hemagglutination tests. This disease affects bird species and has a large economic impact on the domestic animal and poultry industries; furthermore, it is transmissible to humans [122].

Plasma-based inactivation of prions (proteinaceous infectious particles), which belong to one of the most resistant pathogens, is also under research. Most prion diseases affect the nervous system of humans (Creutzfeldt–Jakob disease) and animals (bovine spongiform encephalopathy in cattle, chronic wasting disease in cervids). Prion diseases have long and silent incubation periods, once the symptoms emerge, these disorders are rapidly progressive and usually fatal [16].

Key benefits of utilizing CAPP in the food and agriculture sectors include minimal water and power usage, operation at ambient temperature, and short treatment duration (from seconds to minutes). Furthermore, its use is free of hazardous solvents, it reduces preservative use and it is applicable for both solid as well as liquid phases [10,16]. Currently available data confirm that CAPP technology could be utilized in the agriculture and food industry [22,99]. To achieve broad applicability, an efficient open-air device suitable for the treatment of both large areas and high number of samples is necessary [16]. An ideal industrial scale device allows homogenous disinfection of various products during the sorting process on rolling electrodes [23].

It is important to avoid quality degradation or any undesired effects of plasma treatment. In addition, more intense optimization studies are needed to fully understand the mechanisms behind the pathogen–plasma interactions. There is a need for standardization of the plasma dose (treatment duration is not an appropriate standardized unit because of the diversity of food products and plasma reactors) [11,25]. CAPP treatment limitations are also necessary to account for before consumer acceptance can be achieved [10,11,109].

3.3. Plasma Inactivation Mechanism

As claimed above, CAPP produces different reactive species (RONS, positive and negative ions, atoms, molecules, etc.) playing a crucial role in the inactivation of microbial targets. Bourke et al. reviewed the mechanism of bacteria inactivation via CAPP. The bacteria are eroded by cell bombardment of charged particles, breaking the appropriate chemical bonds and opening the cell membrane to the penetration of reactive agents into the inner volume of bacteria. The etching process (facilitated, in particular, by RONS species) subsequently causes formation of molecular fragments leading to morphological changes of the cell (e.g., formation of deep channels in the bacteria), RONS cause damage by oxidation of cytoplasmic membrane, protein and DNA and thus complete bacterial destruction [57]. To increase the use of CAPP technology in industry, it is important to provide theoretical studies about the pathogen inactivation process. To describe the inactivation mechanism at the atomic level is difficult based on only experimental research [123]. A better understanding of plasma dynamics and chemistry, and the transport of reactive species in the plasma can be achieved using numerical simulations. Most computational studies evaluate the plasma physics and gas phase chemistry (e.g., spatial-temporal profile of the electric field, density of reactive species, radiation intensity). Various kinetic models (classical reactive molecular dynamics, nonreactive molecular dynamics, density functional theory) are used to describe the biomolecular systems at the molecular or atomic scale [124]. These models save time, money and other resources by analyzing a large amount of data at the same time and provide valuable correlations. The study of Cui et al., based on reactive force field molecular dynamics simulation, found that ROS (O, OH, HO_2 and H_2O_2) reacted with the S. cerevisiae glucan structure by hydrogen abstraction reaction to cleave the chemical bonds (C–O and C–C), which resulted in cell wall destruction. Their results showed that O (highest activity) and OH induced the largest number of hydrogen abstraction reactions. The activity of HO_2 and H_2O_2 were lower, however, the number of main chain and branched chain fractures were bigger. Consequently, the destructive effect of H_2O and H_2O_2 was more efficient [123].

The bacterial cell membranes, barriers protecting proteins and nucleic acids can block ROS from entering the interior of cells. However, ROS with high permeability are able to enter the cell interior and cause cell death. Therefore, the permeability of ROS into the bacterial membrane plays a crucial role in the bacterial inactivation mechanism [125] as was shown by Hu et al. Their molecular dynamics simulation described the behavior of various ROS at the membrane–water interface. They showed that the cell membrane acts as a weak barrier to O_2 (hydrophobic ROS), which remains within the lipid bilayer, and plays the most important role in oxidation reactions. On the other hand, the cell membrane serves as a strong barrier to protect internal substances from the hydrophilic ROS (OH, HO_2, H_2O_2). The permeability of the cell membrane to HO_2 was markedly enhanced after the CAPP treatment, which enhanced the bacteria-killing properties of the plasma. They also concluded that the arrangement of phospholipid molecules (the main constituent of the cell membrane having hydrophilic head and hydrophilic tail) in the cell depends on the ROS generated by the plasma. High amount of ROS resulted in decreased cell membrane thickness and disordered phospholipid arrangements [125].

4. Conclusions

Cold atmospheric pressure plasma (CAPP) technology, which is a fast-growing research area due to interdisciplinary cooperation between specialists in various research areas, such as physics, chemistry, biology, medicine, agriculture, etc. Plasma technology operating at atmospheric pressure and near room temperature attracts attention because of its time- and cost-effectivity (no need for vacuum systems) and its ability to process heat sensitive materials (e.g., polymers, plastics, cells, living tissue, food). Furthermore, as a dry process, it is significantly more environmentally friendly than the traditional wet chemistry processes. The environmental benefits of CAPP technology comprise its nontoxic nature, reduced application of chemicals, and a significant reduction in water and energy consumption.

Plasma treatment provides an efficient way to improve various surface properties (wettability, adhesion, etc.) without altering the desired bulk characteristics of the material. Furthermore, CAPP can effectively inactivate various pathogens (e.g., bacteria, fungi, viruses, prions) on/in foods, medical devices, etc. CAPP can also be utilized in agriculture for enhancing seed germination, seed decontamination, plant disease control, water cleaning, etc. Plasma in medicine holds great promise for various therapeutic treatments (disinfection, dermatology, oncology, dentistry). The efficiency of the plasma treatmentdepends on the experimental conditions (reactor design, electrode configuration, feeding gas, operating conditions, substrate type, etc.). However, there is a need to fully understand and evaluate the benefits and risks of cold plasma treatment, taking into consideration economic, consumer, environmental and social aspects. It can be concluded that CAPP has a wide range of possible applications in medicine, agriculture and food industry and is expected to become omnipresent in almost all major industries in the foreseeable future.

Author Contributions: Writing—original draft preparation, M.D.; writing—review and editing, M.D., P.T., J.T. and P.D. All authors have read and agreed to the published version of the manuscript.

Funding: This work was supported by the Technical University in Prague, project No. SGS19/141/OHK1/3T/11.

Institutional Review Board Statement: Not applicable.

Informed Consent Statement: Not applicable.

Conflicts of Interest: The authors declare no conflict of interest.

References

1. Domonkos, M.; Ižák, T.; Varga, M.; Potocky, S.; Demo, P.; Kromka, A. Diamond nucleation and growth on horizontally and vertically aligned Si substrates at low pressure in a linear antenna microwave plasma system. *Diam. Relat. Mater.* **2018**, *82*, 41–49. [CrossRef]
2. Domonkos, M.; Izak, T.; Kromka, A.; Varga, M. Polymer-based nucleation for chemical vapour deposition of diamond. *J. Appl. Polym. Sci.* **2016**, *133*, 133. [CrossRef]
3. Tichá, P.; Domonkos, M.; Demo, P. Fiber reinforced concrete: Residual flexure strength enhancement using surface modified fibers. In *Special Concrete and Composites 2020: 17th International Conference*; AIP Publishing: College Park, MD, USA, 2021; Volume 2322, p. 020030.
4. Steinerova, M.; Matejka, R.; Stepanovska, J.; Filova, E.; Stankova, L.; Rysova, M.; Martinova, L.; Dragounova, H.; Domonkos, M.; Artemenko, A.; et al. Human osteoblast-like SAOS-2 cells on submicron-scale fibers coated with nanocrystalline diamond films. *Mater. Sci. Eng. C* **2021**, *121*, 111792. [CrossRef] [PubMed]
5. Domonkos, M.; Demo, P.; Kromka, A. Nanosphere Lithography for Structuring Polycrystalline Diamond Films. *Crystals* **2020**, *10*, 118. [CrossRef]
6. Cvelbar, U.; Walsh, J.L.; Černák, M.; De Vries, H.W.; Reuter, S.; Belmonte, T.; Corbella, C.; Miron, C.; Hojnik, N.; Jurov, A.; et al. White paper on the future of plasma science and technology in plastics and textiles. *Plasma Process. Polym.* **2018**, *16*, 1700228. [CrossRef]
7. Talviste, R.; Galmiz, O.; Stupavská, M.; Tučeková, Z.; Kaarna, K.; Kováčik, D. Effect of DCSBD plasma treatment on surface properties of thermally modified wood. *Surf. Interfaces* **2019**, *16*, 8–14. [CrossRef]
8. Medvecká, V.; Kováčik, D.; Stupavská, M.; Roch, T.; Kromka, A.; Fajgar, R.; Zahoranová, A.; Černák, M. Preparation and characterization of alumina submicron fibers by plasma assisted calcination. *Ceram. Int.* **2020**, *46*, 22774–22780. [CrossRef]
9. Thomas, S.; Mozetič, M.; Cvelbar, U.; Špatenka, P.; Praveen, K.M. *Non-Thermal Plasma Technology for Polymeric Materials: Applications in Composites, Nanostructured Materials, and Biomedical Fields*; Elsevier: Amsterdam, The Netherlands, 2019; ISBN 978-0-12-813153-4.
10. Ohta, T. Plasma in Agriculture. In *Cold Plasma in Food and Agriculture*; Misra, N.N., Schlüter, O., Cullen, P.J., Eds.; Academic Press: San Diego, CA, USA, 2016; Chapter 8; pp. 205–221, ISBN 978-0-12-801365-6.

11. Cullen, P.J.; Lalor, J.; Scally, L.; Boehm, D.; Milosavljević, V.; Bourke, P.; Keener, K. Translation of plasma technology from the lab to the food industry. *Plasma Process. Polym.* **2017**, *15*, 1700085. [CrossRef]
12. Pinson, J.; Thiry, D. *Surface Modification of Polymers*; WILEY-VCH: Weinheim, Germany, 2020; ISBN 978-3-527-34541-0.
13. Dou, S.; Tao, L.; Wang, R.; El Hankari, S.; Chen, R.; Wang, S. Plasma-Assisted Synthesis and Surface Modification of Electrode Materials for Renewable Energy. *Adv. Mater.* **2018**, *30*, e1705850. [CrossRef]
14. Ollegott, K.; Wirth, P.; Oberste-Beulmann, C.; Awakowicz, P.; Muhler, M. Fundamental Properties and Applications of Dielectric Barrier Discharges in Plasma-Catalytic Processes at Atmospheric Pressure. *Chem. Ing. Tech.* **2020**, *92*, 1542–1558. [CrossRef]
15. Alemán, C.; Fabregat, G.; Armelin, E.; Buendía, J.J.; Llorca, J. Plasma surface modification of polymers for sensor applications. *J. Mater. Chem. B* **2018**, *6*, 6515–6533. [CrossRef] [PubMed]
16. Sakudo, A.; Yagyu, Y.; Onodera, T. Disinfection and Sterilization Using Plasma Technology: Fundamentals and Future Perspectives for Biological Applications. *Int. J. Mol. Sci.* **2019**, *20*, 5216. [CrossRef] [PubMed]
17. Nema, S.K.; Jhala, P.B. *Plasma Technologies for Textile and Apparel*; CRC Press: Boca Raton, FL, USA, 2015; ISBN 978-93-80308-95-1.
18. Stryczewska, H.D. Supply Systems of Non-Thermal Plasma Reactors. Construction Review with Examples of Applications. *Appl. Sci.* **2020**, *10*, 3242. [CrossRef]
19. Dimitrakellis, P.; Gogolides, E. Atmospheric plasma etching of polymers: A palette of applications in cleaning/ashing, pattern formation, nanotexturing and superhydrophobic surface fabrication. *Microelectron. Eng.* **2018**, *194*, 109–115. [CrossRef]
20. Pankaj, S.K.; Wan, Z.; Keener, K.M. Effects of Cold Plasma on Food Quality: A Review. *Foods* **2018**, *7*, 4. [CrossRef]
21. Izadjoo, M.; Zack, S.; Kim, H.; Skiba, J. Medical applications of cold atmospheric plasma: State of the science. *J. Wound Care* **2018**, *27*, S4–S10. [CrossRef]
22. Mandal, R.; Singh, A.; Singh, A.P. Recent developments in cold plasma decontamination technology in the food industry. *Trends Food Sci. Technol.* **2018**, *80*, 93–103. [CrossRef]
23. Hertwig, C.; Meneses, N.; Mathys, A. Cold atmospheric pressure plasma and low energy electron beam as alternative nonthermal decontamination technologies for dry food surfaces: A review. *Trends Food Sci. Technol.* **2018**, *77*, 131–142. [CrossRef]
24. Filipić, A.; Gutierrez-Aguirre, I.; Primc, G.; Mozetič, M.; Dobnik, D. Cold Plasma, a New Hope in the Field of Virus Inactivation. *Trends Biotechnol.* **2020**, *38*, 1278–1291. [CrossRef]
25. Bermúdez-Aguirre, D. *Advances in Cold Plasma Applications for Food Safety and Preservation*, 1st ed.; Bermudez-Aguirre, D., Ed.; Elsevier: Cambridge, UK, 2019; ISBN 978-0-12-814921-8.
26. Laroussi, M. Plasma Medicine: A Brief Introduction. *Plasma* **2018**, *1*, 47–60. [CrossRef]
27. Brandenburg, R. Dielectric barrier discharges: Progress on plasma sources and on the understanding of regimes and single filaments. *Plasma Sources Sci. Technol.* **2017**, *26*, 053001. [CrossRef]
28. Šimončicová, J.; Kryštofová, S.; Medvecká, V.; Ďurišová, K.; Kaliňáková, B. Technical applications of plasma treatments: Current state and perspectives. *Appl. Microbiol. Biotechnol.* **2019**, *103*, 5117–5129. [CrossRef]
29. Subedi, D.P.; Joshi, U.M.; Wong, C.S. Dielectric Barrier Discharge (DBD) Plasmas and Their Applications. In *Plasma Science and Technology for Emerging Economies*; Springer: Singapore, 2017; pp. 693–737.
30. Scholtz, V.; Pazlarova, J.; Souskova, H.; Khun, J.; Julak, J. Nonthermal plasma—A tool for decontamination and disinfection. *Biotechnol. Adv.* **2015**, *33*, 1108–1119. [CrossRef]
31. Matsusaka, S. Control of particle charge by atmospheric pressure plasma jet (APPJ): A review. *Adv. Powder Technol.* **2019**, *30*, 2851–2858. [CrossRef]
32. Morabit, Y.; Hasan, M.I.; Whalley, R.D.; Robert, E.; Modic, M.; Walsh, J.L. A review of the gas and liquid phase interactions in low-temperature plasma jets used for biomedical applications. *Eur. Phys. J. D* **2021**, *75*, 1–26. [CrossRef]
33. Deepak, G.D.; Joshi, N.K.; Prakash, R. Model analysis and electrical characterization of atmospheric pressure cold plasma jet in pin electrode configuration. *AIP Adv.* **2018**, *8*, 055321. [CrossRef]
34. Von Woedtke, T.; Emmert, S.; Metelmann, H.-R.; Rupf, S.; Weltmann, K.-D. Perspectives on cold atmospheric plasma (CAP) applications in medicine. *Phys. Plasmas* **2020**, *27*, 070601. [CrossRef]
35. Shihab, A.M. The study of thermal description for non-thermal plasma needle system. *Iraqi J. Phys.* **2018**, *16*, 66–72. [CrossRef]
36. Julák, J.; Soušková, H.; Scholtz, V.; Kvasničková, E.; Savická, D.; Kříha, V. Comparison of fungicidal properties of non-thermal plasma produced by corona discharge and dielectric barrier discharge. *Folia Microbiol.* **2017**, *63*, 63–68. [CrossRef]
37. Zainal, M.N.F.; Redzuan, N.; Misnal, M.F.I. Brief Review: Cold Plasma. *J. Teknol.* **2015**, *74*. [CrossRef]
38. Khalili, F.; Shokri, B.; Khani, M.-R.; Hasani, M.; Zandi, F.; Aliahmadi, A. A study of the effect of gliding arc non-thermal plasma on almonds decontamination. *AIP Adv.* **2018**, *8*, 105024. [CrossRef]
39. Dasan, B.G.; Onal-Ulusoy, B.; Pawlat, J.; Diatczyk, J.; Sen, Y.; Mutlu, M. A New and Simple Approach for Decontamination of Food Contact Surfaces with Gliding Arc Discharge Atmospheric Non-Thermal Plasma. *Food Bioprocess. Technol.* **2017**, *10*, 650–661. [CrossRef]
40. Tabibian, S.; Labbafi, M.; Askari, G.; Rezaeinezhad, A.; Ghomi, H. Effect of gliding arc discharge plasma pretreatment on drying kinetic, energy consumption and physico-chemical properties of saffron (*Crocus sativus* L.). *J. Food Eng.* **2020**, *270*, 109766. [CrossRef]
41. Brany, D.; Dvorská, D.; Halašová, E.; Škovierová, H. Cold Atmospheric Plasma: A Powerful Tool for Modern Medicine. *Int. J. Mol. Sci.* **2020**, *21*, 2932. [CrossRef]

42. Wiegand, C.; Fink, S.; Hipler, U.-C.; Beier, O.; Horn, K.; Pfuch, A.; Schimanski, A.; Grünler, B. Cold atmospheric pressure plasmas exhibit antimicrobial properties against critical bacteria and yeast species. *J. Wound Care* **2017**, *26*, 462–468. [CrossRef]
43. Chen, Z.; Wirz, R. Cold Atmospheric Plasma for COVID-19. *Preprints* **2020**, 2020040126. [CrossRef]
44. Avellar, H.K.; Williams, M.R.; Brandão, J.; Narayanan, S.; Ramachandran, A.; Holbrook, T.C.; Schoonover, M.J.; Bailey, K.L.; Payton, M.E.; Pai, K.K.; et al. Safety and efficacy of cold atmospheric plasma for the sterilization of a *Pasteurella multocida*–contaminated subcutaneously implanted foreign body in rabbits. *Am. J. Vet. Res.* **2021**, *82*, 118–124. [CrossRef]
45. Kampf, G.; Todt, D.; Pfaender, S.; Steinmann, E. Persistence of coronaviruses on inanimate surfaces and their inactivation with biocidal agents. *J. Hosp. Infect.* **2020**, *104*, 246–251. [CrossRef] [PubMed]
46. Rutala, W.A.; Weber, D.J. Disinfection, sterilization, and antisepsis: An overview. *Am. J. Infect. Control.* **2019**, *47*, A3–A9. [CrossRef]
47. Liu, D.; Zhang, Y.; Xu, M.; Chen, H.; Lu, X.; Ostrikov, K. Cold atmospheric pressure plasmas in dermatology: Sources, reactive agents, and therapeutic effects. *Plasma Process. Polym.* **2020**, *17*, 1900218. [CrossRef]
48. Weltmann, K.-D.; Von Woedtke, T. Plasma medicine—Current state of research and medical application. *Plasma Phys. Control. Fusion* **2017**, *59*, 014031. [CrossRef]
49. Laroussi, M. Cold Plasma in Medicine and Healthcare: The New Frontier in Low Temperature Plasma Applications. *Front. Phys.* **2020**, *8*, 74. [CrossRef]
50. Bekeschus, S.; Lin, A.; Fridman, A.; Wende, K.; Weltmann, K.-D.; Miller, V. A Comparison of Floating-Electrode DBD and kINPen Jet: Plasma Parameters to Achieve Similar Growth Reduction in Colon Cancer Cells Under Standardized Conditions. *Plasma Chem. Plasma Process.* **2018**, *38*, 1–12. [CrossRef]
51. Friedman, P.C. Cold atmospheric pressure (physical) plasma in dermatology: Where are we today? *Int. J. Dermatol.* **2020**, *59*, 1171–1184. [CrossRef]
52. Misra, N.; Yepez, X.; Xu, L.; Keener, K. In-package cold plasma technologies. *J. Food Eng.* **2019**, *244*, 21–31. [CrossRef]
53. Kaushik, N.K.; Kaushik, N.; Adhikari, M.; Ghimire, B.; Linh, N.N.; Mishra, Y.K.; Lee, S.-J.; Choi, E.H. Preventing the Solid Cancer Progression via Release of Anticancer-Cytokines in Co-Culture with Cold Plasma-Stimulated Macrophages. *Cancers* **2019**, *11*, 842. [CrossRef]
54. Ozcan, A.; Öğün, M. Biochemistry of Reactive Oxygen and Nitrogen Species. In *Basic Principles and Clinical Significance of Oxidative Stress*; IntechOpen: London, UK, 2015.
55. Dayem, A.A.; Hossain, M.K.; Bin Lee, S.; Kim, K.; Saha, S.K.; Yang, G.-M.; Choi, H.Y.; Cho, S.-G. The Role of Reactive Oxygen Species (ROS) in the Biological Activities of Metallic Nanoparticles. *Int. J. Mol. Sci.* **2017**, *18*, 120. [CrossRef]
56. Guo, L.; Xu, R.; Gou, L.; Liu, Z.; Zhao, Y.; Liu, D.; Zhang, L.; Chen, H.; Kong, M.G. Mechanism of Virus Inactivation by Cold Atmospheric-Pressure Plasma and Plasma-Activated Water. *Appl. Environ. Microbiol.* **2018**, *84*, 00726. [CrossRef]
57. Bourke, P.; Ziuzina, D.; Han, L.; Cullen, P.; Gilmore, B.F. Microbiological interactions with cold plasma. *J. Appl. Microbiol.* **2017**, *123*, 308–324. [CrossRef]
58. Dai, X.; Bazaka, K.; Thompson, E.W.; Ostrikov, K. Cold Atmospheric Plasma: A Promising Controller of Cancer Cell States. *Cancers* **2020**, *12*, 3360. [CrossRef]
59. Xu, H.; Zhu, Y.; Du, M.; Wang, Y.; Ju, S.; Ma, R.; Jiao, Z. Subcellular mechanism of microbial inactivation during water disinfection by cold atmospheric-pressure plasma. *Water Res.* **2021**, *188*, 116513. [CrossRef]
60. Gaur, N.; Kurita, H.; Oh, J.-S.; Miyachika, S.; Ito, M.; Mizuno, A.; Cowin, A.J.; Allinson, S.; Short, R.D.; Szili, E.J. On cold atmospheric-pressure plasma jet induced DNA damage in cells. *J. Phys. D Appl. Phys.* **2021**, *54*, 035203. [CrossRef]
61. Waskow, A.; Betschart, J.; Butscher, D.; Oberbossel, G.; Klöti, D.; Büttner-Mainik, A.; Adamcik, J.; Von Rohr, P.R.; Schuppler, M. Characterization of Efficiency and Mechanisms of Cold Atmospheric Pressure Plasma Decontamination of Seeds for Sprout Production. *Front. Microbiol.* **2018**, *9*, 3164. [CrossRef]
62. Karaman, D.Ş.; Ercan, U.K.; Bakay, E.; Topaloğlu, N.; Rosenholm, J.M. Evolving Technologies and Strategies for Combating Antibacterial Resistance in the Advent of the Postantibiotic Era. *Adv. Funct. Mater.* **2020**, *30*, 1908783. [CrossRef]
63. Rapacka-Zdonczyk, A.; Wozniak, A.; Nakonieczna, J.; Grinholc, M. Development of Antimicrobial Phototreatment Tolerance: Why the Methodology Matters. *Int. J. Mol. Sci.* **2021**, *22*, 2224. [CrossRef]
64. Theinkom, F.; Singer, L.; Cieplik, F.; Cantzler, S.; Weilemann, H.; Cantzler, M.; Hiller, K.-A.; Maisch, T.; Zimmermann, J.L. Antibacterial efficacy of cold atmospheric plasma against Enterococcus faecalis planktonic cultures and biofilms in vitro. *PLoS ONE* **2019**, *14*, e0223925. [CrossRef]
65. Dijksteel, G.S.; Ulrich, M.M.W.; Vlig, M.; Sobota, A.; Middelkoop, E.; Boekema, B.K.H.L. Safety and bactericidal efficacy of cold atmospheric plasma generated by a flexible surface Dielectric Barrier Discharge device against Pseudomonas aeruginosa in vitro and in vivo. *Ann. Clin. Microbiol. Antimicrob.* **2020**, *19*, 1–10. [CrossRef]
66. Brun, P.; Bernabè, G.; Marchiori, C.; Scarpa, M.; Zuin, M.; Cavazzana, R.; Zaniol, B.; Martines, E. Antibacterial efficacy and mechanisms of action of low power atmospheric pressure cold plasma: Membrane permeability, biofilm penetration and antimicrobial sensitization. *J. Appl. Microbiol.* **2018**, *125*, 398–408. [CrossRef]
67. Wang, L.; Xia, C.; Guo, Y.; Yang, C.; Cheng, C.; Zhao, J.; Yang, X.; Cao, Z. Bactericidal efficacy of cold atmospheric plasma treatment against multidrug-resistant *Pseudomonas aeruginosa*. *Futur. Microbiol.* **2020**, *15*, 115–125. [CrossRef]
68. Bunz, O.; Mese, K.; Funk, C.; Wulf, M.; Bailer, S.M.; Piwowarczyk, A.; Ehrhardt, A. Cold atmospheric plasma as antiviral therapy–Effect on human herpes simplex virus type. *J. Gen. Virol.* **2020**, *101*, 208–215. [CrossRef]

69. Zhang, L.; Liu, Y. Potential interventions for novel coronavirus in China: A systematic review. *J. Med. Virol.* **2020**, *92*, 479–490. [CrossRef]
70. Guo, L.; Yao, Z.; Yang, L.; Zhang, H.; Qi, Y.; Gou, L.; Xi, W.; Liu, D.; Zhang, L.; Cheng, Y.; et al. Plasma-activated water: An alternative disinfectant for S protein inactivation to prevent SARS-CoV-2 infection. *Chem. Eng. J.* **2020**, 127742. [CrossRef]
71. Chen, Z.; Garcia, G., Jr.; Arumugaswami, V.; Wirz, R.E. Cold atmospheric plasma for SARS-CoV-2 inactivation. *Phys. Fluids* **2020**, *32*, 111702. [CrossRef]
72. Somsen, G.A.; van Rijn, C.; Kooij, S.; Bem, R.A.; Bonn, D. Small droplet aerosols in poorly ventilated spaces and SARS-CoV-2 transmission. *Lancet Respir. Med.* **2020**, *8*, 658–659. [CrossRef]
73. Bisag, A.; Isabelli, P.; Laurita, R.; Bucci, C.; Capelli, F.; Dirani, G.; Gherardi, M.; Laghi, G.; Paglianti, A.; Sambri, V.; et al. Cold atmospheric plasma inactivation of aerosolized microdroplets containing bacteria and purified SARS-CoV-2 RNA to contrast airborne indoor transmission. *Plasma Process. Polym.* **2020**, *17*, 2000154. [CrossRef]
74. Gao, H.; Wang, G.; Chen, B.; Zhang, Y.; Liu, D.; Lu, X.P.; He, G.; Ostrikov, K. Atmospheric-pressure non-equilibrium plasmas for effective abatement of pathogenic biological aerosols. *Plasma Sources Sci. Technol.* **2021**. [CrossRef]
75. Ibáñez-Cervantes, G.; Alcantara, J.C.B.; Nájera-Cortés, A.S.; Meneses-Cruz, S.; Delgado-Balbuena, L.; Cruz-Cruz, C.; Durán-Manuel, E.M.; Cureño-Díaz, M.A.; Gómez-Zamora, E.; Chávez-Ocaña, S.; et al. Disinfection of N95 masks artificially contaminated with SARS-CoV-2 and ESKAPE bacteria using hydrogen peroxide plasma: Impact on the reutilization of disposable devices. *Am. J. Infect. Control* **2020**, *48*, 1037–1041. [CrossRef] [PubMed]
76. Osman, I.; Ponukumati, A.; Vargas, M.; Bhakta, D.; Ozoglu, B.; Bailey, C. Plasma-Activated Vapor for Sanitization of Hands. *Plasma Med.* **2016**, *6*, 235–245. [CrossRef]
77. Attri, P.; Koga, K.; Shiratani, M. Possible impact of plasma oxidation on the structure of the C-terminal domain of SARS-CoV-2 spike protein: A computational study. *Appl. Phys. Express* **2021**, *14*, 027002. [CrossRef]
78. Šrámková, P.; Zahoranová, A.; Kelar, J.; Tučeková, Z.K.; Stupavská, M.; Krumpolec, R.; Jurmanová, J.; Kováčik, D.; Černák, M. Cold atmospheric pressure plasma: Simple and efficient strategy for preparation of poly (2-oxazoline)-based coatings designed for biomedical applications. *Sci. Rep.* **2020**, *10*, 9478. [CrossRef]
79. Laroussi, M.; Lu, X.; Keidar, M. Perspective: The physics, diagnostics, and applications of atmospheric pressure low temperature plasma sources used in plasma medicine. *J. Appl. Phys.* **2017**, *122*, 020901. [CrossRef]
80. Jungbauer, G.; Moser, D.; Müller, S.; Pfister, W.; Sculean, A.; Eick, S. The Antimicrobial Effect of Cold Atmospheric Plasma against Dental Pathogens—A Systematic Review of In-Vitro Studies. *Antibiotics* **2021**, *10*, 211. [CrossRef]
81. Ranjan, R.; Krishnamraju, P.V.; Shankar, T.; Gowd, S. Nonthermal Plasma in Dentistry: An Update. *J. Int. Soc. Prev. Community Dent.* **2017**, *7*, 71–75.
82. Borges, A.; Kostov, K.; Pessoa, R.; de Abreu, G.; Lima, G.; Figueira, L.; Koga-Ito, C. Applications of Cold Atmospheric Pressure Plasma in Dentistry. *Appl. Sci.* **2021**, *11*, 1975. [CrossRef]
83. Lee, M.-J.; Kwon, J.-S.; Jiang, H.B.; Choi, E.H.; Park, G.; Kim, K.-M. The antibacterial effect of non-thermal atmospheric pressure plasma treatment of titanium surfaces according to the bacterial wall structure. *Sci. Rep.* **2019**, *9*, 1–13. [CrossRef]
84. Tanaka, H.; Bekeschus, S.; Yan, D.; Hori, M.; Keidar, M.; Laroussi, M. Plasma-Treated Solutions (PTS) in Cancer Therapy. *Cancers* **2021**, *13*, 1737. [CrossRef]
85. Yadav, D.K.; Adhikari, M.; Kumar, S.; Ghimire, B.; Han, I.; Kim, M.-H.; Choi, E.-H. Cold atmospheric plasma generated reactive species aided inhibitory effects on human melanoma cells: An in vitro and in silico study. *Sci. Rep.* **2020**, *10*, 1–15. [CrossRef]
86. Metelmann, H.-R.; Seebauer, C.; Miller, V.; Fridman, A.; Bauer, G.; Graves, D.B.; Pouvesle, J.-M.; Rutkowski, R.; Schuster, M.; Bekeschus, S.; et al. Clinical experience with cold plasma in the treatment of locally advanced head and neck cancer. *Clin. Plasma Med.* **2018**, *9*, 6–13. [CrossRef]
87. Pereira, S.; Pinto, E.; Ribeiro, P.; Sério, S. Study of a Cold Atmospheric Pressure Plasma jet device for indirect treatment of Squamous Cell Carcinoma. *Clin. Plasma Med.* **2019**, *13*, 9–14. [CrossRef]
88. Mateu-Sanz, M.; Tornín, J.; Brulin, B.; Khlyustova, A.; Ginebra, M.-P.; Layrolle, P.; Canal, C. Cold Plasma-Treated Ringer's Saline: A Weapon to Target Osteosarcoma. *Cancers* **2020**, *12*, 227. [CrossRef]
89. Toyokuni, S. The origin and future of oxidative stress pathology: From the recognition of carcinogenesis as an iron addiction with ferroptosis-resistance to non-thermal plasma therapy. *Pathol. Int.* **2016**, *66*, 245–259. [CrossRef] [PubMed]
90. Rana, S.; Mehta, D.; Bansal, V.; Shivhare, U.S.; Yadav, S.K. Atmospheric cold plasma (ACP) treatment improved in-package shelf-life of strawberry fruit. *J. Food Sci. Technol.* **2020**, *57*, 102–112. [CrossRef] [PubMed]
91. Ozen, E.; Singh, R. Atmospheric cold plasma treatment of fruit juices: A review. *Trends Food Sci. Technol.* **2020**, *103*, 144–151. [CrossRef]
92. El Kadri, H.; Costello, K.M.; Thomas, P.; Wantock, T.; Sandison, G.; Harle, T.; Fabris, A.L.; Gutierrez-Merino, J.; Velliou, E.G. The antimicrobial efficacy of remote cold atmospheric plasma effluent against single and mixed bacterial biofilms of varying age. *Food Res. Int.* **2021**, *141*, 110126. [CrossRef]
93. Varilla, C.; Marcone, M.; Annor, G.A. Potential of Cold Plasma Technology in Ensuring the Safety of Foods and Agricultural Produce: A Review. *Foods* **2020**, *9*, 1435. [CrossRef]
94. Mir, S.A.; Shah, M.A.; Mir, M.M. Understanding the Role of Plasma Technology in Food Industry. *Food Bioprocess Technol.* **2016**, *9*, 734–750. [CrossRef]

95. Hosseini, S.M.; Rostami, S.; Samani, B.H.; Lorigooini, Z. The effect of atmospheric pressure cold plasma on the inactivation of Escherichia coli in sour cherry juice and its qualitative properties. *Food Sci. Nutr.* **2020**, *8*, 870–883. [CrossRef]
96. Go, S.-M.; Kim, H.-S.; Park, M.-R.; Jeong, R.-D. Antibacterial effect of non-thermal atmospheric plasma against soft rot bacteria on paprika. *LWT* **2020**, *117*, 108600. [CrossRef]
97. Bauer, A.; Ni, Y.; Bauer, S.; Paulsen, P.; Modic, M.; Walsh, J.; Smulders, F. The effects of atmospheric pressure cold plasma treatment on microbiological, physical-chemical and sensory characteristics of vacuum packaged beef loin. *Meat Sci.* **2017**, *128*, 77–87. [CrossRef]
98. Bourke, P.; Ziuzina, D.; Boehm, D.; Cullen, P.J.; Keener, K. The Potential of Cold Plasma for Safe and Sustainable Food Production. *Trends Biotechnol.* **2018**, *36*, 615–626. [CrossRef]
99. Thirumdas, R.; Sarangapani, C.; Annapure, U. Cold Plasma: A novel Non-Thermal Technology for Food Processing. *Food Biophys.* **2015**, *10*, 1–11. [CrossRef]
100. López, M.; Calvo, T.; Prieto, M.; Múgica-Vidal, R.; Muro-Fraguas, I.; Alba-Elías, F.; Alvarez-Ordóñez, A. A Review on Non-thermal Atmospheric Plasma for Food Preservation: Mode of Action, Determinants of Effectiveness, and Applications. *Front. Microbiol.* **2019**, *10*, 622. [CrossRef] [PubMed]
101. Giannoglou, M.; Stergiou, P.; Dimitrakellis, P.; Gogolides, E.; Stoforos, N.G.; Katsaros, G. Effect of Cold Atmospheric Plasma Processing on Quality and Shelf-Life of Ready-to-Eat Rocket Leafy Salad. *Innov. Food Sci. Emerg. Technol.* **2020**, *66*, 102502. [CrossRef]
102. Yadav, B.; Spinelli, A.C.; Misra, N.N.; Tsui, Y.Y.; McMullen, L.M.; Roopesh, M. Effect of in-package atmospheric cold plasma discharge on microbial safety and quality of ready-to-eat ham in modified atmospheric packaging during storage. *J. Food Sci.* **2020**, *85*, 1203–1212. [CrossRef]
103. Pina-Perez, M.; Martinet, D.; Palacios-Gorba, C.; Ellert, C.; Beyrer, M. Low-energy short-term cold atmospheric plasma: Controlling the inactivation efficacy of bacterial spores in powders. *Food Res. Int.* **2020**, *130*, 108921. [CrossRef]
104. Attri, P.; Han, J.; Choi, S.; Choi, E.H.; Bogaerts, A.; Lee, W. CAP modifies the structure of a model protein from thermophilic bacteria: Mechanisms of CAP-mediated inactivation. *Sci. Rep.* **2018**, *8*, 1–10. [CrossRef]
105. Beyrer, M.; Smeu, I.; Martinet, D.; Howling, A.; Pina-Pérez, M.C.; Ellert, C. Cold Atmospheric Plasma Inactivation of Microbial Spores Compared on Reference Surfaces and Powder Particles. *Food Bioprocess Technol.* **2020**, *13*, 827–837. [CrossRef]
106. Nasiru, M.M.; Frimpong, E.B.; Muhammad, U.; Qian, J.; Mustapha, A.T.; Yan, W.; Zhuang, H.; Zhang, J. Dielectric barrier discharge cold atmospheric plasma: Influence of processing parameters on microbial inactivation in meat and meat products. *Compr. Rev. Food Sci. Food Saf.* **2021**, *20*, 2626–2659. [CrossRef]
107. Ekonomou, S.I.; Boziaris, I.S. Non-Thermal Methods for Ensuring the Microbiological Quality and Safety of Seafood. *Appl. Sci.* **2021**, *11*, 833. [CrossRef]
108. Adhikari, B.; Adhikari, M.; Park, G. The Effects of Plasma on Plant Growth, Development, and Sustainability. *Appl. Sci.* **2020**, *10*, 6045. [CrossRef]
109. Adhikari, B.; Pangomm, K.; Veerana, M.; Mitra, S.; Park, G. Plant Disease Control by Non-Thermal Atmospheric-Pressure Plasma. *Front. Plant Sci.* **2020**, *11*, 77. [CrossRef]
110. Attri, P.; Ishikawa, K.; Okumura, T.; Koga, K.; Shiratani, M. Plasma Agriculture from Laboratory to Farm: A Review. *Processes* **2020**, *8*, 1002. [CrossRef]
111. Takaki, K.; Takahashi, K.; Hamanaka, D.; Yoshida, R.; Uchino, T. Function of plasma and electrostatics for keeping quality of agricultural produce in post-harvest stage. *Jpn. J. Appl. Phys.* **2021**, *60*, 010501. [CrossRef]
112. Feizollahi, E.; Iqdiam, B.; Vasanthan, T.; Thilakarathna, M.S.; Roopesh, M.S. Effects of Atmospheric-Pressure Cold Plasma Treatment on Deoxynivalenol Degradation, Quality Parameters, and Germination of Barley Grains. *Appl. Sci.* **2020**, *10*, 3530. [CrossRef]
113. Tamošiūnė, I.; Gelvonauskienė, D.; Haimi, P.; Mildažienė, V.; Koga, K.; Shiratani, M.; Baniulis, D. Cold Plasma Treatment of Sunflower Seeds Modulates Plant-Associated Microbiome and Stimulates Root and Lateral Organ Growth. *Front. Plant Sci.* **2020**, *11*, 568924. [CrossRef]
114. Attri, P.; Koga, K.; Okumura, T.; Shiratani, M. Impact of atmospheric pressure plasma treated seeds on germination, morphology, gene expression and biochemical responses. *Jpn. J. Appl. Phys.* **2021**, *60*, 040502. [CrossRef]
115. Wang, J.; Cui, D.; Wang, L.; Du, M.; Yin, Y.; Ma, R.; Sun, H.; Jiao, Z. Atmospheric pressure plasma treatment induces abscisic acid production, reduces stomatal aperture and improves seedling growth in Arabidopsis thaliana. *Plant Biol.* **2021**, 13245. [CrossRef]
116. Kučerová, K.; Henselová, M.; Slováková, Ľ.; Bačovčinová, M.; Hensel, K. Effect of Plasma Activated Water, Hydrogen Peroxide, and Nitrates on Lettuce Growth and Its Physiological Parameters. *Appl. Sci.* **2021**, *11*, 1985. [CrossRef]
117. Hashizume, H.; Kitano, H.; Mizuno, H.; Abe, A.; Yuasa, G.; Tohno, S.; Tanaka, H.; Ishikawa, K.; Matsumoto, S.; Sakakibara, H.; et al. Improvement of yield and grain quality by periodic cold plasma treatment with rice plants in a paddy field. *Plasma Process. Polym.* **2021**, *18*, 2000181. [CrossRef]
118. Nguyen, T.T.; Rosello, C.; Bélanger, R.; Ratti, C. Fate of Residual Pesticides in Fruit and Vegetable Waste (FVW) Processing. *Foods* **2020**, *9*, 1468. [CrossRef]
119. Ali, M.; Cheng, J.-H.; Sun, D.-W. Effect of plasma activated water and buffer solution on fungicide degradation from tomato (*Solanum lycopersicum*) fruit. *Food Chem.* **2021**, *350*, 129195. [CrossRef]

120. Volkov, A.G.; Bookal, A.; Hairston, J.S.; Roberts, J.; Taengwa, G.; Patel, D. Mechanisms of multielectron reactions at the plasma/water interface: Interfacial catalysis, RONS, nitrogen fixation, and plasma activated water. *Electrochim. Acta* **2021**, *385*, 138441. [CrossRef]
121. Kwon, T.; Chandimali, N.; Lee, N.-H.; Son, Y.; Yoon, S.-B.; Lee, J.-R.; Lee, S.; Kim, K.J.; Lee, S.-Y.; Kim, S.-Y.; et al. Potential Applications of Non-thermal Plasma in Animal Husbandry to Improve Infrastructure. *In Vivo* **2019**, *33*, 999–1010. [CrossRef]
122. Su, X.; Tian, Y.; Zhou, H.; Li, Y.; Zhang, Z.; Jiang, B.; Yang, B.; Zhang, J.; Fang, J. Inactivation Efficacy of Nonthermal Plasma-Activated Solutions against Newcastle Disease Virus. *Appl. Environ. Microbiol.* **2018**, *84*, 02836. [CrossRef]
123. Cui, J.; Zhao, T.; Zou, L.; Wang, X.; Zhang, Y. Molecular dynamics simulation of *S. cerevisiae* glucan destruction by plasma ROS based on ReaxFF. *J. Phys. D Appl. Phys.* **2018**, *51*, 355401. [CrossRef]
124. Babaeva, N.Y.; Naidis, G.V. Modeling of Plasmas for Biomedicine. *Trends Biotechnol.* **2018**, *36*, 603–614. [CrossRef] [PubMed]
125. Hu, Y.; Zhao, T.; Zou, L.; Wang, X.; Zhang, Y. Molecular dynamics simulations of membrane properties affected by plasma ROS based on the GROMOS force field. *Biophys. Chem.* **2019**, *253*, 106214. [CrossRef] [PubMed]

MDPI
St. Alban-Anlage 66
4052 Basel
Switzerland
Tel. +41 61 683 77 34
Fax +41 61 302 89 18
www.mdpi.com

Applied Sciences Editorial Office
E-mail: applsci@mdpi.com
www.mdpi.com/journal/applsci

www.ingramcontent.com/pod-product-compliance
Lightning Source LLC
LaVergne TN
LVHW070625100526
838202LV00012B/725